# Exercise for Older Adults

## ACE'S GUIDE FOR FITNESS PROFESSIONALS
### Second Edition

**American Council on Exercise®**

**Cedric X. Bryant, Ph.D.**
**Daniel J. Green**
**Editors**

AMERICAN COUNCIL ON EXERCISE

Library of Congress Control Number: 2005920330

Second edition
ISBN: 1-58518-927-8
Copyright © 2005, 1998  American Council on Exercise® (ACE®)

A  B  C  D

Distributed by:
American Council on Exercise
P. O. Box 910449
San Diego, CA 92191-0449
800-825-3636
www.acefitness.org

**Second Edition:**
*Managing Editor:* Daniel J. Green
*Technical Editor:* Cedric X. Bryant, Ph.D.
*Publications Director:* Christine J. Ekeroth
*Cover Design & Art Direction:* Karen McGuire
*Assistant Editor:* Jennifer Schiffer
*Production:* Sandra Pennock
*Photography:* Dennis Dal Covey
*Index:* Bonny McLaughlin
*Models:* James Alesi, Mary Alesi,
John L. Boyer, M.D., Donna Boyer,
Roger Martin, Gerry Martin, and Andrea Wells

**First Edition:**
*Editor:* Richard T. Cotton, M.A.
*Associate Editors:* Christine J. Ekeroth, Holly Yancy
*Design & Production:* Nancy S. Simerly
*Art Direction:* Steve Lux
*Photographer (interior):* Rick Starkman
*Glossary:* Karen Nelson
*Copy Editors/Proofreaders:* Christina Gandolfo, Gail Katz

*Acknowledgements:*
Thanks to the entire American Council on Exercise staff for their support and guidance through the process of creating this manual.

P04-043

# TABLE OF
# contents

# reviewers

**Susan J. Bartlett, Ph.D.,** *is an assistant professor in the School of Medicine at Johns Hopkins Medical Institutions in Baltimore, Md. Dr. Bartlett's research focuses on the effects of weight loss and exercise in persons with chronic medical conditions such as arthritis. She has authored more than 30 scientific papers, as well as chapters in both the* ACE Lifestyle & Weight Management Consultant Manual *and* ACE Clinical Exercise Specialist Manual.

**Jennifer S. Bolger, M.S.,** *has a master's degree in exercise physiology from San Diego State University. She is the senior program manager and director of YMCA initiatives for FitLinxx, the industry leader in integrated fitness technology. Prior to coming to FitLinxx she served as the health and fitness director for the Mission Valley YMCA in San Diego, Calif., where she was responsible for developing and managing programs designed to help under-active adults make regular physical activity a part of their lives.*

**John L. Boyer, M.D.,** *is a past president of the American College of Sports Medicine and an Emeritus Professor in the College of Professional Studies at San Diego State University. He has a 35-year background in medicine and cardiology with emphasis on risk-factor modification in the prevention and rehabilitation of cardiovascular disorders.*

**Lawrence J. Cheskin, M.D., F.A.C.P.,** *is an associate professor of international health and director of the Johns Hopkins Weight Management Center.*

*He is the author of* Losing Weight for Good: Developing Your Personal Plan of Action *(Johns Hopkins Press).*

**Laura A. Gladwin, M.S., A.F.P.,** *is the director of You're in Charge! health promotions at Preferred Care, which provides preventive and health education programs and support services for older adults in Rochester, N.Y. Gladwin is a member of the American Senior Fitness Association's National Coalition to Develop Recommended Curriculum Standards for Preparing Senior Fitness Specialists and former advisor to the California Governor's Council on Physical Fitness and Sports. She also teaches Physical Activity and Aging for the LIFESPAN/St. John Fisher College Gerontology Certificate program.*

**Jeanne F. Nichols, Ph.D., F.A.C.S.M.,** *is a professor of exercise physiology in the Department of Exercise and Nutritional Sciences at San Diego State University. She also served as the director of the Adult Fitness Program at San Diego State University.*

**Brenda L. Wolfe, Ph.D.,** *is a clinical psychologist who specializes in the treatment of obesity and eating disorders, and substance abuse. In addition to her private practice, Dr. Wolfe is involved in research collaborations at the University of New Mexico, serves as a consultant to business enterprises developing psychologically based services, and is active in various professional organizations. Her books and articles have appeared in both the professional and popular press.*

# foreword

It seems that every piece of research that applies to aging or disease prevention includes a statement regarding the role that physical activity plays in the maintenance of lifelong health. From diabetes, arthritis, and osteoporosis to depression and anxiety, regular exercise programs have proven effective in the prevention and control of a myriad of diseases. So why aren't more people getting even the recommended minimum amount of exercise? If we know the "miracle cure," why aren't more people taking it?

We also face a rapidly aging society in which, for the first time ever, people over age 65 outnumber teenagers, and will constitute 20% of Americans by the year 2030. In addition, the number of people in that same age bracket in the work force will increase by 30% by 2010. Baby Boomers will work for a greater part of their lives than any previous generation, creating an ever-increasing need to be healthy and productive later in life. Improving the functional health of older adults, as well as the ability to perform beyond the activities of daily living, has never been more important.

That's my challenge to you! I am not talking about preparing clients for the Senior Olympics—though that's a fantastic goal for very fit members of this population. Instead, your role is to help prepare older adults to be healthy, fulfilled, and productive each and every day.

The personal and professional success available in the fitness industry is boundless, but it is even more so when working with older adults. The sense of satisfaction derived from improving a client's ability to enjoy new experiences cannot be overstated. But to effectively and safely train older adults you must be educated not only in proper exercise technique and contraindications, for example, but also appropriate motivation strategies and teaching tools. This manual provides the essential knowledge you will need when working with older adults, and I hope you take advantage of the challenge this opportunity presents and enjoy making such an important difference in the lives of so many people.

*Ken Germano*
*President*

# introduction

In the seven years since the publication of the first edition of this manual, older adults have emerged as the fastest-growing group of potential clients for fitness professionals. A quick review of the statistics presented in the introduction to Chapter 1 reveals just how enormous the demographic shift has become, and you can easily surmise the impact these trends can have on the fitness industry.

In 1998, ACE brought together top experts from the fields of exercise physiology and psychology who specialize in the specific needs of older adults to develop a manual that met the demand for clear and comprehensive guidelines for fitness professionals who serve this community.

This second edition of ACE's *Exercise for Older Adults* builds upon the foundation of the first, which quickly became a go-to resource for the fitness industry. All of the original authors returned to update their chapters based on the research of the past seven years. In addition, four new experts were called upon to lend their specific expertise to the project.

Chapter 1 details the physiology of the aging process and how those functional changes affect exercise within this population. In addition to the statistical information mentioned above, updates were made to reflect changes in our understanding of cognitive functioning. Chapter 2, which covers communication and motivation techniques specific to older adults, was augmented by the work of Drs. David Williams and Bess Marcus. This chapter explains how to take theoretical research regarding behavior change and apply it to your exercise leadership.

Chapter 3 outlines many of the most common health challenges faced by older adults and offers advice on how to modify exercise programs to meet special needs. Everything from hypertension and asthma to Parkinson's disease and visual problems is covered. Chapter 4 presents a comprehensive assessment protocol, with a broad range of tools to improve information gathering. An all-new Appendix that details various functional ability tests accompanies this chapter.

Chapter 5 presents a variety of exercise modes and techniques appropriate for an older population. From warm-up to cool-down, this chapter includes comprehensive guidelines and ideas for modifications, and includes options for both chair-based and water-based exercises.

Chapter 6, Basic Strength-training Guidelines for Older Adults, is completely new, and was added to address the increased focus on the effectiveness of this type of training. Drs. James Peterson and Barry Franklin address the many barriers to participation and give advice on how overcome those barriers with your clients. Basic principles are also covered, as well as information on organizing a strength-training program. Finally, four full-body workouts were added, each utilizing a different form of resistance. Cueing and training tips are included alongside photographs and descriptions of each exercise.

Chapter 7 explains how to use the pre-exercise assessment results to structure both individual and group exercise programs for older adults, as well as how to lead older clients and class members in cardiovascular, strength, and flexibility training.

Whether you are a group fitness instructor, personal trainer, health educator, or fitness facility manager, you will benefit from this valuable resource. If you currently work with the older adult population, you already understand the challenges and rewards that come from focusing on the individuals in this diverse group. In addition to enriching and expanding your career, the rewards come from helping older adults not only achieve their personal fitness goals, but live healthier and happier lives as well.

*Cedric X. Bryant, Ph.D.*
*Chief Exercise Physiologist/Vice*
*President of Educational Services*

*Daniel J. Green*
*Managing Editor*

CHAPTER ONE

# PHYSIOLOGY OF
# Aging and Exercise

## Wojtek J. Chodzko-Zajko

Wojtek J. Chodzko-Zajko, Ph.D., is head of the Department of Kinesiology at the University of Illinois at Urbana-Champaign. For the past 15 years he has focused his research on the effects of exercise and physical activity on sensory, motor, and cognitive functioning in old age. Dr. Chodzko-Zajko chairs the National Active Aging Partnership, a national coalition in the area of healthy aging linking the American College of Sports Medicine, the National Institute on Aging, the Centers for Disease Control and Prevention, the American Geriatrics Society, the National Council on the Aging, the American Association for Retired Persons, and the Robert Wood Johnson Foundation.

Dr. Chodzko-Zajko served on the Scientific Advisory Committee of the World Health Organization and as the founding editor of the Journal of Aging and Physical Activity (1992–2002). He currently serves as president of the International Society on Aging and Physical Activity.

Aging is a universal phenomenon that affects us all. Provided we live long enough, we will eventually experience significant sensory, motor, and cognitive changes in response to advancing age. However, although we are all aging, we do not age at the same rate. While some people experience relatively rapid declines in physiological and psychological functioning as they grow older, others undergo significantly less-pronounced changes over time (Fries & Crapo, 1981).

A major focus of **gerontologists** continues to be on increasing our understanding of the factors responsible for individual differences in the rate and extent at which we age. Clearly, hereditary factors play an important role in determining the pattern of changes observed in **senescence.** This genetic component of human aging is largely beyond our control and gerontologists often joke that the single best way to ensure longevity and healthful old age is to choose one's parents wisely! However, in addition to the genetic factors influencing human aging, there is now strong evidence that many aspects of the aging process are related to environmental factors, such as nutrition, stress, smoking, and physical activity (Bokovy & Blair, 1994; Armstrong et al., 2001).

The need to develop effective lifestyle interventions that have the potential to improve the quality of life for older persons is especially apparent when one considers the growing proportion of older adults in today's society. The following statistics illustrate some aspects of the enormous demographic shift in the United States (Armstrong et al., 2001).

✓ In the year 2000 an estimated 35 million people, 13% of the population, were age 65 and older.

✓ By 2030, 20% of Americans, about 70 million people, will have passed their 65th birthday.

✓ The "Baby Boomer" generation will begin to turn 65 in 2009 and the number of people age 65 and older is expected to nearly triple to 93 million within the next 50 years.

✓ The youngest of the "Baby Boomer" generation will reach the age of 65 in 2030.

✓ People age 85 and above currently represent the fastest growing segment of the older population.

✓ By 2050 the size of the 85-plus age group will increase to almost 5% of our population.

✓ There were about 65,000 people age 100 or older in 2000, and the number of centenarians is projected to grow so quickly that there may be as many as 381,000 by 2030.

There is little doubt that such a dramatic increase in the number of older adults will have far-reaching consequences for society. The past two decades have witnessed a remarkable expansion of interest in the physical activity needs of older persons. The major medical and scientific organizations endorse the importance of physically active lifestyles for older adults (American College of Sports Medicine, 2000; U.S. Department of Health and Human Services, 1996; World Health Organization, 1997; Armstrong et al., 2001). It is now possible for students to specialize in the study of physical activity and aging, both through traditional academic programs offered at universities (Jones & Rikli, 1994), and specialized educational programs such as those offered by the American Council on Exercise.

This chapter examines some of the key issues influencing the relationship between physical activity and the aging process. We begin with a discussion of underlying biological mechanisms responsible for aging, including: (1) What is aging? (2) What causes us to age? (3) What are the consequences of aging? and (4) Why do some people appear to age faster than others? We then examine the role regular physical activity plays in physiological, psychological, and social functioning, and the extent to which lifestyle change promotes healthy aging. Finally, we discuss issues related to exercise programming for older persons. Throughout the chapter a broad definition of physical activity is adopted, and the acute, or short-term, effects of a single bout of activity and the chronic, or long-term, benefits of extended participation are considered.

## THE PHYSIOLOGY OF THE AGING PROCESS

### Aging Defined

It may seem unnecessary to define aging. Age is typically defined as the number of years, months, or days that have elapsed since a particular point in time, usually birth. Similarly, the *aging process* is almost always defined by the passage of calendar time. However, many gerontologists believe definitions of aging that focus exclusively on calendar time are incomplete, and that more complex definitions of both "age" and "aging" are needed to understand the intricacies associated with human aging.

**Chronological age** is the length of time—expressed by the number of years or months since birth—a person has lived. Its measurement is independent of physiological, psychological, and sociocultural factors. The presence of large differences in functional performance between individuals of the same chronological age, however, suggests that chronological age alone is an insufficient measure of senescence.

Many gerontologists believe that to increase our understanding of senescence, chronological age must be supplemented by other measures of aging designed to differentiate between individuals of the same chronological age. These measures are often described as indices of **functional age.** The most common measure of functional age is biological age, although other functional ages, including psychological age and social age, have been identified (Schroots & Birren, 2001).

**Biological age** characterizes senescence in terms of discrete biological, rather than chronological, processes. Research designs that emphasize chronological age typically focus on elements of calendar time (years, decades, etc.) as the principal units of analysis, whereas biological-age research focuses on senescent changes in biological or physiological processes and their subsequent effects on behavior. A common goal of all biological age inventories is to determine **relative age,** or the extent to which an individual is aging faster or slower than an average person of the same chronological age. For example, an individual who is aging successfully may have a biological age 10 years younger than their chronological age. Conversely, a person experiencing multi-

ple medical problems in old age may be older biologically than chronologically.

Because there is little consensus as to how biological age should be measured, it is difficult to summarize the research on the effects of physical activity on biological age. However, most studies suggest that, on average, people who exercise regularly have lower biological ages than people of the same chronological age who do not exercise (Chodzko-Zajko & Ringel, 1987; Heikkinen et al., 1994; Kim & Tanaka, 1995; Shephard, 1998).

In much the same way that people of the same chronological age can differ biologically, it also is possible for people to have different psychological ages (Schroots & Birren, 2001). **Psychological age** refers to an individual's capabilities along a number of dimensions of mental or cognitive functioning, including self-esteem and self-efficacy, as well as learning, memory, and perception (Birren, 1959). Birren suggests that some older persons demonstrate psychological adjustments typical for their chronological age, whereas others behave as though they were psychologically younger or older than their contemporaries. The concept of psychological age and its relationship to quality of life is an important area of exercise science research. Recognizing the importance of regular physical activity in the psychological, social, and physiological health of older persons, the World Health Organization (WHO) published the *Guidelines for Promoting Physical Activity Among Older Persons* in 1997.

**Social age** refers to the notion that society often has fairly rigid expectations of what is and is not appropriate behavior for a person of a particular age (Rose, 1972; McGrath & Kelly, 1985). Socialization is a tremendously complex process, and it is difficult to make broad generalizations about the acquisition of social roles in later life (McPherson, 1990). However, the impact that social roles and expectations have on the lifestyle choices of older persons is of considerable interest in experimental gerontology. A number of studies have examined the extent to which later-life physical activity choices are dependent on an individual's perception of what is, or is not, age-appropriate behavior (Cousins & Vertinsky, 1995; Cousins, 1997). For example, many older persons consider it undignified to be seen physically exerting themselves in public. The WHO guidelines encourage older people to break away from such stereotypical perspectives about aging. Instead of encouraging seniors to "take it easy," the WHO promotes a more vigorous and healthful model of aging in which older persons are invited to play a more active role in their own senescence (World Health Organization, 1997).

Unfortunately, despite many years of research, there is no consensus on how best to quantify any of these alternative measures of aging. Thus, although it is apparent that chronological age is an inadequate measure of senescence and that alternative definitions of aging are necessary, no single unified definition of biological, psychological, or social aging exists (Balin, 1994). Nonetheless, it is clear that an appreciation of chronological, biological, and psychosocial perspectives on aging is essential to grasp the true essence of aging.

A central tenet underlying physical fitness and aging research is that physically fit individuals may be functionally younger than less-fit individuals of the same chronological age. From this point of view, research studies examining the relationship between age, physical fitness, and behavior focus on both chronological and functional perspectives on aging.

## Biological Theories of Aging

Biological theories of aging examine the underlying mechanisms responsible for the structural and functional changes that characterize advancing age. Researchers have attempted to specify a single causal element responsible for age-related declines in physiological functioning but, to date, little progress has been made toward identifying a unified theory of biological aging (Hayflick, 1985; Baker & Martin, 1994).

Aging is probably not a single biological process, but rather a wide variety of age-related changes that occur simultaneously in many different systems throughout the body. Together, these changes decrease the body's ability to respond appropriately to the stresses of everyday life (Chodzko-Zajko & Ringel, 1987).

The complex nature of aging is reflected by the wide variety of theories proposed to account for the underlying mechanisms of aging. While many different classification schemes exist (Arking, 1998), the model proposed by the renowned biologist Leonard Hayflick is among the most straightforward (Hayflick, 1985). Hayflick was one of the first to demonstrate conclusively that cellular aging is influenced by both genetic and environmental factors. In his model of biological aging, Hayflick proposes that aging theories can be subdivided into three major classes: cellular theories, genetic theories, and control theories.

## CELLULAR THEORIES OF AGING

Cellular theories of aging focus on the degenerative changes that occur at the level of the individual cell. The most commonly proposed mechanism of cellular aging is **free-radical oxidation** (Harman, 1956). A free radical is a highly unstable molecule of oxygen with an uneven number of electrons in its outer shell. The presence of an unpaired electron causes the free radical to be both unstable and highly chemically reactive. To obtain the electron it needs to achieve stability, the free radical attempts to link up with other molecules. This process initiates a cascade of destructive chain reactions that may number in the thousands.

In healthy individuals, free radicals coexist in a state of equilibrium with a series of mixed-function oxidases that neutralize the destructive effects. The disruption of this equilibrium may be caused by a wide variety of intrinsic biological processes, as well as in response to environmental factors, such as exposure to radiation and chemical carcinogens. It is now well established that advancing age is associated with a reduction in the expression of mixed-function oxidases, which in turn leads to a progressive increase in free-radical oxidation (Balin, 1983; Baker & Martin, 1994). Alterations to the structure of collagen and elastin, the destruction of DNA, and a progressive breakdown of the immune system are among the damages attributed to free radicals (Arking, 1998).

The formation of covalent and hydrogen bond cross-links between adjacent molecules is a consequence of age-related increases in free-radical oxidation (Bjorksten, 1968). The bonding of adjacent molecules alters their configuration and has significant functional consequences. For example, age-related changes in skin elasticity may be the result of the formation of cross-links caused by increases in free-radical oxidation (Partridge, 1970). Aging also is associated with significant declines in flexibility and range of motion (Vandervoort et al., 1992), and it is likely that these changes are due, in part, to intrinsic changes brought about by cellular aging.

## GENETIC THEORIES OF AGING

Genetic theories of aging focus on the role of heredity in the regulation of senescence. Studies of identical twins reveal that a significant portion of age-related changes in physiological variables can be attributed to genetic mechanisms (Kallman & Sander, 1948). Medvedev (1981) proposed that aging is the result of a breakdown in the integrity of DNA nucleotide sequences. This breakdown in DNA sequencing disrupts the ability of the cell to reproduce. Although some degree of DNA mutation occurs at all stages of the life cycle, the adverse consequences of these mutations are seldom realized until later in life.

Hayflick proposed that senescence is controlled by a purposeful sequence of events written into the genetic code (Hayflick, 1965; 1985). He showed that cells cultured in vitro exhibit a finite ability to reproduce. The **Hayflick limit** has been replicated in numerous tissues from a wide variety of species (Hayflick, 1985), and suggests that cellular aging is, at least to some extent, preprogrammed.

Hayflick's finding indicates that, although important, lifestyle changes alone will not allow us to overcome the genetically programmed factors responsible for human aging. We cannot escape the aging process indefinitely.

## CONTROL THEORIES OF AGING

A third class of theories explains aging in terms of the function of specific systems known to be vital for the control of physiological functioning. For example, it is now accepted that advancing age often compromises immune system functioning. Older persons not only exhibit a significant decline in T-cell activity, but they also are more susceptible to **autoimmune disease** (Walford, 1987).

The **Major Histocompatibility Complex (MHC)** is a complex series of genes that provides a viable link between the cellular, genetic, and control theories of aging. The MHC not only controls immunologic functioning, but also regulates the expression of mixed-function oxidases, which protect cells against damaging free-radical oxidation (Walford, 1983). Walford showed that genetic control of the immune system occurs in the MHC, the integrity of which typically deteriorates with advancing age (Walford, 1987). In addition to the immune system, the neuroendocrine and central nervous systems also have been implicated in the regulation of degenerative changes in aging (Arking, 1998; Baker & Martin, 1994). Future research will likely confirm the importance of several different control systems in the regulation of aging at the molecular, cellular, and intact-organ levels.

Available evidence suggests that biological aging is a complex process regulated by numerous, redundant mechanisms. It is unlikely that a single biological mechanism can be identified as the principal factor responsible for senescence. Rather, it is more probable that a complex combination of mechanisms, acting at several different levels throughout the body, brings about the structural and functional changes that characterize old age. Since biological aging does not appear to be caused by a single mechanism, it is extremely unlikely that we will develop a "cure" for the aging process in the foreseeable future.

## The Structural and Functional Consequences of Aging

The structural and functional consequences of aging are surprisingly consistent across a broad range of physiological systems. A General Model of Aging (Figure 1.1) summarizes the common structural and functional changes that are characteristic of aging throughout the body (Chodzko-Zajko & Ringel, 1987).

With advancing age, most physiological systems eventually exhibit atrophy, dystrophy, and edema at the cellular level. These disruptions in the integrity of the cell are, in turn, precursors of more gross morphological changes, such as decreased elasticity and compliance, **demyelinization,** and **neoplastic** growth. As expected, these structural changes are almost always associated with profound behavioral consequences.

In much the same way that structural changes exhibit similarities across physiological systems, the functional consequences also are fairly consistent across different systems of the body. Aging organ systems, which are usually slower and less accurate, exhibit not only reduced strength and stability, but also decreased coordination and endurance.

Although structural decay and functional decline are an inescapable consequence

Figure 1.1

General Model of Aging

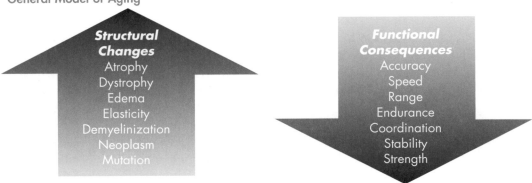

Chodzko-Zajko, W.J. & Ringel, R.L. (1987). Physiological fitness measures and sensory and motor performance in aging. *Experimental Gerontology, 22,* 5, 317–328. Reprinted with permission from Elsevier.

of aging, both the rate and extent of this decline vary widely between individuals. Individuals may deviate from expected patterns of aging and, at least for some period of time, postpone the consequences of aging (Fries & Crapo, 1981). For example, while measures of cardiovascular functioning usually decline with age (Lakatta, 1990), physically fit and active individuals sometimes exhibit slower declines in function than less healthy people of the same age (Goldberg & Hagberg, 1990). Researchers at San Diego State University studied a group of regular exercisers for several decades. Declines in maximal oxygen consumption were considerably less than the 10%-per-decade decrease that is usually observed in the general population (Kasch et al., 1990).

The physiological consequences of aging cannot be offset indefinitely. Nonetheless, there is increasingly strong evidence to suggest that aging need not occur at a uniform rate. Indeed, many age-related changes may be modified by specific lifestyle interventions, including regular physical activity.

## LIFESTYLE INTERVENTIONS— REGULAR PHYSICAL ACTIVITY

### The Benefits of Exercise for Older Adults

A good deal of attention has focused on the importance of regular physical activity as a means of enhancing health and effective functioning in old age. While most early research has focused on relatively young and healthy adults, there is now a conscious effort to extend our knowledge to a broader cross-section of the population. As an understanding of the physiological, psychological, and sociocultural significance of exercise grows, an increasing proportion of adults are opting to participate in some form of structured physical activity. Physicians and other health-care professionals are now recommending exercise as an adjunct to more traditional therapy for a variety of physical and psychological disorders.

Two often cited reports strongly endorse participation in physical activity for individuals of all ages. In 1996, the *Surgeon General's Report on Physical Activity and Health* concluded that regular physical activity has important positive effects on the musculoskeletal, cardiovascular, respiratory, and endocrine systems (U.S. Department of Health and Human Services, 1996). Furthermore, the effect of exercise on these systems is associated with a number of health benefits, including a decreased risk of premature mortality and reduced risks of coronary heart disease, hypertension, colon cancer, and diabetes. In addition, regular participation in physical activity also appears to reduce depression and anxiety, improve mood, and enhance our ability to perform daily tasks throughout the life span (U.S. Department of Health and Human Services, 1996).

The World Health Organization's (WHO) *Guidelines for Promoting Physical Activity Among Older Persons* (1997) offer a similarly strong endorsement. The guidelines conclude that there is compelling evidence that regular physical activity can assist in avoiding, minimizing, and/or reversing many of the physical, psychological, and social hazards that often accompany advancing age.

On May 1, 2001, a coalition of national organizations released a major planning document designed to develop a national strategy for the promotion of physically active lifestyles among the mid-life and older adult population. *The National Blueprint: Increasing Physical Activity Among Adults Age 50 and Older* was developed with input from 46 organizations with expertise in health, medicine, social and behavioral sciences, epidemiology, gerontology/geriatrics, clinical science, public policy, marketing, medical systems, community organization, and environmental issues (Armstrong et al., 2001). The National Blueprint Steering Committee consisted of representatives of the National Institute on Aging, the National Council on Aging, the Centers for Disease Control and Prevention, the American Geriatrics Society, the American College of Sports Medicine, and the Robert Wood Johnson Foundation.

*The National Blueprint* concludes that there is a substantial body of scientific evidence that indicates that regular physical activity can bring dramatic health benefits to people of all ages and abilities, and that this benefit extends over the entire life span. Physical activity offers one of the greatest opportunities to extend years of active independent life, reduce disability, and improve the quality of life for mid-life and older persons (Atienza, 2001; Eakin, 2001; Linnan & Marcus, 2001; Stewart,

2001; U.S. Department of Health and Human Services, 1996).

The following sections provide a brief overview of some of the physiological, psychological, and social benefits of regular exercise. Whenever possible, an attempt is made to address both the acute effects of a single bout of physical activity, as well as the more persistent and long-term effects of sustained participation in exercise and physical activity. Because physical activity has been defined in many different ways, in this section we will adopt the WHO's broad and inclusive definition of physical activity, which includes all movements in everyday life, including work, recreation, exercise, and sporting activities (World Health Organization, 1997).

## PHYSIOLOGICAL BENEFITS OF PHYSICAL ACTIVITY

The physiological benefits of participation in regular physical activity are well established (Table 1.1). Among the short-term benefits attributed to regular

---

Table 1.1

**A Summary of the Physiological Benefits of Physical Activity for Older Persons**

*Immediate Benefits:*

✓ Glucose Levels: Physical activity helps regulate blood glucose levels.

✓ Catecholamine Activity: Both adrenalin (epinephrine) and noradrenalin (norepinephrine) levels are stimulated by physical activity.

✓ Improved Sleep: Physical activity has been shown to enhance sleep quality and quantity in individuals of all ages.

*Long-term Effects:*

✓ Aerobic/Cardiovascular Endurance: Substantial improvements in almost all aspects of cardiovascular functioning have been observed following appropriate physical training.

✓ Resistive Training/Muscle Strengthening: Individuals of all ages can benefit from muscle-strengthening exercises. Resistance training can have a significant impact on the maintenance of independence in old age.

✓ Flexibility: Exercise that stimulates movement throughout the range of motion assists in the preservation and restoration of flexibility.

✓ Balance/Coordination: Regular activity helps prevent and/or postpone the age-associated declines in balance and coordination that are a major risk factor for falls.

✓ Velocity of Movement: Behavioral slowing is a characteristic of advancing age. Individuals who are regularly active can often postpone age-related declines.

World Health Organization (1997). The Heidelberg guidelines for promoting physical activity among older persons. *Journal of Aging and Physical Activity, 5,* 1, 2–8.

exercise are improved sleep (Brassington & Hicks, 1995), improved glucose regulation (Giacca et al., 1994), and increases in catecholamine activity (Richter & Sutton, 1994). Long-term adaptation to extended exercise participation includes improved cardiovascular performance, increased muscular strength and endurance, enhanced flexibility and range of motion, decreased adiposity, and improved lipid status (Spirduso, Francis, & MacRae, 2005). Goldberg and Hagberg (1990) suggest that the physiological responses of older adults to exercise training are essentially the same as those experienced by younger individuals. Several of the more common physiological adaptations associated with regular physical activity are discussed below.

## Cardiovascular Function

**Maximal oxygen consumption ($\dot{V}O_2max$)** during exercise is an excellent measure of cardiovascular fitness (McArdle, Katch, & Katch, 2000). $\dot{V}O_2max$ was previously thought to decline at a constant rate with advancing age (about 10% per decade). This decline was considered to be relatively stable across subjects and, to a large degree, independent of physical activity status (Hodgson, 1971; Dehn & Bruce, 1972). However, a number of studies suggest that age-related changes in $\dot{V}O_2max$ may be more variable (Heath et al., 1981; Rogers et al., 1990). For example, highly trained individuals who maintain high activity levels often experience little or no decline in $\dot{V}O_2max$ over periods of a decade or more (Kasch, Wallace, & VanCamp, 1985; Pollock et al., 1987).

Although the mechanisms by which exercise influences cardiovascular performance in older adults are complex, there is evidence to suggest that both central (increased **cardiac output**) and peripheral (increased oxidative capacity of the skeletal muscle) factors are involved (Goldberg & Hagberg, 1990). It is not possible to postpone age-related declines

in aerobic capacity forever. Nonetheless, there is increasingly strong evidence to suggest even modest levels of physical activity can result in significant increases in cardiovascular efficiency in old age.

## Pulmonary Function

Pulmonary efficiency declines with age, resulting in compromised lung elasticity and compliance (McKeown, 1965). Degenerative changes in the vertebral discs alter the shape of the thoracic cavity with a resultant reduction in pulmonary volume (McKeown, 1965). Decreased strength and mass of the thoracic muscles further compromise pulmonary efficiency (Dhar, Shastri, & Lenora, 1976), as do **calcification** and **ossification** of the **costovertebral** and **costochondral** joints (Grant, 1999).

In young and middle-aged individuals, aerobic exercise has minimal effects on vital capacity, expiratory volumes, and other measures of pulmonary performance (Shephard, 1993). However, because regular exercise is associated with reduced vertebral degeneration rates and increased thoracic muscle strength, physical activity may help preserve adequate levels of pulmonary function in older adults (Shephard, 1993). The results of a 25-year follow-up study indicate that physical activity is associated with a slower decline in pulmonary function in middle-aged and older adults (Pelkonen et al., 2003).

## Blood Pressure

More than two-thirds of people over age 65 have hypertension (National Institutes of Health, 2003). While both systolic and diastolic blood pressure increase significantly with advancing age (Spirduso, Francis, & MacRae, 2005), several exercise-training studies have shown that physical activity can reduce systolic and diastolic blood pressure in individuals of all ages with mild hypertension (Hagberg & Goldberg, 1990; Kokkinos, 2001; Whelton et al., 2002). For example, Motoyama et al. found that low-intensity aerobic training significantly reduced blood pressure in elderly hypertensive patients who were receiving medication to treat their high blood pressure. The study demonstrated that "blood pressure decreased significantly after three months of training and the blood pressure of all participants stabilized at a significantly lower level by the end of nine months in the training group, whereas no significant changes in blood pressure were found in the control group" (Motoyama et al., 1998).

### Blood Lipids

Aging is associated with increases in both total cholesterol and serum triglycerides (Buskirk, 1985). **Hypercholesterolemia** and **hyperlipidemia** are major medical problems that lead to the premature development of coronary artery disease (Castelli et al., 1977). Exercise training is now commonly associated with a reduction of coronary heart disease risk, and the American Heart Association (AHA) recognizes sedentary living as an independent risk factor for the development of **atherosclerosis** (Fletcher et al., 1992). A number of studies have shown that highly trained masters athletes exhibit favorable biochemical profiles (reduced low-density lipoprotein cholesterol, elevated high-density lipoprotein cholesterol) when compared with sedentary individuals of the same chronological age (Seals et al., 1984; Tamai et al., 1988). Because almost all instances of favorable improvements in biochemical profiles are associated with coincident decreases in body weight, it is frequently difficult to dissociate the effects of exercise from the effects of weight loss (Goldberg & Hagberg, 1990). This problem notwithstanding, there is sufficient evidence to suggest that regular exercise is associated with a decrease in body fat, which, in turn, is associated with a decrease in circulating lipids. However, the effect of exercise on blood lipids appears to be transient, and blood lipids return to pre-exercise values within a few days of cessation of physical activity (World Health Organization, 1997).

### Muscle Strength and Endurance

Muscle strength and endurance decline significantly with advancing age (Spirduso, Francis, & MacRae, 2005). In the past, strength training was seldom emphasized as a component of exercise programs designed for older adults. The lifting of heavy weights requires maximal or near-maximal muscular contractions that, if incorrectly performed, can result in sharp increases in blood pressure due to a physiological mechanism known as the **Valsalva maneuver** (McArdle, Katch, & Katch, 2000). Since these acute elevations in blood pressure are potentially dangerous for hypertensive individuals, most professional organizations did not advocate strength training for older adults. However, a number of studies have examined the effect of dynamic strength training in older adults. Morgan et al. (1995) demonstrated that older adults who trained with weights for 12 months were able to gain appreciable increases in muscular strength and endurance. No adverse consequences associated with weight training were reported in this study. Fiaterone et al. (1990) demonstrated that men and women as old as 90 years can safely lift heavy weights (80% of one repetition maximum). Remarkable strength gains in excess of 100% were reported for some of the muscle groups trained in this study.

Since the maintenance of adequate levels of muscular strength is critical for successfully performing many activities of daily living, exercise scientists are reevaluating the importance of strength training as a component of exercise programs for elderly adults. The American College of Sports Medicine recommends the inclusion of low- to moderate-intensity strength exercises in exercise-training regimens for older adults (American College of Sports Medicine, 2000).

## Flexibility

Aging is associated with changes in the elasticity and compliance of connective tissue (Spirduso, Francis, & MacRae, 2005), resulting in significant decreases in flexibility and range of motion. Although declines in flexibility and active range of motion are observed in most seniors, there is some evidence to suggest that declines in these areas are due in part to decreased physical activity, and that not all older individuals lose flexibility at the same rate (Campanelli, 1996). Stretching exercises that emphasize range of motion and flexibility have been shown to increase ankle, knee joint, and lower-back flexibility in older adults (Frekany & Leslie, 1975). Almost all structured

exercise programs advocate the inclusion of calisthenic exercises prior to aerobic exercise (Spirduso, Francis, & MacRae, 2005).

## PSYCHOLOGICAL BENEFITS OF PHYSICAL ACTIVITY

In addition to its effects on physiological variables, physical activity also can have significant psychological consequences. A summary of the long- and short-term benefits of physical activity for psychological functioning is included in Table 1.2.

Among the short-term psychological benefits attributed to regular exercise are improved relaxation (Landers & Petruzzello, 1994), reduced stress and anxiety (Petruzzello et al., 1991), and improved mood state (Nieman et al., 1993). Long-term benefits include improved life satisfaction (Berger &

---

Table 1.2

**A Summary of the Psychological Benefits of Physical Activity for Older Persons**

*Immediate Benefits:*

✓ Enhanced Relaxation: Appropriate physical activity enhances relaxation.

✓ Reduced Stress and Anxiety: There is evidence that regular physical activity can reduce stress and anxiety.

✓ Enhanced Mood State: Numerous people report elevations in mood state following appropriate physical activity.

*Long-term Effects:*

✓ General Well-being: Improvements in almost all aspects of psychological functioning have been observed following extended periods of physical activity.

✓ Improved Mental Health: Regular exercise can make an important contribution in the treatment of several mental illnesses, including depression and anxiety neuroses.

✓ Cognitive Improvements: Regular physical activity may help postpone age-related declines in central nervous system processing speed and improve reaction time.

✓ Motor Control and Performance: Regular activity helps prevent and/or postpone the age-associated declines in both fine and gross motor performance.

✓ Skill Acquisition: New skills can be learned and existing skills refined by all individuals regardless of age.

World Health Organization (1997). The Heidelberg guidelines for promoting physical activity among older persons. *Journal of Aging and Physical Activity, 5,* 1, 2–8.

Hecht, 1990), enhanced self-esteem and heightened self-efficacy (McAuley & Rudolph, 1995), and fewer mood state disturbances (O'Connor, Aenchbacher, & Dishman, 1993). Some of the more common psychological benefits associated with regular physical activity are discussed below.

### General Psychological Well-being

Although psychological health consists of both positive and negative components, previous research in the exercise sciences has focused predominantly on the effects of physical activity on negative components of psychological health, such as depression, anxiety, and other stress-related disorders. McAuley and his colleagues argued the importance of examining the relationship between physical activity and more positive elements of psychological functioning, including self-esteem, **self-efficacy,** and general well-being (McAuley, 1994; McAuley & Rudolph, 1995).

A review of 38 studies examining the relation between regular physical activity and general psychological well-being in older adult populations indicates that the vast majority of studies report a positive association between physical activity and well-being (McAuley & Rudolph, 1995). While this relationship appears to be independent of the mode of exercise employed (Mihalko & McAuley, 1996), the strength of the association is greatest for programs lasting 10 weeks or longer.

### Depression and Anxiety

The incidence of depression increases significantly with age (LaRue, Dessonville, & Jarvik, 1985). However, several studies suggest that the association between chronological age and depression may be confounded by decreases in physical activity levels that usually accompany advancing age (Parent & Whall, 1986; Berkman et al., 1986). When statistical procedures are used to control for individual differences in fitness, the association between advancing age and depression is substantially reduced (Chodzko-Zajko, 1990).

Accordingly, data suggesting depression increases with age may be at least partially due to the tendency for physical activity levels to decline with age and not simply due to the passage of time.

A number of studies have shown that participation in regular exercise reduces depression in patients with mild-to-moderate levels of clinical depression (Greist et al., 1979; Martinsen, Medhus, & Sandvik, 1985). Similarly, studies with non-clinical populations also indicate beneficial effects of exercise on mood state and anxiety (Morgan & O'Connor, 1987). There is mounting evidence that exercise plays an important role in helping individuals of all ages in managing anxiety and depression (Buckworth & Dishman, 2002).

### Cognitive Functioning

Age-related declines in **cognitive** performance are well established. However, cognition is not a unitary phenomenon and there are wide variations in the magnitude of changes in cognitive performance tasks observed with advancing age. Age-related changes in cognitive performance appear to be maximized for tasks that require rapid and complex processing, and are minimized for tasks that are more automatic or can be performed at a self-paced rate (Chodzko-Zajko & Moore, 1994).

Despite the fact that both processing resources and cognitive performance decline with advancing age, there are often considerable differences between subjects in both the rate and extent of this decline. There is substantial evidence to support the hypothesis that physically fit older adults often process cognitive information more efficiently than less-fit individuals of the same chronological age (Chodzko-Zajko, 1991). However, it is clear that the relationship between physical fitness and cognition is highly task-dependent. Physical fitness effects are observed more often during tasks requiring rapid cognitive processing than during self-paced or automatic processing tasks (Chodzko-Zajko & Moore, 1994). Because numerous task- and subject-related factors can influence the relationship between fitness and cognition, extreme caution is warranted before making generalizations about the influence of physical fitness on cognitive performance.

Despite the presence of a cross-sectional association between fitness and cognitive performance, the effect of exercise on cognitive performance remains unclear. Several well-controlled studies successfully demonstrated improvement in cognitive performance following training (Dustman et al., 1984; Hawkins, Kramer, & Capaldi, 1992; Moul, Goldman, & Warren, 1995). However, at least as many studies have been unable to replicate these findings (Blumenthal et al., 1989; 1991; Panton et al., 1990). Both the magnitude of improvement in aerobic capacity and the demand-level of the cognitive task may be important factors in determining the presence or absence of training effects. It is important to point out that the magnitude of changes in cognitive performance observed following exercise training has always been small.

In an attempt to clarify the confusion in the exercise training and cognition literature, Kramer and his colleagues (1999) have proposed that the benefits of exercise training may vary as a function of the demand level of the cognitive task. To test this hypothesis, they more recently conducted a meta-analysis of the 18 Randomized Clinical Trials and were able to identify which examined the effect of exercise training on cognitive functioning (Colcombe & Kramer, 2003). They characterized the cognitive tasks employed in these studies into four categories: (1) speeded tasks, which are simple tasks requiring rapid responses presumed to be relatively uncontaminated by high-level cognition; (2) visuospatial tasks, which require rotating real or imaginary objects in three dimensional space; (3) controlled processing tasks, which are dependent upon effortful processing strategies and which gradually become automatic with extended practice; and (4) executive control tasks, such as coordination, inhibition,

and working memory, which also depend on effortful processing but which do not become automatic over time. The meta-analysis found that effect sizes were strongest for the executive control tasks (.68), followed by the controlled processing tasks (.46), visuospatial (.42) and speeded (.27) tasks.

Kramer and colleagues concluded that there is clear evidence that both aerobic exercise and combined aerobic and strength exercise are associated with improvements in cognitive functioning relative to sedentary controls. However, they conclude that fitness effects are largest for tasks that require complex processing requiring executive control. Interestingly, combined aerobic and strength training was found to be slightly more effective in changing cognitive performance than aerobic exercise alone. Although the mechanisms responsible for training-induced improvements in cognitive performance are not well understood, Kramer and his colleagues have proposed that patterns of brain activation may vary between active and sedentary seniors. Future research using functional magnetic resonance imaging (fMRI) may be able to shed light on this possibility (Kramer et al., 2002).

Although much remains to be learned about the exact nature of the relationship between exercise training and cognitive performance, the most recent evidence is promising to the extent that reliable effects are consistently identified for at least certain aspects of cognitive processing.

A number of mechanisms have been proposed to explain the relationship between physical fitness and cognitive performance in old age (Chodzko-Zajko & Moore, 1994). Some evidence suggests that highly fit adults process information in the central nervous system faster and more efficiently than less-fit individuals of the same chronological age. This increased efficiency may be secondary to improvements in cerebral circulation, nerve cell regeneration, and/or changes in neurotransmitter synthesis and degradation.

## Social Implications of Regular Physical Activity

The vast majority of research studies examining the effects of exercise on the aging process have focused on the physiological and psychological benefits of activity. However, it would be inappropriate to conclude this section without a brief comment about the importance of physical activity for the social functioning of older persons.

In the WHO *Guidelines for Promoting Physical Activity Among Older Persons* (1997), a number of significant short- and long-term effects of physical activity on sociocultural variables are discussed (Table 1.3). Empowering older individuals and assisting them in playing a more active role in society are among the social benefits attributed to physical activity.

Aging is associated with a need to adjust to changing roles. Factors such as the deaths of friends and loved ones, retirement, financial hardship, ill-health, and isolation force many older people to systematically relinquish more and more of the roles that are a meaningful part of their identity (McPherson, 1990). Physical activity can help older persons better adjust to these changing roles. Activity programs provide seniors with the opportunity to widen their social networks, to stimulate new friendships, and to acquire positive new roles in their retirement (McPherson, 1990; 1994).

# EXERCISE PROGRAMMING FOR OLDER ADULTS

In the past, physical activity programming for older adults typically focused on a relatively small and healthy subgroup of

---

Table 1.3

**A Summary of the Social Benefits of Physical Activity for Older Persons**

*Immediate Benefits:*

✓ Empowering Older Individuals: A large proportion of the older adult population voluntarily adopts a sedentary lifestyle, which eventually threatens to reduce independence and self-sufficiency. Participation in appropriate physical activity can help empower older individuals and assist them in playing a more active role in society.

✓ Enhanced Social and Cultural Integration: Physical activity programs, particularly when carried out in small groups and/or in social environments, enhance social and intercultural interactions for many older adults.

*Long-term Effects:*

✓ Enhanced Integration: Regularly active individuals are less likely to withdraw from society and more likely to actively contribute to the social milieu.

✓ Formation of New Friendships: Participation in physical activity, particularly in small groups and other social environments, stimulates new friendships and acquaintances.

✓ Widened Social and Cultural Networks: Physical activity frequently provides individuals with an opportunity to widen available social networks.

✓ Role Maintenance and New Role Acquisition: A physically active lifestyle helps foster the stimulating environments necessary for maintaining an active role in society, as well as for acquiring positive new roles.

✓ Enhanced Intergenerational Activity: In many societies, physical activity is a shared activity that provides opportunities for intergenerational contact, thereby diminishing stereotypical perceptions about aging and the elderly.

World Health Organization (1997). The Heidelberg guidelines for promoting physical activity among older persons. *Journal of Aging and Physical Activity, 5,* 1, 2–8.

the older adult population (Chodzko-Zajko, 1995). However, it is now clear that the beneficial effects of regular physical activity are observable in almost all older persons regardless of their physical health. Several excellent and well-publicized studies have focused attention on the benefits of regular physical activity for seniors who were previously thought to be "too old" or "too frail" to partake in structured exercise programming (Spirduso, Francis, & MacRae, 2005). The World Health Organization (1997) suggests that most older adults fall along a Health-Fitness Gradient, with good health and fitness at one end of the continuum, and physical frailty and dependence at the other (Figure 1.2).

Within the WHO scheme, the physical activity needs of older persons differ substantially depending on their position along the Health-Fitness Gradient. The differing physical activity needs of the three groups are described below.

## Group III: Physically Fit—Healthy

These individuals regularly engage in physical activity, are described as physically fit and healthy, and have few limits in performing activities of daily living. Older adults in this group can participate in most physical activity programs, often exercising alongside individuals many years their junior.

## Group II: Physically Unfit—Unhealthy Independent

These individuals do not engage in adequate physical activity. While they still live independently in the community, they are at high risk for developing multiple chronic medical conditions that threaten their independence. Regular physical activity can help maintain independence and prevent regression into full dependency. However, physical activity programming must be individualized to account for special limitations and disabilities. The *Surgeon General's Report on Physical Activity and Health* estimates that at least 60% of the older adult population falls into this category (U.S. Department of Health and Human Services, 1996).

## Group I: Physically Unfit—Unhealthy Dependent

These individuals are no longer able to function independently in society due to a variety of physical and/or psychological reasons. Appropriate physical activity can significantly enhance the quality of life and restore independence in some areas of functioning. Physical activity programs have been developed for application in nursing homes and other residential facilities (Campanelli, 1996). A wide variety of chair and bed exercises can be performed on an individualized basis (Barry, Rich, & Carlson, 1993).

Figure 1.2
**World Health Organization Health-Fitness Gradient**

| | *Physically Fit* | *Physically Unfit* | *Physically Unfit Frail* |
|---|---|---|---|
| Healthy | GROUP III | | |
| Unhealthy Independent | | GROUP II | |
| Unhealthy Dependent | | | GROUP I |

World Health Organization (1997). The Heidelberg guidelines for promoting physical activity among older persons. *Journal of Aging and Physical Activity, 5,* 1, 2–8.

# Principles of Exercise Programming for Older Adults

It is inappropriate to apply generic exercise programs across the board for all older adults. Individual differences in health status, physical fitness, and previous exercise experience require that an exercise program be tailored to meet the specific needs of each person.

Older adults should be encouraged to seek advice from a health or exercise professional who can design a program to meet their individual needs. Previously sedentary men over 45 and women over 55 should obtain a thorough medical examination before embarking on an exercise program (American College of Sports Medicine, 2000). In cases where a physician's examination is not possible, pre-exercise screening questionnaires can assist in identifying contraindications to exercise (Cardinal & Cardinal, 1995).

A large percentage of the elderly population has remained sedentary due to the mistaken belief that they were not candidates for participation in regular physical activity. While there is an extremely small number of individuals for whom exercise is medically contraindicated (Stone, 1987), the vast majority of the elderly population can benefit from participation in some form of physical activity (World Health Organization, 1997). The emergence of specialized programs for specific clinical populations, such as cardiac rehabilitation programs, the Arthritis Foundation's PACE program, and programs for people with diabetes, is a testament to the fact that the benefits of physical activity need not be restricted to "jocks" and exercise fanatics.

The WHO *Guidelines for Promoting Physical Activity Among Older Persons* acknowledge the wide diversity of exercise regimens for older adults. Exercise, which can be an individual or group activity, can be performed in supervised or unsupervised settings. The guidelines stress that it is not necessary to have expensive facilities and equipment, and that successful programs are possible with limited resources (World Health Organization, 1997).

The sixth edition of the American College of Sports Medicine's *Guidelines for Exercise Testing and Prescription* (2000) notes that the general principles of exercise programming apply to individuals of all ages. However, due to the wide range of health and fitness levels observed among seniors, special care is needed when recommending exercise to older persons. The guidelines recognize that, for most older persons, a well-rounded exercise program consists of a cardiovascular component, resistance training, and flexibility exercises. For specific exercises and program design strategies, see Chapters 5, 6, and 7.

While recognizing the importance of individualized exercise programming, it is possible to make some comments about general principles of exercise programming for older adults.

## ACTIVITY MODE

Low-intensity, rhythmic activities that utilize large muscle groups, such as walking, jogging, bicycling, and swimming, are optimal for enhancing aerobic capacity. While personal preference typically dictates the type of activity chosen, orthopedic and/or other medical factors may restrict the number of available options. An increasing number of older adults participate in other activities such as various forms of dance and weight training. While these activities may not be appropriate for all older individuals, many people can obtain significant physiological benefits and much enjoyment from them (American College of Sports Medicine, 2000).

## TRAINING FREQUENCY

To obtain a reliable training effect, two to three training sessions per week are required (American College of Sports Medicine, 2000). However, habitual exercisers often exercise five or six days per week without adverse consequences (American College of Sports Medicine, 2000). It is important to note that many of the physiological, psychological, and social benefits of physical activity require regular and continuous participation and can rapidly be reversed by a return to inactivity.

## DURATION OF EXERCISE

Most structured exercise programs are designed to last about 45 minutes to one hour. This time is typically divided into 15 to 20 minutes of warm-up and stretching, 20 to 30 minutes of aerobic activity, and five to 10 minutes of cool-down. While this format is flexible, some evidence suggests that the aerobic component of exercise programs should last at least 20 minutes to obtain optimal cardiovascular benefits (Spirduso, Francis, & MacRae, 2005).

For the sedentary and frail individuals in Groups I and II of the WHO Health-Fitness Gradient, continuous activity for 45 to 60 minutes may be an unrealistic goal, at least at the onset of an exercise program. More modest exercise targets should be set for these individuals. As they slowly become reaccustomed to physical activity, exercise programs may be adjusted accordingly.

## EXERCISE INTENSITY

It is a popular misconception that high-intensity exercise is required for significant physiological gain. The saying "no pain, no gain" is simply not true. Such misconceptions perpetuate inappropriate attitudes about exercise and result in large numbers of individuals avoiding potentially beneficial and enjoyable behaviors. Many older adults first learned to exercise at a time when high-intensity exercise was widely considered more effective than more modest levels of activity. There has been extensive debate regarding the utility of traditional exercise programs when applied to the sedentary population (Blair, 1994).

Rather than adopt a hard-and-fast stance regarding the minimum frequency, duration, and intensity of exercise necessary to achieve a training effect, individuals should be encouraged to simply increase their activity level without setting rigid (and frequently intimidating) exercise programming guidelines.

## CONCLUSION

Advancing age is characterized by a progressive and insidious decline in the functional capacity of most physiological systems. While these declines in functional capacity are, to a large extent, inevitable and inescapable, considerable differences exist between individuals in the rate and extent of this decline. Several lines of research suggest that individuals who engage in healthful behaviors can often postpone or reduce these adverse consequences and, thus, deviate from expected patterns of aging.

The *Surgeon General's Report on Physical Activity and Health* recommends incorporating regular physical activity, which has significant physiological, psychological, and sociocultural benefits, into the everyday lives of all Americans of all ages (U.S. Department of Health and Human Services, 1996). The World Health Organization (1997) concludes that there is ample evidence that physical activity is associated with improvements in functional ability and health status and may frequently prevent or diminish the severity of certain diseases.

The benefits of physical activity are not restricted to the healthiest segment of the older adult population. On the contrary, there are significant benefits of physical activity for even the most frail members of society. As the advantages of physical activity for older adults become more widely appreciated, it is likely that a growing proportion of the population, regardless of age, will begin to include exercise as an integral component of their everyday routines.

# REFERENCES AND SUGGESTED READING

American College of Sports Medicine (2000). *ACSM's Guidelines for Exercise Testing and Prescription* (6th ed.). Baltimore: Lippincott Williams & Wilkins.

Armstrong, S. et al. (2001). National blueprint: Increasing physical activity among adults age 50 and older. *Journal of Aging and Physical Activity*, 9(Suppl.), 5–13.

Arking, R. (1998). *Biology of Aging: Observations and Principles* (2nd ed.). Englewood Cliffs, N.J.: Prentice-Hall, Inc.

Atienza, A.A. (2001). Home-based physical activity programs for middle-aged and older adults: Summary of empirical research. *Journal of Aging and Physical Activity*, 9(Suppl.), 38–58.

Baker, G.T. & Martin, G.R. (1994). Biological aging and longevity: Underlying mechanisms and potential intervention strategies. *Journal of Aging and Physical Activity*, 2, 4, 304–328.

Balin, A.K. (1994). *Practical Handbook of Human Biologic Age Determination*. Boca Raton, Fla.: CRC Press.

Balin, A.K. (1983). Testing the free radical theory of aging. In R.C. Adelman & G.S. Roth (Eds.) *Testing the Theories of Aging*. Boca Raton, Fla.: CRC Press.

Barry, H., Rich, B., & Carlson, T. (1993). How exercise can benefit older patients: A practical approach. *The Physician and Sportsmedicine*, 21, 2, 124–140.

Berger, B.G. & Hecht, L.M. (1990). Exercise, aging and psychological well-being: The mind-body question. In A.C. Ostrow (Ed.) *Aging and Motor Behavior* (307–323). Indianapolis: Benchmark Press.

Berkman, L.F. et al. (1986). Depressive symptoms in relation to physical health and functioning in the elderly. *American Journal of Epidemiology*, 124, 372–388.

Birren, J.E. (1959). Principles of research on aging. In J.E. Birren (Ed.) *Handbook of Aging and the Individual* (3–32). Chicago, Ill.: University of Chicago Press.

Bjorksten, J. (1968). The cross linkage theory of aging. *Journal of the American Geriatric Society*, 16, 408–427.

Blair, S.N. (1994). Physical activity, fitness, and coronary heart disease. In C. Bouchard, R.J. Shephard, & T. Stephens (Eds.) *Physical Activity, Fitness, and Health*. Champaign, Ill.: Human Kinetics.

Blumenthal, J.A. et al. (1991). Long-term effects of exercise on psychological functioning in older men and women. *Journal of Gerontology*, 46, 352–361.

Blumenthal, J.A. et al. (1989). Cardiovascular and behavioral effects of aerobic exercise training in healthy older men and women. *Journal of Gerontology*, 44, 147–157.

Bokovy, J.L. & Blair, S.N. (1994). Aging and exercise and health perspective. *Journal of Aging and Physical Activity*, 2, 3, 243–260.

Brassington, G.S. & Hicks, R.A. (1995). Aerobic exercise and self-reported sleep quality in elderly individuals. *Journal of Aging and Physical Activity*, 3, 2, 120–134.

Buckworth, J. & Dishman, R.K. (2002). *Exercise Psychology*. Champaign, Ill.: Human Kinetics.

Buskirk, E.R. (1985). Health maintenance and longevity: Exercise. In E.L. Schneider et al. (Eds.). *The Handbook of the Biology of Aging* (2nd ed.). New York: Van Nostrand Reinhold.

Campanelli, L.C. (1996). Mobility changes in older adults: Implications for practitioners. *Journal of Aging and Physical Activity*, 4, 2, 105–118.

Cardinal, B.J. & Cardinal, M.K. (1995). Screening efficiency of the revised physical activity readiness questionnaire in older adults. *Journal of Aging and Physical Activity*, 3, 3, 299–308.

Castelli, W.P. et al. (1977). HDL cholesterol and other lipids in coronary heart disease: The Cooperative Lipoprotein Phenotyping Study. *Circulation*, 55, 767–772.

Chodzko-Zajko, W.J. (1995). Editorial: Addressing the physical activity needs of the physically frail and the oldest old. *Journal of Aging and Physical Activity*, 3, 3, 221–222.

Chodzko-Zajko, W.J. (1994). A multivariate approach to the quantification of biologic age. In A.K Balin. (Ed.) *Practical Handbook of Human Biologic Age Determination* (157–171). Boca Raton, Fla.: CRC Press.

Chodzko-Zajko, W.J. (1993). Editorial: Great beginnings for JAPA. *Journal of Aging and Physical Activity,* 1, 1, 1.

Chodzko-Zajko, W.J. (1991). Physical fitness, cognitive performance and aging. *Medicine and Science in Sports and Exercise,* 23, 868–872.

Chodzko-Zajko, W.J. (1990). The influence of general health status on the relationship between chronological age and depressed mood state. *Journal of Geriatric Psychiatry,* 23, 13–22.

Chodzko-Zajko, W.J. & Moore, K.A. (1994). Physical fitness and cognitive functioning in aging. *Exercise and Sport Science Reviews,* 22, 195–220.

Chodzko-Zajko, W.J. & Ringel, R.L. (1987). Physiological fitness measures and sensory and motor performance in aging. *Experimental Gerontology,* 22, 5, 317–328.

Colcombe, S. & Kramer, A.F. (2003). Fitness effects on the cognitive function of older adults: A meta analytic study. *Psychological Science,* 14, 125–130.

Cousins, S.O. (1997). Elderly tomboys? Sources of self-efficacy for physical activity in late life. *Journal of Aging and Physical Activity,* 5, 229–243.

Cousins, S.O. & Vertinsky, P.A. (1995). Recapturing the physical activity experiences of the old: A study of three women. *Journal of Aging and Physical Activity,* 3, 2, 146–162.

Dehn, M.M. & Bruce, R.A. (1972). Longitudinal variations in maximal oxygen intake with age and activity. *Journal of Applied Physiology,* 33, 6, 805–807.

Dhar, S., Shastri, S.R., & Lenora, R.A.K. (1976). Aging and the respiratory system. *Medical Clinics of North America,* 60, 1121–1139.

Dustman, R.E. et al. (1984). Aerobic exercise training and improved neuropsychological function of older individuals. *Neurobiology of Aging,* 5, 35–42.

Eakin, E. (2001). Promoting physical activity among middle-aged and older adults in health care settings. *Journal of Aging and Physical Activity,* 9(Suppl.), 29–37.

Fiaterone, M.A. et al. (1990). High-intensity strength training in nonagenarians. *Journal of the American Medical Association,* 263, 3029–3034.

Fletcher, G.F. et al. (1992). Statement on exercise: Benefits and recommendations for physical activity programs for all Americans. A statement for health professionals by the Committee on Exercise and Cardiac Rehabilitation of the Council on Clinical Cardiology, American Heart Association. *Circulation,* 86, 340–344.

Frekany, G.A. & Leslie, D.K. (1975). Effects of an exercise program on selected flexibility measurements of senior citizens. *Gerontologist,* 15, 182–183.

Fries J.F. & Crapo L.M. (1981). *Vitality and Aging.* San Francisco: Freeman.

Giacca, A. et al. (1994). Physical activity, fitness, and type 1 diabetes. In: C. Bouchard, R.J. Shephard, & T. Stephens (Eds.) *Physical Activity, Fitness and Health: International Proceedings and Consensus Statement* (656–668). Champaign, Ill.: Human Kinetics.

Goldberg, A.P. & Hagberg, J.M. (1990). Physical exercise and the elderly. In: E.L. Schneider & J.W. Rowe (Eds.) *Handbook of the Biology of Aging* (407–423). San Diego: Academic Press.

Grant, J.C.B. (1999). *Grant's Atlas of Anatomy* (10th ed.). Baltimore: Lippincott Williams & Wilkins.

Greist, J.H. et al. (1979). Running as a treatment for depression. *Comprehensive Psychiatry,* 20, 41–54.

Hagberg, J.M. et al. (1985). A hemodynamic comparison of young and older endurance athletes during exercise. *Journal of Applied Physiology,* 58, 2041–2046.

Harman, D. (1956). Aging: A theory based on free radical and radiation chemistry. *Journal of Gerontology,* 11, 298–300.

Hawkins, H., Kramer, A.F, & Capaldi, D. (1992). Aging, exercise, and attention. *Psychology and Aging,* 7, 643–653.

Hayflick, L. (1985). Theories of biological aging. *Experimental Gerontology*, 20, 145–159.

Hayflick, L. (1965). The limited in vitro lifespan of human diploid cell strains. *Experimental Cellular Respiration*, 37, 614–635.

Heath, G.W. et al. (1981). A physiological comparison of young and older endurance athletes during exercise. *Journal of Applied Physiology*, 58, 6, 2041–2046.

Heikkinen, E. et al. (1994). Variations in aging parameters, their sources, and possibilities of predicting physiological age. In A.K. Balin (Ed.) *Practical Handbook of Human Biologic Age Determination* (71–92). Boca Raton, Fla.: CRC Press.

Hodgson, J.L. (1971). *Age and aerobic capacity of urban midwestern males.* Ph.D. Dissertation, University of Minnesota.

Jones, C.J. & Rikli, R.E. (1994). The revolution in aging: Implications for curriculum development and professional preparation in physical education. *Journal of Aging and Physical Activity*, 2, 3, 261–272.

Kallman, F.J. & Sander, G. (1948). Twin studies on aging and longevity. *Journal of Heredity*, 39, 349–357.

Kasch, F.W. et al. (1990). The effects of physical activity and inactivity on aerobic power in older men: A longitudinal study. *The Physician and Sportsmedicine*, 18, 73–83.

Kasch, F.W., Wallace, J.P., & VanCamp, S.P. (1985). Effects of 18 years endurance exercise on the physical work capacity of older men. *Journal of Cardiopulmonary Rehabilitation*, 5, 308–312.

Kim, H.S. & Tanaka, K. (1995). The assessment of functional age using Activities of Daily Living Performance Tests: A study of Korean women. *Journal of Aging and Physical Activity*, 3, 1, 39–48.

Kokkinos, P.F. (2001). Exercise as hypertension therapy. *Hellenic Journal of Cardiology*, 42, 182–192.

Kramer, A.F. et al. (2002). Effects of aerobic fitness training on human cortical functioning. *Journal of Molecular Neuroscience*, 19, 227–231.

Kramer, A.F. et al. (1999). Aging, fitness, and neurocognitive function. *Nature*, 400, 418–419.

Lakatta, E.G. (1990). Changes in cardiovascular function with aging. *European Heart Journal*, 11, 22–29.

Landers, D.M. & Petruzzello, S.J. (1994). Physical activity, fitness, and anxiety. In C. Bouchard, R.J. Shephard, & T. Stephens (Eds.) *Physical Activity, Fitness and Health: International Proceedings and Consensus Statement* (868–882). Champaign, Ill.: Human Kinetics.

LaRue, A., Dessonville, C., & Jarvik, L.F. (1985). Aging and mental disorders. In J.E. Birren & K.W. Schaie (Eds.) *Handbook of the Psychology of Aging.* New York: Van Nostrand Reinhold.

Linnan, L.A. & Marcus, B. (2001). Worksite-based physical activity programs and older adults: Current status and priorities for the future. *Journal of Aging and Physical Activity*, 9(Suppl.), 59–70.

Martinsen, E.W., Medhus, A., & Sandvik, L. (1985). Effects of aerobic exercise on depression: A controlled study. *British Medical Journal*, 291, 109.

McArdle, W.D., Katch, F.I., & Katch, V.L. (2000). *Essentials of Exercise Physiology* (2nd ed.). New York: Lippincott Williams & Wilkins.

McAuley, E. (1994). Physical activity and psychosocial outcomes. In C. Bouchard, R.J. Shephard, & T. Stephens (Eds.) *Physical Activity, Fitness and Health: International Proceedings and Consensus Statement* (551–568). Champaign, Ill.: Human Kinetics.

McAuley, E. & Rudolph, D. (1995). Physical activity, aging, and psychological well-being. *Journal of Aging and Physical Activity*, 3, 1, 67–98.

McGrath, J.E. & Kelly, J.R. (1985). *Time and Human Interaction: Toward a Social Psychology of Time.* New York: Guildford.

McKeown, F. (1965). *Pathology of the Aged.* London: Butterworths.

McPherson, B.D. (1994). Sociocultural perspectives on aging and physical activity. *Journal of Aging and Physical Activity*, 2, 4, 329–353.

McPherson, B.D. (1990). *Aging as a Social Process.* Toronto: Butterworths.

Medvedev, Z.A. (1981). Age changes and the rejuvenation processes related to reproduction. *Mechanisms of Aging and Development,* 17, 331–359.

Mihalko, S.L. & McAuley, E. (1996). Strength training effects on subjective well-being and physical function in the elderly. *Journal of Aging and Physical Activity,* 4, 1, 56–68.

Morgan, A.L. et al. (1995). The supplemental benefits of strength training for aerobically active postmenopausal women. *Journal of Aging and Physical Activity,* 3, 332–339.

Morgan, W.P. & O'Connor, P.J. (1987). Exercise and mental health. In R.K. Dishman (Ed.) *Exercise Adherence* (91–121). Champaign, Ill.: Human Kinetics.

Motoyama, M. et al. (1998). Blood pressure lowering effect of low-intensity aerobic training in elderly hypertensive patients. *Medicine and Science in Sports and Exercise,* 30, 6, 818–823.

Moul, J.L., Goldman, B., & Warren, B. (1995). Physical activity and cognitive performance in the older population. *Journal of Aging and Physical Activity,* 3, 2, 135–144.

National Institutes of Health (2003). The Seventh Report of the Joint National Committee on Prevention, Detection, Evaluation, and Treatment of High Blood Pressure: The JNC 7 Report. *Journal of the American Medical Association,* 298, 2560–2571.

Nieman, D.C. et al. (1993). Physical activity, psychological well-being, and mood state in elderly women. *Journal of Aging and Physical Activity,* 1, 1, 22–33.

O'Connor, P.J., Aenchbacher, L.E., & Dishman, R.K. (1993). Physical activity and depression in the elderly. *Journal of Aging and Physical Activity,* 1, 1, 34–58.

Panton, L.B. et al. (1990). Effect of aerobic resistance training on fractionated reaction time and speed of movement. *Journal of Gerontology,* 45, 26–31.

Parent, C.J. & Whall, A.L. (1986). Are physical activity, self-esteem and depression related? *Journal of Geriatric Nursing,* 10, 8–11.

Partridge, S.M. (1970). Biological role of cutaneous elastin. In W. Montagna, J.P. Bentley, & R.L. Dobson (Eds.) *Advances in Biology of Skin* (69–87). New York: Meredith.

Pelkonen, M. et al. (2003). Delay and decline in pulmonary function with physical activity: A 25-year follow up. *American Journal of Respiratory and Critical Care Medicine,* 168, 494–499.

Petruzzello, S.J. et al. (1991). A meta-analysis on the anxiety reducing effects of acute and chronic exercise. *Sports Medicine,* 11, 143–182.

Pollock, M.L. et al. (1987). Effect of age and training on aerobic capacity and body composition of masters athletes. *Journal of Applied Physiology,* 62, 725–731.

Richter, E.A. & Sutton, J.A. (1994). Hormonal adaptations to physical activity. In C. Bouchard, R.J. Shephard, & T. Stephens (Eds.) *Physical Activity, Fitness and Health: International Proceedings and Consensus Statement* (331–342). Champaign, Ill.: Human Kinetics.

Rogers, M.A. et al. (1990). Decline in $VO_2$max with aging in master athletes and sedentary men. *Journal of Applied Physiology,* 68, 5, 2195–2199.

Rose, C.L. (1972). The measurement of social age. *Aging and Human Development,* 3, 153–168.

Schroots, J.J. & Birren, J.E. (2001). Concepts of time and aging in science. In J.E. Birren & K.W. Schaie (Eds.) *The Handbook of the Psychology of Aging* (5th ed.) (45–66). San Diego: Academic Press.

Seals, D.R. et al. (1984). Elevated high-density lipoprotein levels in older endurance athletes. *American Journal of Cardiology,* 54, 390–393.

Shephard, R.J. (1998). Aging and exercise, In T.D. Fahey (Ed.) *Encyclopedia of Sports Medicine and Science.* Internet Society for Sports Science. www.sportsci.org

Shephard, R.J. (1997). *Aging, Physical Activity and Health.* Champaign, Ill.: Human Kinetics.

Shephard, R.J. (1993). Aging respiratory function and exercise. *Journal of Aging and Physical Activity,* 1, 1, 59–83.

Spirduso, W.W., Francis, K.L., & MacRae, P.G. (2005). *Physical Dimensions of Aging* (2nd ed.). Champaign, Ill.: Human Kinetics.

Stewart, A.L. (2001). Community-based physical activity programs for adults age 50 and older. *Journal of Aging and Physical Activity,* 9(Suppl.), 71–91.

Stone, W.J. (1987). *Adult Fitness Programs.* Glenview, Ill.: Scott Foresman.

Tamai, T. et al. (1988). The effects of physical exercise on plasma lipoprotein and apolipoprotein metabolism in elderly men. *Journal of Gerontology,* 43, 4, M75–79.

United States Department of Health and Human Services (1996). *Physical Activity and Health: A Report of the Surgeon General.* Atlanta, Ga.: U.S. Department of Health and Human Services, Centers for Disease Control and Prevention, National Center for Chronic Disease Prevention and Health Promotion.

Vandervoort, A.A. et al. (1992). Age and sex effects on the mobility of the human ankle. *Journal of Gerontology: Medical Sciences,* 47, M17–M24.

Walford, R.L. (1987). MHC regulation of aging: An extension of the immunologic theory of aging. In H.R. Warner et al. (Eds.) *Modern Biological Theories of Aging.* New York: Raven Press.

Walford, R.L. (1983). Supergenes: Histocompatibility, immunologic and other parameters in aging. In W. Regelson & F.M. Sinex (Eds.) *Intervention in the Aging Process, Part B: Basic Research and Preclinical Screening.* New York: Alan R. Liss.

Whelton, S.P. et al. (2002). Affect of aerobic exercise on blood pressure: A meta-analysis of randomized, controlled trials. *Annals of Internal Medicine,* 136, 493–503.

World Health Organization (1997). The Heidelberg guidelines for promoting physical activity among older persons. *Journal of Aging and Physical Activity,* 5, 1, 2–8.

# CHAPTER TWO

# Understanding and Motivating

## OLDER ADULTS

Sheri Thompson
Susan J. Hoekenga

David M. Williams
Bess H. Marcus

*Sheri Thompson, Ph.D., is a licensed clinical psychologist with more than 14 years of experience in the field of behavioral health research and intervention development. She has worked on a variety of behavioral health research projects and programs, including a longitudinal health outcome study of 700 frail elders, multiple projects as part of the San Diego State University Institute for Public Health, and on a physical activity intervention project for college students. Since the early 1990s, Dr. Thompson has worked with the PACE projects, which offer tailored physical activity and nutrition interventions for various populations, and was a co-editor of the PACE provider manuals. Dr. Thompson trained healthcare providers on how to counsel patients to make physical activity and dietary changes for several PACE projects and for the San Diego Center for Health Interventions, LLC.*

*Susan J. Hoekenga, M.P.A., M.S.G., has worked in the field of aging for more than 20 years. She has been involved with aging policy issues at the federal, state, and local levels, and is currently building programs to reach under-served, frail, and low-income elders for a non-profit agency. Hoekenga completed her graduate degrees in public administration and gerontology at the University of Southern California in 1995.*

*David M. Williams, Ph.D., is a postdoctoral fellow in clinical psychology at the Centers for Behavioral and Preventive Medicine, Brown Medical School/The Miriam Hospital. Dr. Williams has developed and implemented physical activity interventions and has expertise in critical analysis and integration of theoretical variables from various health behavior models that are particularly relevant to physical activity motivation.*

*Bess H. Marcus, Ph.D., is Professor of Psychiatry and Human Behavior at the Brown University School of Medicine and Director of Physical Activity Research at the Brown University Centers for Behavioral and Preventive Medicine at The Miriam Hospital. Dr. Marcus is a clinical health psychologist who has spent the last 18 years conducting research on physical activity behavior and has published more than 100 papers and book chapters as well as three books on this topic. She has developed a series of assessment instruments to measure psychosocial mediators of physical activity behavior and has developed low-cost interventions to promote physical activity behavior in community, workplace, and primary care settings.*

How can you learn to address individual needs and facilitate positive changes in health and physical activity behaviors? This can be a difficult task, especially when your viewpoint may differ from that of your clients. As a fitness professional, your role extends beyond the scope of technical instruction and demonstrating proper form for a stretch or the operation of strength-training equipment. Health behaviors such as physical activity are simply one aspect of a complex life, so attempts to promote health-behavior changes must take into account the individual's unique lifestyle. While competent technical instruction is crucial, fitness professionals also must collaborate with each client to develop and implement a physical activity program that complements the individual's objectives, personality, and life demands.

The ability to adapt your work to the individual needs of each client is particularly important when working with older adults, as diversity is the theme that best characterizes this population.

Imagine trying to describe all 30-year-olds in a few sentences. You probably would be quick to note vast differences between people of that age group. Why would we expect those same diverse individuals to become more similar to one another by the time they reach their senior years? Older Americans vary widely in terms of physical and psychological health, cultural and ethnic backgrounds, economic means, living conditions, availability of social support, and perspectives on aging and physical activity. In addition, while some older adults have retired, others continue working well past what is often considered typical retirement age. In short, older adults vary in just about every aspect of life.

Individuals of similar ages may share some common perspectives, as they have gone through some of the same historical events and life experiences. It is important to learn about issues and viewpoints commonly shared by older adults. A basic understanding of the aging process can help you listen for and understand common themes that may emerge. With these issues in mind, you can apply sound behavior-change principles to promote positive, sustainable gains in your clients' physical activity and health. This chapter covers some common issues related to aging and physical activity, as well as specific behavior-change, leadership, and communication strategies to use while working with older adults. Combined with your fitness expertise, this knowledge of how the aging process relates to physical activity and recommended strategies will enable you to better serve your older clients.

## UNDERSTANDING THE CONTEXT OF EXERCISE AMONG OLDER ADULTS

### Impact of Stereotypes on Exercise Programs for Older Adults

Stereotypes are problematic because they restrict our ways of seeing and interacting with members of the stereotyped groups. Ageism describes stereotypes of, or discrimination against, peo-ple in a certain age group, such as older adults (Butler et al., 2000). Those with ageist views often see older adults as homogeneous. Rowe and Kahn (1998) discuss a number of fundamental myths of aging, including:

✓ To be old is to be sick.
✓ You can't teach an old dog new tricks.
✓ It is too late to benefit from lifestyle change.
✓ The secret to successful aging is to choose your parents wisely.
✓ Older adults cannot pull their own weight.

Although many people accept some of these statements as common knowledge, each of these myths has been refuted by empirical evidence (Rowe & Kahn, 1998).

Older adults are often aware of these stereotypes. They receive messages that growing older should go hand-in-hand with decreased physical activity, and that older adults should slow down and "take it easy." Exposure to negative stereotypes can lead to reduced **self-efficacy** (defined as self-confidence in one's ability to perform a certain task) and a heightened cardiovascular response to stress (Levy et al., 2000). Moreover, people who believe that exercise is inappropriate or unnatural for older adults will not be inclined to develop or support exercise programming for this group, restricting the scope of exercise options for those who are motivated to be physically active.

Unfortunately, stereotyping also has led many health professionals—and the public in general—to view the elderly as less worthy of investment than the young. There is a temptation to encourage older persons to tolerate even reversible conditions rather than take a proactive approach to their well-being. Such treatment may convey the message that seniors should adjust to the circumstances of their lives without actively attempting to alter them (Steuart, 1993).

## Factors Related to Exercise Among Older Adults

Americans are aging, but aging does not create a homogeneous group. Older Americans are wealthy and poor, young-old and old-old, healthy and living with chronic ailments. There are probably more dissimilarities than common traits among the elderly. These differences significantly impact the profiles of older persons who typically seek out formal exercise programs, and are most evident when viewed by gender, ethnicity, and income.

Demographic factors associated with higher rates of physical activity among those 65 years of age or older include male gender, younger age, higher levels of education, and being unmarried (Kaplan et al., 2001). In addition, older adults who do not have chronic health conditions, injuries, or functional limitations are more likely to be physically active. This is also true of those who have a lower body mass index, do not smoke, or have lower levels of psychological distress (Kaplan et al., 2001). Among older women, those of Native-American and African-American ethnicity are less likely to be physically active than women of other ethnicities (King et al., 2000). For low-income and minority seniors in particular, the biggest deterrents are lack of access to exercise programs and lack of knowledge about the benefits of exercise for older adults. These seniors also may not be aware of (or have access to) financial and community resources that might enable them to practice healthy habits such as proper nutrition and preventive healthcare.

Also, in the United States, women live significantly longer than men. The life expectancy of men is 74.4 years, while for women it is 79.8 (Arias & Smith, 2003). Because life expectancy is greater for women than for men, exercise programs will continue to be needed by more older women than men, particularly those older than 75.

## Meeting the Needs of a Diverse Older Adult Population

A growing number of seniors have recognized the benefits of physical activity, and exercise programs must be developed to address their needs and encourage increased participation. Effective exercise promotion for older adults should include the following elements:

✓ Consideration of the exercise attitudes and behaviors of each individual
✓ Explanation of the risks and complications of exercise
✓ A medical assessment to determine fitness level
✓ Exercise programs tailored to each individual
✓ Monitored effects of exercise
✓ Use of motivational tools to increase compliance
✓ Referral to other professionals for nutritional evaluation or counseling, if necessary

Programs that include each of the above elements will be best-suited to meeting diverse needs.

# THE FUNCTIONS OF EXERCISE FOR OLDER ADULTS

## Exercise to Improve or Maintain Fitness or Health

The Surgeon General has summarized data on the numerous health benefits of physical activity (U.S. Department of Health and Human Services, 1996), some of which are specific to older adults. For example, in a review of studies in this area, Keysor (2003) found that physical activity increases muscle strength and aerobic capacity and can help reduce functional limitations, such as being unable to do household chores. Moreover, resistance training, in addition to aerobic exercise such as walking, can build muscle or prevent loss of existing muscle mass, which can help preserve bone mineral density and prevent osteoporosis, heart disease, and type 2 diabetes (Seguin & Nelson, 2003).

## Exercise to Improve Emotional and Mental Status

A number of studies of middle-aged and younger adults have shown that physical activity also has a number of psychological benefits, including improved mood and decreased risk of depression (for a review see Morgan, 1997; Buckworth & Dishman, 2002). Although there is less research on the psychological benefits of physical activity specifically for older adults, existing studies also show beneficial effects in terms of reducing risk of depression (Blumenthal et al., 1999) and anxiety (Lavie et al., 1999). A more recent study provided evidence that resistance training, in addition to aerobic exercise, also reduces risk of depression (Seguin & Nelson, 2003). In addition, exercise is associated with improved cognitive functioning in older adults, including enhanced memory (Rebok & Plude, 2001).

## THEORIES OF HEALTH BEHAVIOR CHANGE

Beginning or modifying an exercise program requires change on the part of your clients, an often difficult task to undertake. A regular exerciser may have to increase intensity, duration, or frequency, or add another type of exer-

cise to their program to address a new component of fitness. Non-active individuals may have to incorporate a brand new set of activities into their lifestyle, which may require decreasing sedentary pursuits like watching television or reading, and/or setting aside time for exercise despite a schedule filled with active tasks (i.e., volunteer work, caring for friends or family members, or paid work).

To help others make desired behavior changes, you must first understand those factors that encourage or hinder exercise behaviors. Although the field of exercise psychology is relatively new, various health, exercise, and psychology researchers already have developed useful theories about how and why people engage in physical activity.

## The Health Belief Model

The Health Belief Model (Rosenstock, 1966) suggests that the major factors influencing physical activity include perceptions of vulnerability to illness or negative health outcomes, combined with the perception of the seriousness of these outcomes. A person with a strong family history of heart disease, for example, might be highly motivated to improve their cardiovascular fitness as a means of decreasing their chance of having a heart attack. The individual must believe the preventive action (such as regularly running on a treadmill) will help prevent the health problem. Additionally, the perceived benefits of physical activity must outweigh the perceived costs of changing. The person also must have a minimum degree of confidence in their ability to start and maintain the healthy behavior. Lastly, this model suggests the use of cues as reminders to be active, such as placing jogging shoes by the front door.

## Social Cognitive Theory

According to social cognitive theory, physical activity is determined by self-regulation of behavior over time, which is accomplished through goal-setting and feelings of personal efficacy, as well as perceiving and structuring the physical and social environment in ways that provide rewards for continuing physical activity. Self-efficacy is an important determinant of physical activity. Expectations about the outcomes of physical activity are also important. Indeed, a review of outcome expectancies suggests that expected health benefits of physical activity may be especially important among older adults (Williams, Anderson, & Winett, 2005). One possible explanation for this is that older adults, more than younger adults, may view the protective effects of physical activity, such as preventing heart attack and some forms of cancer, as more relevant and urgent. However, this hypothesis has not yet been directly tested (Williams, Anderson, & Winett, 2005).

## The Theory of Planned Behavior

The theory of planned behavior posits that a person's intention to be physically active and their belief that they are able to be consistently active determines their level of physical activity (Ajzen, 1991). People's intentions are based on the expected outcomes of physical activity, the perceived importance of those outcomes, and the perceived expectations or norms of other people, such as family or friends, who are considered to be important. Meta-analyses have shown that the theory of planned behavior has been successful in predicting and explaining physical activity behavior (Hagger, Chatzisarantis, &

Biddle, 2002; Hausenblas, Carron, & Mack, 1997).

## Relapse Prevention Model

The Relapse Prevention Model was derived from research on why people stop abstaining from undesirable behaviors such as cigarette smoking or substance abuse (Marlatt & Gordon, 1980; 1985). The concept of relapse prevention also has been applied to understanding why individuals stop healthy habits. Factors such as negative emotional states, limited coping skills, social pressure to cease desired behaviors, interpersonal conflicts, limited social support, stress, and encountering "high-risk" situations can contribute to the cessation of desired behaviors.

When individuals do experience a setback (a temporary lapse in activity), they often believe it will lead to complete failure. Belief in their ability to succeed may be lost after only one slip-up, leaving them feeling out of control, guilty, discouraged, and ashamed. This negative thinking can interfere with resuming the desired behaviors (Marlatt & Gordon, 1985). Preparing clients to cope with high-risk situations can prevent relapses. Helping clients to understand that relapses are normal, and even likely, can help them to better cope with setbacks when they do occur, and to resume physical activity as soon as possible. Research has shown that relapse-prevention strategies increase adherence to physical activity programs (Belisle, Roskies, & Levesque, 1987).

## Transtheoretical Model

The transtheoretical model is different from previous models discussed in that it suggests an individual's readiness to engage in behaviors can be described on a continuum of stages, known as the Stages of Change (Prochaska &

DiClemente, 1982; 1983). Although this theory was originally developed to refer to psychotherapy processes (Prochaska & DiClemente, 1982) and later, to smoking cessation (Prochaska & DiClemente, 1983), other researchers have adapted the model specifically to physical activity (Marcus & Forsyth, 2003).

A number of processes of change are important in moving people from one stage to the next. These processes were incorporated into the transtheoretical model by looking at important mechanisms from a number of other theoretical models. Therefore, the transtheoretical model can be thought of as an integration of a number of different motivational theories, and it incorporates many of the theorized determinants described in the prior models. For example, self-efficacy and outcome expectancies are also thought to be important determinants of physical activity in the transtheoretical model.

Stages of readiness to be physically active include:

**Precontemplation**—an absence of serious consideration of changing the behavior within the next six months or so (e.g., "I have never exercised before and I have no desire to start now.")

**Contemplation**—not engaging in the behavior but seriously considering doing so (e.g., "I know I should start getting more exercise to help lose weight. Maybe I should join my neighbors on their morning walks.")

**Preparation**—have decided to initiate a change within a month's time and have begun the change process (e.g., have begun taking daily 10-minute walks, meet friends to walk at least once a week)

**Action**—consistently engaging in the behavior at the recommended frequency and intensity (e.g., brisk walking for 30 minutes per day five or more days per week) but for less than six consecutive months, and thus still at a high risk of relapse

**Maintenance**—have made a successful, sustained lifestyle change and are consistently engaging in the behavior at the recommended frequency and intensity for at least six months

This model is especially helpful to fitness professionals because it acknowledges individual differences in readiness to exercise at any particular point in time. Marcus and Forsyth (2003) suggest that goals and program strategies must be tailored to the readiness of each individual. It would be inappropriate, for example, to expect a person in the precontemplation stage to commit to an exercise program. Instead, interventions with a person in this stage would ideally encourage them to consider starting an exercise plan, perhaps by educating them about the benefits of exercise.

In contrast, a person who has been in the maintenance stage of physical activity for three years has already discovered the benefits of exercise. This exercise "maintainer" might be quite interested in discussing ways to add excitement to their well-established routine, a topic that clearly would not be appropriate for a person just beginning a physical activity program. Because people can move back and forth between stages, always remain alert for possible changes in your clients' stages and adjust interventions accordingly.

Barke and Nicholas (1990) specifically studied older adults in terms of these Stages of Change. Although we may be tempted to view older people as set in their ways and unwilling to be active, their sample of 59 adults between ages 59 and 80 were more likely to be in the contemplation, action, or maintenance stages than in precontemplation. Even among the least active older adults, there were fewer people in the precontemplation stage than any other stage of readiness. This suggests that even the least active older adults were thinking about engaging in physical activity or were already preparing or attempting to be active. These results suggest that we should recognize the continuing growth potential of older adults, rather than believe stereotypes that imply older adults are unable or unwilling to change.

## Summary

These are just a few of the models that help us to understand motivation for physical activity. Generally, models of physical activity behavior change take into account some combination of expected outcomes (including benefits and costs), perceived ability to engage in the physical activity, and positive and negative social influences. The transtheoretical model can be especially useful because it incorporates ideas from a number of other models and considers when and for whom each of these potential determinants is important, based on the individual's stage of readiness.

# FROM THEORY TO ACTION

Motivation generally refers to factors that determine "why people initiate, choose, or persist in specific actions in specific circumstances" (Mook, 1996). Often, people talk about motivation as if it were a completely stable, enduring characteristic. Some people just seem motivated to accomplish great things and appear to stay motivated against all odds. In reality, motivation varies over time and according to the task.

Motivation impacts decisions to exercise as well as the likelihood of stopping or maintaining exercise over the long run. It is estimated that approximately half of the people who start exercise programs stop within six months (Willis & Campbell, 1992; Dishman, 1988; Wankel, 1987). Common barriers to continuing physical activity among older adults include

personal symptoms, bad weather, lack of sidewalks, and having no place to sit down to take breaks during the activity (Clark, 1999). In addition, older adults often believe that exercise must be strenuous to yield health benefits (Lee, 1993). Misconceptions such as this can prevent older adults from initiating or continuing a physical activity program. Therefore, consistent maintenance of physical activity at the desired level is a major concern.

On the other hand, older adults are more likely to be motivated to be physically active when the activity is at a moderate intensity, inexpensive, convenient, and, especially for older women, includes a social aspect (Brawley, Rejeski, & King, 2003). Physical activity research suggests that there are behavior-change strategies that can help people initiate exercise and stay motivated to continue. Physical activity programs often employ behavioral strategies, such as goal-setting, self-monitoring, feedback on progress in the program, and setting up a reward system for continuing physical activity behavior (Barone, Maddux, & Snyder, 1997). The approach outlined below includes many of these same aspects. However, it is important to understand not only what, but also when certain aspects of behavior change programs are appropriate. Consistent with the transtheoretical model, some strategies are more effective at different stages of motivational readiness. (For a more comprehensive explanation of effective strategies at each stage see Marcus & Forsyth, 2003.) Each strategy is followed by an example of how the strategy might be implemented with an individual older adult.

The behavior-change strategies described below are useful in promoting exercise adherence among all clients. Some, however, may be particularly helpful when working with older adults. As you read the descriptions and examples of these behavior-change strategies, think about your own experiences as a fitness professional, and about times that you employed—or could have employed—these strategies with your clients. How would you introduce these behavior-change topics to your clients? What recommendations would you make to those clients based upon these behavior-change principles? Visualizing yourself using these techniques will help you to become comfortable with them and incorporate them into your work.

## Strategies for Older Adults in Precontemplation

Clients in the precontemplation stage have not yet begun to think about starting a program of physical activity. Therefore, teaching them ways to set goals or strategies for reminding them to exercise is not appropriate. Instead, these clients can benefit from discussions about the pros and cons of physical activity to help motivate them to be physically active. Once they are motivated, then more specific strategies about how to increase physical activity are relevant. Individuals in the precontemplation stage may encounter fitness professionals during a routine physical or stress test or while accompanying or transporting friends or family to exercise programs. However, encounters with these potential clients can be rare; therefore, it is important to make the most of these opportunities. In addition, the strategies discussed in this section may be used in advertising campaigns to encourage potential clients to set up an initial appointment.

### POTENTIAL COSTS AND BENEFITS OF BEGINNING AN EXERCISE PROGRAM

It is basic human nature to want to engage in activities that produce more benefits than costs. Who wants to slave away at a job that offers no pay and no other rewards? The "costs" of physical activity vary from person to person, but could include the time it takes to exercise; the hassle of getting to the exercise location; muscle soreness; feeling self-conscious about exercising in front of other people; the expense of a fitness facility membership, special equipment, or clothing; having to miss out on preferred activities; feeling tired after exercise; or sweating.

The benefits of physical activity also vary with the individual. Although certain physiological benefits might be expected for most or all people, only the benefits that are personally valued will serve as motivators. If Sally does not care about her improved ability to climb stairs without losing her breath, reminding her of this benefit will not be helpful. If Sally values being able to sleep better and having to take less medication to control her high blood pressure, these are more potent motivators worth discussing.

Why discuss anything negative such as the costs of exercise with clients? To help clients maintain physical activity over the long run, it is necessary to be realistic about their negative expectations about physical activity. Ignoring the drawbacks of engaging in an exercise program will not make these costs disappear. In fact, negative expectations that are never addressed may eventually lead clients to drop out of their program. By discussing clients' objections to their exercise routine up front, it is possible to work with them to decrease or eliminate the costs before they give up on exercise. Although people in the precontemplation stage are not currently engaging in any exercise, it is likely that they have done so before, or at least exerted themselves physically at some time in the past. If a client hates working out alone, for example, perhaps they can find an exercise partner to join them or try some group activities. If feeling tired after exercise is a complaint, perhaps they could schedule exercise sessions in the evening, when feeling relaxed would encourage better sleep.

Many people do not like to have to expend physical effort when it is not necessary. Discussing this drawback of exercise lets clients know that their perception of exercise as requiring excessive effort is not abnormal, but a natural step in developing new, healthy exercise habits. This is important, since many sedentary people mistakenly assume that people who exercise regularly are fundamentally different from themselves—that regular exercisers stick with it because they love every minute of working out. The realization that even physically active people encounter difficulties—but have learned ways to overcome them—will help clients see that they can learn skills that will help them stay active.

While addressing client concerns over the costs of exercise, it is also necessary to discuss the benefits they may reap from being active. Some of these may be immediate, such as feeling more alert or experiencing a boost in self-esteem after an exercise session. Others may be long-term, such as living longer or decreasing the loss of bone density associated with osteoporosis. Helping clients to maximize their expected benefits improves the ratio of expected benefits to costs, which will make them more likely to initiate physical activity. If a client identifies increased energy and weight management as the greatest benefits of exercise, he could consider scheduling his workout in the morning on his busiest days to help him to tackle those days with more energy. Perhaps he'll want to save his occasional high-calorie treats (like ice cream) for his exercise days when he burns more calories.

Following is an example of how a fitness professional might help a client improve the ratio of expected exercise benefits to costs:

FITNESS PROFESSIONAL (FP): Loretta, you mentioned that it's hard for you to go to the gym to exercise because you don't like other people looking at you when you exercise. Is that right?

LORETTA: That's right. I get embarrassed when more athletic people see me try to exercise.

FP: So for you, one cost of exercising is feeling embarrassed in front of others. Can you think of any ways to deal with the situation?

LORETTA: Well, I guess I could try to go to the gym when no one else is there.

FP: That sounds like a good idea. Maybe you could find out when the peak hours are and try to avoid those times. I also have another idea. Have you considered doing some physical activity that does not require going to the gym? Maybe you could start walking around your neighborhood for exercise, rather than going to the gym. You could even ask a friend to walk with you.

LORETTA: I never thought of that. My neighbor has been thinking about starting a physical activity program, too. Maybe she would be interested in walking with me. Plus, then I wouldn't have to pay for a gym membership.

FP: Would you like to ask her about starting a walking routine together?

LORETTA: Yes, I'll ask her about it tonight.

Directly addressing a client's concerns can help them eliminate or minimize expected costs. It is also helpful to remember the positive aspects of their exercise program and to increase expected benefits. Once a client believes that the potential benefits of physical activity outweigh the potential costs, they will be more likely to begin a physical activity program. Discussing the benefits and barriers to exercise can also be helpful in the contemplation and preparation stages.

## Strategies for Older Adults in Contemplation

Clients in the contemplation stage have begun thinking about participating in physical activity and intend to begin a physical activity program, but have not yet started. These clients may understand some of the benefits of physical activity, but may need further encouragement with respect to how physical activity might be beneficial for them in the short-term. Continued discussion of the pros and cons of physical activity (as discussed in the previous section) is warranted. In addition, introducing the concept of social support as a potential motivator for physical activity is important at this stage. Again, do not discuss specific goal-setting strategies at this point, as too much specific planning may overwhelm clients, sending them back to the precontemplation stage.

## THE SOCIAL CONNECTION: USING SOCIAL SUPPORT TO ASSIST WITH MOTIVATION FOR EXERCISE

Support from other people is an important tool that may help clients of all ages maintain physical activity. Many older adults are faced with the challenge of coping with multiple losses that often restrict the amount and nature of social contact. Spouses, siblings, or treasured friends now may be deceased, while others may have moved away to retirement or assisted-living communities. Physical disabilities or illnesses may prevent friends or other family members from being able to engage in previously enjoyed activities, such as long walks or shopping excursions. Retired individuals who relied upon the work setting as a primary source of social contact may now experience distress over the loss of that environment. Children and other relatives may live in distant cities and be unable to visit regularly.

However, rather than disengaging from society, many older adults desire to rebuild and keep nurturing social connections. If older clients want to maintain social connections with others and do not already have sufficient opportunities to do so, their physical activity programs can serve a dual function by meeting both exercise and social needs. Exercise programs that take into account the psychological value of social interaction, in addition to the physical benefits of exercise, can become especially prized by older adults.

How can social support be employed to help clients? One way is to teach them that encouragement will help them comply with their exercise program, and suggest that they seek support from others on an ongoing basis. Here are some social support strategies to suggest to clients:

✓ Find an enjoyable and reliable exercise partner. If partners are not readily available in the exercise setting, look to community agencies or programs offered by churches, social groups, university-based senior programs, etc.

✓ Ask friends and family members to be encouraging and positive about the exercise program.

✓ Ask for reminders from friends and family members about physical activity goals or appointments.

✓ Set up fun "contests" with a friend as well as rewards based upon meeting an exercise goal, such as attending a water aerobics class 10 times without an absence. (The friend's goal does not have to be exercise-related, although mutual support for exercise is beneficial for everyone. The main objective is to use accountability to someone else as a motivational tool for meeting exercise goals.)

✓ Add a social element to the exercise program. For example, arrive at class a little early if it affords the opportunity to chat with other class members.

Fitness instructors can facilitate social support for exercise by fostering interaction in their programs. Speak with as many clients as possible, even in a large class or group. Introduce clients to one another. Incorporate brief exercise activities that require a partner or small groups. Allow clients the space to meet before or after classes to socialize, and encourage participants to plan social events if they desire to do so. Over time, older clients may develop rewarding friendships with other exercise participants, thereby enhancing their sense of belonging and improving their commitment to the program.

It also should be noted that social influences sometimes can make exercise more difficult. Common examples include a spouse who makes negative comments about an exercise program or friends who always try to persuade a client to go to lunch rather than exercise. A client's participation in an exercise program may require adaptation on the part of others, which may or may not be forthcoming.

Although friends and family ultimately may only want the best for the client, they may be experiencing some feelings of neglect or jealousy, or other interpersonal issues that need to be resolved. If you hear a client discussing negative influences, work with them to evaluate the impact of such instances on their exercise motivation level. Help clients take greater control over the situation by suggesting that they:

✓ Schedule their contact with unsupportive people *after* they exercise for the day.
✓ Try to balance out time with unsupportive people by increasing time with supporters.

✓ Set clear limits for how much time they will spend with unsupportive people, or avoid such contact altogether.
✓ Mentally prepare themselves to respond to negative comments.
✓ Mentally review why their exercise program is important, prior to spending time with unsupportive peers.
✓ Explain to an unsupportive person why their exercise is important to them, and ask for the person's encouragement. If the person is willing to try to be more supportive, the client should tell them specifically what they would and would not like them to do. (For example, "It would help me a lot if you wouldn't say, 'Are you off to the gym again?' each time I leave the apartment for a while. But asking how I am progressing in my program every now and then would be nice.")

Helping clients recognize the impact that others' responses may have on their motivation can prepare them to use positive social support to their advantage, and to decrease the impact of discouraging influences. Recruiting social support is almost always an effective strategy for physical activity promotion; however, it can be most effective during the contemplation and preparation stages when clients are attempting to establish regular patterns of physical activity.

## Strategies for Older Adults in Preparation

Clients in the preparation stage have decided that they want to begin a physical activity program and have begun to engage in some activity. However, they are not yet regularly active. This is a good time to reinforce the benefits of starting regular physical activity, and

## SETTING EXERCISE GOALS WITH OLDER ADULTS

Goal-setting is important for anyone attempting to change a behavior. You can play a pivotal role in teaching clients how to set and evaluate their physical-activity goals. It is crucial, however, that clients' goals be their own. This means that each client should fully agree with the selection of goals and how progress will be measured. Remember that most people quickly lose enthusiasm for meeting others' expectations when those expectations are not compatible with their own motivations and lifestyle. Although terms such as "fitness prescriptions" suggest that an exercise plan can be imposed by an expert upon an accepting client, exercise programs are unlikely to be maintained if the client does not feel they have played a primary role in choosing their own goals and developing the fitness program.

To illustrate, Mary is a 68-year-old woman who has not engaged in formal exercise for 20 years, but has recently been attending a yoga class once each week. She has a busy schedule that includes volunteer work and caring for a seriously ill friend, but she wants to begin exercising regularly. She makes an appointment with a fitness professional to discuss using exercise to manage her weight, as well as to improve her energy level and overall health. The fitness professional may conclude that, ideally, she should be participating in a water aerobics class three times a week, as well as performing strength training and flexibility exercises at least twice a week. Initially, however, Mary may feel overwhelmed by a program that includes all the physical activities deemed appropriate. The challenge is to identify one or two goals that match Mary's current needs and abilities.

The only way to evaluate the compatibility between the proposed goals and the individual client is to ask all clients how they feel about the proposed goals, and how long they think they can continue to meet these goals. Their responses will help identify the level and types of activities that are appropriate for them. Initial goals may fall far below what might be recommended for health or fitness benefits, but remember that early success can help clients gradually work toward more advanced goals. A client may choose to maintain a physical activity level that seems too low or appears to neglect a component of fitness. Do not lose sight, however, of the fact that sustained moderate-intensity physical activity is infinitely more beneficial than a complete withdrawal from activity, which could be caused by feeling pushed into a program that was too aggressive.

For Mary, participating in a water aerobics class two times a week may initially be the most challenging goal she feels she can fit into her schedule. In conjunction with this goal, encouraging her to increase lifestyle activity by 15 minutes per day may be appropriate. For example, would Mary be willing and able to climb the stairs to her apartment rather than taking the elevator, or walk down the street to pick up small items at the grocery store? In a month or two, she may be willing to consider making time for increased fitness activities such as strength training or flexibility exercises. For now, however, acknowledge the motivation that Mary demonstrated initially and applaud her for setting realistic goals.

The previous example illustrates the primary rule of effective goal-setting for fitness professionals: Listen carefully when helping a client set goals, and ensure that the goals are appropriate for their current lifestyle, motivations, and stage of readiness for physical

also move into setting specific physical-activity goals.

activity. This is especially important when working with older adults, who may differ from younger clients in all of these respects. Taking the time to understand an older adult's concerns, motivation, and comfort level with proposed goals will help you collaborate on setting encouraging and constructive program goals.

An important note about health, fitness, and exercise goals: Goal-setting with clients should be contingent upon whether they are seeking health or fitness benefits, or both. Although vigorous activity may be desirable for certain fitness gains, moderate-intensity physical activity is quite sufficient for attaining health benefits. Most older adults (and most clients in general) will need to be educated that the "no pain, no gain" theory is not accurate, and that moderate activity provides substantial health benefits. Similarly, unrealistic weight-loss goals should be addressed early on so that clients are less likely to quit exercising if they do not experience significant weight loss. While exercise is certainly a key to long-term weight loss, it is necessary to decrease calorie intake below calorie expenditure to lose weight. Therefore, for most people an adjustment in dietary intake also is necessary to achieve weight-loss goals.

Clients may need some education about activity guidelines to assist them with goal setting. The *Surgeon General's Report on Physical Activity and Health* recommends that for health benefits—many older adults are seeking health, not fitness, gains—people of all ages should engage in at least 30 minutes of moderate-intensity physical activity (such as brisk walking) on most, if not all, days of the week (U.S. Department of Health and Human Services, 1996). There are several options for attaining the recommended amount of moderate-intensity physical activity, ranging from single 30-minute sessions, to breaking up activity into multiple short bouts (of at least 10 minutes each) at least five days per week. Make program recommendations appropriate to the type of benefits sought, as well as client interests and lifestyle. Be sensitive to the fact that for some older adults, goal-setting may need to revolve exclusively around increasing lifestyle activity—a very worthy goal in its own right.

The specific steps of goal-setting are described below. An example of the implementation of each step with an older client accompanies each description.

*Step One: Identify the client's primary objective(s).* Ask what they want to accomplish over the long run (months or years) by engaging in an exercise program. They may want to decrease blood pressure, lose weight, improve appearance, perform daily tasks such as carrying groceries or climbing stairs with more ease, decrease stress, meet new people, relieve boredom, improve balance, prevent or manage certain medical problems, improve mood, or obtain other positive outcomes. Often, a person's reasons for developing an exercise plan will be discussed at the beginning of the first meeting. In this case, it is appropriate to review their primary long-term objectives when developing specific goals.

FITNESS PROFESSIONAL (FP): Bill, I'd like to be sure I understand what you want to accomplish over the long run so we set goals that meet your needs. Your main reason for beginning exercise is to improve your golf game, right?

BILL: Yes, that's right. I also wouldn't mind being in better shape so I'm not so sore after doing home-repair projects.

*Step Two: Identify one or two short-term goals that will move the client toward their primary objectives.* Although it is fine to have long-term goals (such as losing 100 pounds or transforming from a sedentary person to a marathon runner), it is difficult to stay motivated with only long-term goals in mind. Work with clients to set daily or weekly goals so they can experience smaller, motivating successes on the way to meeting their long-term objective.

Even though the client may want to set multiple goals right away, it is advisable to initially focus on only one or two short-term goals. If necessary, explain to the client that new habits—even healthy ones like exercise—take time to develop. Encourage focusing energy on one or two main goals, allowing clients to succeed in meeting them for a period of time, before adding new goals. This is far more productive than having an overly ambitious client try to do too much and then experience the frustration and disappointment of failing.

An important note about selecting short-term goals: It can be very motivating to track and record physical outcomes, such as changes in body measurements. However, try to ensure that a client's short-term goals focus on the actual *behaviors* they are doing, rather than solely on outcomes. This is especially important for older adults who may no longer experience rapid physiological improvements. If the primary focus is on the process of completing their exercise routine properly and regularly, clients can feel good about this very important accomplishment, even if they do not see rapid gains in stamina or strength. Of course, tangible physical or physiological measurements are valuable tools for assessing a client's response to the program and for helping clients to improve health and/or fitness. But for motivation reasons, always have clients set some small, short-term goals focused on personal behaviors under their control (e.g., participating in their walking program or completing their flexibility exercises), rather than out-

comes, which can vary widely from one person to the next.

FP: It sounds as though some exercises to generally improve your flexibility and muscle strength could help you with your golf game and prepare your muscles for home-repair projects. How would you feel about setting a goal to complete a 45-minute strengthening and flexibility routine in the gym three times a week?

BILL: I think I can do that, as long as you teach me how.

FP: That's what I'm here for. Together, we'll go through each exercise and you can ask me any questions you have. We also will write notes about the exercises that you can keep.

*Step Three: Once general short-term goals have been agreed upon, define them in measurable, realistic, and specific terms.* Goals must be measurable so that there is a clear, objective way to determine whether they have been met. Take vague goals and find one or two quantifiable ways to measure progress. For instance, a goal of "working out" is hard to measure, but a goal of completing a pre-planned workout routine in the gym six times over the next two weeks is measurable. It is crucial to have clients track their exercise behaviors, either in a personal notebook or on structured forms.

Goals also must take into account the client's current fitness level, stage of readiness to increase physical activity, and lifestyle. Chapter 4 details the specifics of pre-exercise screening and fitness assessment. It is imperative to collect high-quality screening and assessment data from clients and use it to determine whether their goals are realistic. It is helpful to develop short-term goals that are slightly challenging, so the person feels a genuine sense of accomplishment when they are met. At the same time, these goals should be designed to produce success and, as such, be within the client's ability. Early successes help to increase client confidence in their ability (both their physical ability and the ability to incorporate the exercise routine into their life), thereby encouraging adherence to exercise programs.

Goals also must be specific so plans for meeting them are not left to chance. Vaguely stated intentions such as "mall walking three times this week" are easy to forget or put off (indefinitely). In contrast, people often feel much more committed to meeting specifically defined goals such as "mall walking at XYZ Mall at 8:30 a.m., Monday, Wednesday, and Friday, for at least 30 minutes each day." To encourage clients to think through their plans and increase their commitment, supportively ask them to explain the "what, when, where, and how" of meeting their exercise goals.

It also is important that clients explicitly agree to meet their exercise goals. This may take the form of a verbal commitment. Some exercise professionals prefer to put such commitments into writing with a "behavioral contract" that defines physical activity goals and states that the client agrees to make every effort to meet the goals. Written contracts should be signed both by the fitness professional and the client, and each should keep copies for subsequent reference. Such contracts assist in keeping track of client goals, and underscore the importance of their exercise plans.

FP: Now that we have gone through your exercise routine, let's make concrete plans for the next two weeks. People usually are more successful at sticking to exercise programs when they determine how they will meet their goals. You said you can do the exercise routine you just learned three times a week. What days and times will you come to the gym to do this routine?

BILL: Well, I golf on Mondays, Wednesdays, and Fridays, so I don't think those days would be good. I think I should try coming on Tuesdays, Thursdays, and Saturdays.

FP: OK. Is there a particular time you can come on those days?

BILL: I usually feel more energetic in the morning, so I guess morning would be good.

FP: Sounds like a good idea. An exact time doesn't have to be etched in stone, but can you tentatively plan the time you'll come on those mornings?

BILL: Let's say I'll leave my house around 9:00. That will give me time to eat breakfast and read the morning paper.

FP: Great. Even if you end up having to change the time, now you have your exercise session in your schedule. So you will leave for the gym at 9:00 a.m. on Tuesdays, Thursdays, and Saturdays, right?

BILL: Yeah, that's what I'll do.

FP: OK. I suggest writing it on your calendar, just like a doctor's appointment or any other important event. When we meet again after your first two weeks, we can discuss how this schedule worked for you.

Goal setting is a vitally important strategy for clients in the preparation, action, and maintenance stages. However, as clients move into the action and maintenance stages, and learn how to set and readjust goals on their own, you may end up spending less in-session time with them on goal-setting.

## Strategies for Older Adults in Action

Clients in the action stage have been engaging in regular physical activity, but for less than six months. At this stage it is helpful to review the initial goals and adjust them as necessary. In addition, clients may be looking for additional ways to motivate themselves, especially on days when social support is unavailable. Now that the client has some experience with exercise, introducing the use of environmental cues and self-talk strategies can be helpful and is appropriate at this stage.

## REVISE SHORT-TERM GOALS AS NEEDED

This is a critical step often overlooked by clients and fitness professionals. Patterns of exercise successes and difficulties contain a wealth of information that can be used to help clients. Try to review goals with clients on a weekly or biweekly basis. Congratulate them on all successes, including partially met goals. Too often clients feel like failures when they do not meet 100% of their stated goals, and they don't give themselves credit for what was accomplished. Clients should understand that all effort put toward meeting their long-term objectives and improving their health or fitness is valuable.

Ask successful clients what helped them to succeed. Did they discover especially helpful strategies such as exercising with a friend or attending fitness classes at a certain time of day? Congratulate them on their ingenuity and note the strategies that were helpful for them. If a client begins to have difficulties with exercise at a later date, encourage them to employ these strategies again.

Unsuccessful clients can share valuable personal experiences that will facilitate problem-solving. In an understanding manner, ask what factors made it difficult for them to meet their goals. Listen for possible patterns. Once major problems have been identified, work to generate solutions or modify goals. Remember that it is critical to praise clients for coming back in to talk with you, even if they do not meet their goals—remind them that this is a critical step toward eventual success with behavior change.

The first concern should be helping the client feel good about what they have accomplished. This will give them the confidence to meet future activity goals. Explain that it is only through trying to meet exercise goals that they can discover which strategies do or do not help them succeed. Explain that instances they see as failures can be helpful if they learn from the experience.

After evaluating successes and problems, clients should commit to a new set of short-term goals. They may opt to keep the same exercise goals, decrease goals that were overly ambitious, or challenge themselves with new or intensified goals. In any case, all the previous goal-setting steps still apply. You may make recommendations for revision, but the final selection of the next short-term goals should ultimately rest with the client. As they become regular exercisers, a formal review of goals may occur less often (perhaps monthly or every two to three months, depending on the client). Ideally, clients will become quite good at tracking their own progress and revising their own goals.

(At the second meeting, after Bill has been in his exercise program for two weeks.)

FP: Hello, Bill. It's good to see you. How did the first two weeks of your exercise program go?

BILL: I did pretty well the first week. I came to the gym and completed the routine three times, just like we planned. But the second week, I only got to the gym twice.

FP: I want to congratulate you on your successful first week. A lot of people find that beginning a new program is the hardest part. How do you feel about your first week?

BILL: Really good, especially because I had friends in from out of town and didn't get as much sleep as I'm used to.

FP: But you managed to come to the gym and do your routine even though you were tired?

BILL: Yeah.

FP: That's great. What motivated you to exercise even when you were tired?

BILL: I remembered what you said about exercise sessions being just as important as a doctor's appointment—I thought, I shouldn't cancel on myself! I guess I didn't want to feel like a quitter, either.

FP: Your exercise time is important and you deserve to take it. I'm glad you decided to keep your appointments during the first week. What made it more difficult during the second week?

BILL: Things just kept getting in the way. I didn't come in on Tuesday because the washing machine broke and my wife wanted me to fix it.

FP: I can see how that might interfere with your plans. Let's think about what you can do when a situation like this comes up again so you'll be able to exercise, but still have time to do the other things you need to do.

BILL: OK. It was kind of an unusual week, but I guess things can always come up at the last minute.

FP: That's right. No matter how much you may want to do your workout, other things are bound to interfere with your plans.

BILL: What do you suggest?

FP: Well, let's look at your experience when the washing machine needed to be fixed. Is there any way you could have taken care of that and still worked out that day?

BILL: I guess I could have done my routine at the gym first, then gone home to fix the washer. It's just that my wife asked me if I could fix it so she could do laundry; I didn't want to make her wait.

FP: And did you mention to her that you had planned to go to the gym that morning?

BILL: No, and I don't think she remembered it, either.

FP: That's not surprising since you recently added this to your schedule. How does she feel about you going to the gym three times a week?

BILL: Oh, she's all for it.

FP: That's great. Do you think she would have understood if you said you'd like to go to the gym before fixing the washer?

BILL: Uh-huh. I guess I should have reminded her about my plans. She wouldn't have minded waiting.

FP: It's good that she's supportive of your exercise program. Support from family and friends can really help people stick to their regimens. Maybe later we can talk about ways she can help you adhere to your plan. For now, though, what will you do next time something like a household repair comes up before your workout?

BILL: If it's not an emergency, I'll just exercise first.

FP: Good. This experience probably will help you a lot in the future. Now, what goals do you want to set for the next two weeks?

BILL: I'd like to stick with this same routine until I really get the hang of it.

FP: That's a smart idea. I'll note that doing your current routine three times a week is your new goal. Do you want to change the times, or is Tuesday, Thursday, and Saturday around 9:00 a.m. still best for you?

BILL: I like that schedule. Let's leave those as the times I'll come.

## USE REMINDERS TO EXERCISE

"Cues" are simply influences—either planned or coincidental—that remind people to engage in certain kinds of behaviors. Seeing walking shoes by the front door can remind a client of plans to walk that day, or keeping a fitness facility ID card on one's key ring can provide an ongoing reminder about an exercise commitment. Setting an alarm clock or wrist watch alarm as a reminder to leave for an exercise class can be quite helpful.

Unfortunately, some influences also make it harder to exercise. Starting an engaging new book can make it difficult to get to a water aerobics class. Having friends drop by unexpectedly to play cards can make it hard to go for a walk. Teach your clients to intentionally use cues to remind them to exercise. Whenever possible, also encourage them to avoid cues that make it difficult to exercise until after they have met their physical activity goal for the day.

## USE SELF-TALK AS AN EXERCISE MOTIVATOR

Self-talk can help clients meet exercise goals if it is positive or otherwise motivating. Statements such as "I can do it" or "I'll feel much less stiff once I've done my exercises" can help clients to begin or continue exercising. Self-talk also can be discouraging, as in the case of a person who says to himself, "I don't know why I should bother with all of this work; it's never going to pay off" or "I'll never be able to keep up with the rest of this class." Help clients stay motivated by teaching them how to identify and take control of self-talk related to their exercise goals.

The first step is to identify (i.e., to hear) self-talk. This will be easy for some clients; others may find it difficult. Encourage clients to ask themselves what is "going through their minds" when they are feeling discouraged about exercise or having difficulty meeting physical activity goals. This should help them pinpoint the negative thinking that is interfering with their success. They also can learn from positive experiences. Thoughts that help them feel good about exercising can be recalled at times they feel discouraged.

Next, negative self-talk should be corrected. This doesn't require becoming oblivious to reality or trying to think only "happy thoughts." Instead, encourage clients to try to make their self-talk realistic, rather than unduly harsh, by assessing the accuracy of self-talk. Acknowledging that such statements as "I always mess up" or "I'll never be able to succeed" are exaggerations will help clients to regain a more realistic perspective.

Sometimes, negative statements will be accurate. (Perhaps your client is not in the mood to exercise or does find a particular exercise difficult.) In these cases, suggest that they work to find solutions, such as determining a way to make their program more appealing or substituting other good exercises for ones that are currently frustrating. When realistic negative thoughts do occur, however, ask clients to try shifting their attention to motivating self-talk. Motivating self-talk often emphasizes the positive effects of exercise: "This will help me to improve my balance" or "I will be so proud of myself when I finish my workout today." Using self-talk to their advantage is a way for clients to motivate themselves to adhere to their exercise routine. As with goal setting, positive self-talk can be an effective strategy at any time. However, you may spend more time on it with your clients during the action and maintenance stages, when negative self-talk about exercise is likely to occur.

## Strategies for Older Adults in Maintenance

Clients in the maintenance stage have been exercising regularly for at least six months. Relapse prevention strategies, such as planning for potential barriers and recognizing minor lapses, can help prevent these lapses (brief periods of inactivity) from turning into relapses (extended periods of inactivity). Clients in the maintenance stage should find ways to reward themselves for continuing to exercise even when the exercise is not intrinsically rewarding. Clients at this stage can also benefit from strategies that keep physical activity interesting, such as using humor and music.

## PLAN FOR THE FUTURE: RELAPSE PREVENTION SKILLS

Knowing the factors that contribute to a relapse can help individuals predict and plan for future high-risk situations. Factors such as illness or injury, social pressure to not engage in activity, a lack of support from friends or family, highly stressful or busy times, and an inability to cope with high-risk situations are just a few of the problems that may hinder progress toward activity goals. Such factors can be difficult for exercisers of all ages.

Fitness professionals should prepare clients to cope with tough situations that are likely to interfere with their exercise programs. Clients must first learn to identify their own high-risk situations. Then they can develop the crucial skills of predicting potential problems and proactively develop plans to deal with them. For example, Mike has difficulty swimming regularly and knows that this will become even harder for him when his family arrives for a three-week visit. He realizes there will be plenty of distractions. Nevertheless, he wants to try to stick with his swimming routine.

A fitness instructor could help Mike turn this challenge into a victory by developing an action plan. Perhaps Mike can reschedule his swim sessions at the time of day when his grandchildren typically nap, so he won't miss out on time with them. Maybe he could arrange to meet a friend at the pool at predetermined times, so he will feel obligated to go. Mike is likely to have some good ideas about what will help

him to keep swimming. Encourage him to generate his own ideas and to rate their value. He should try the most highly rated strategies first.

Exercise researchers also have suggested that teaching clients to distinguish between a lapse and a relapse can be extremely helpful (Dishman, 1991; Marcus & Stanton, 1993). The reason is simple: After missing one or more planned activity sessions, it is common for people to start feeling guilty and ashamed, and to experience decreased self-confidence in their ability to exercise regularly. Additionally, some people will engage in all-or-none thinking, labeling themselves as "quitters" or failures. But if a person has acknowledged in advance that lapses are common, natural, and temporary setbacks rather than catastrophic failures, they can more easily forgive themselves and get back on track with their activity plan. Encourage clients to "get back on the horse" as soon as possible after a lapse, even if they must again start slowly. The sooner they resume some sort of physical activity, the better they will feel about themselves, and the easier it will be to get back into their desired exercise routine.

## USING REWARDS TO MOTIVATE LONG-TERM ADHERENCE

Eventually, clients may find exercise rewarding in and of itself. Internal rewards, such as improved self-esteem and a sense of personal satisfaction from developing new skills, can be highly motivating (Deci & Ryan, 1985). Note that these motivators reside within clients and their personal perspective; this "intrinsic motivation" to exercise is extremely conducive to long-term maintenance of physical activity or exercise (Ryan et al., 1997).

Long-term exercisers typically find many inherent aspects of physical activity give them pleasure and motivate future exercise behaviors (e.g., a sense of accomplishment as they are exercising or post-workout relaxation). Fitness professionals sometimes expect clients to enjoy the intrinsic rewards of exercise, just as they do. The reality, however, is that it often takes time to begin enjoying exercise for its inherent benefits. Until clients sufficiently develop their physical abilities to focus on pleasurable aspects of their workout rather than how difficult their exertion feels, they cannot be expected to love working out. Even motivational, desirable outcomes such as improved muscle strength or weight loss may not occur until the person has continued their program long enough to experience these benefits. For some clients, a genuine, internally generated love of exercise may never develop.

Until clients begin to report internal rewards, it is crucial to employ external rewards to keep motivation levels high. Such rewards should be planned in conjunction with setting physical-activity goals. Clients who do not find exercise to be internally rewarding still can develop and maintain regular exercise routines, but they will need to continue using external rewards.

External rewards for exercise can take many forms. Clients can establish their own reward systems, such as allowing themselves to enjoy a relaxing soak in the spa immediately after they exercise, or treating themselves to a movie each week they meet their exercise goals. Fitness professionals can provide external rewards in the form of praise for achievements or tangible rewards such as prizes for meeting short-term goals. Rewards also can be linked to program monitoring, as in the case of a prominently posted attendance chart documenting each client's attendance, with a gift certificate given for every 10 classes attended.

One word of caution: Remember that the goal is to foster the growth of a client's awareness of internal rewards and intrinsic motivation to exercise. Too much focus on external rewards can foster a reliance upon such rewards (Deci, 1977). To minimize this risk, provide more external rewards when clients are new at exercise behaviors, and gradually decrease them when clients begin to express internal motivation to exercise.

Creating external rewards can also be helpful during earlier stages, such as preparation and action. Rewards should be designed to coincide with the accomplishment of goals. Rewards can also vary in size based on the duration and perceived difficulty of the goal.

## BALANCING CONVENIENCE AND ENJOYMENT

As mentioned earlier, it is easier to quit an activity that carries more costs than benefits. If an activity is too inconvenient, it will be stopped as soon as the effort outweighs the rewards (Epstein, 1998). Many of us do engage in highly inconvenient activities with some regularity. There are snow skiers, for example, who buy expensive and specialized equipment, drive for hours to reach a ski area, wait in line for lift tickets, brave even the harshest of weather conditions on the slopes, ski to the point of exhaustion, and willingly opt to do it all again as soon as they have another chance. This inconvenient exercise occurs because the people who engage in it are having fun. But if every trip to the fitness facility or every daily walk were as inconvenient as a ski trip, most people simply would not bother. The difference is that people are willing to deal with hassle if an activity is extremely enjoyable or rewarding in other ways.

Therefore, there are two very important lessons to teach clients:

1. Engage in exercise plans that are convenient. This applies to a regular exercise routine that can be done even on days when clients have little time or energy for elaborate plans. Going to a nearby fitness facility for a regular class held at a convenient time, or exercising with a videotape at home are good examples of such activities. Hopefully these will be somewhat enjoyable, too, but they don't have to be blissfully fun if they are relatively easy to do.

2. Engage in inconvenient but fun exercise activities, but be realistic about how often they can be done. For example, one client may love to dress in formal attire and go ballroom dancing, while another is willing to drive for an hour to their favorite hiking spot. Clients should be taught to engage in inconvenient but treasured activities when it is realistic to do so, but also to have a set of very convenient exercise options to employ on a daily basis.

Consider enjoyment and convenience when reviewing client progress. Clients who are having trouble meeting exercise goals may need help to increase convenience. If they hate traffic and driving to the fitness center, perhaps they can carpool with someone. If they dislike early-morning obligations, they should attempt to take fitness classes in the afternoon or evening.

Here is an example of a fitness professional guiding a client through a discussion about balancing convenience and enjoyment:

FP: Anna, you say that you are having trouble getting to your stretching class because it is too hard to rush home from your job, change clothes, and get to the class on time. Is that right?

ANNA: Yes. I hate to arrive late, so if I get there and they've already started I just go back home.

FP: I know it's frustrating to join a class in progress, and most people find it hard to exercise when getting to a class becomes a big ordeal. Is there any way we can make your exercise plans more convenient for you?

ANNA: I don't know what to do. I mean, they aren't going to change the class time for me.

FP: Let's consider a few ideas. Some may work and some may not, but at least we can come up with a few possible solutions for you to try.

ANNA: OK. What can I change?

FP: Well, the first thing that comes to my mind is the time you leave your job. Can you leave earlier?

ANNA: I don't know. We set that schedule when I started. I guess it's worth asking to see if I could leave 30 minutes earlier. I wouldn't mind going in earlier to make up the time.

FP: Great. That might be the solution right there, but in case that doesn't work, let's come up with a few more ideas. Is there a way to avoid having to go home to change your clothes before class?

ANNA: I certainly can't work in the clothes I wear for class, and I'd feel silly changing into workout clothes at my volunteer job.

FP: OK. How would you feel about changing clothes here in the locker room?

ANNA: I guess that might be alright. I see other women changing clothes there all the time. I've just never been in the habit of packing up all my things to bring with me.

FP: Well, if you're comfortable with trying it, that may be another solution. You could pack the clothes you'll need for class in the morning, put them in a bag in your car, and then come straight here after work to change clothes. Would that give you enough time to get to class?

ANNA: I think it would.

FP: OK. If these things don't work, maybe we can see if another class starts at a better time for you.

ANNA: Oh, I really like that class. The instructor is great and I like the people in it. I'll see if these other things will work first.

FP: That makes sense. If you really enjoy an exercise class, sometimes it's worth going through a little inconvenience. This week, are you willing to try changing clothes here and asking your supervisor about leaving your job earlier?

ANNA: I'll do both.

FP: Great. I'll look forward to hearing how things turned out when we meet next week.

As this example illustrates, people often do not consider convenience issues when arranging exercise plans, and may not realize which aspects of the program will be inconvenient until it has begun. Clients may not recognize that it is OK to expect their activity plans to be convenient. They may even chide themselves for not being dedicated enough to their exercise goals when inconvenience gets in the way of goal attainment. You can help them understand the balance between enjoyment and convenience, and to plan their program accordingly.

## COMMUNICATION AND LEADERSHIP SKILLS

In both group and individual formats, your leadership skills can significantly affect your older clients' attitudes toward physical activity. First and foremost, it must be clear to all of your clients that you enjoy working with them and are genuinely interested in their well-being. Sincere warmth plus enthusiasm for the exercise skills you are teaching will go a long way toward gaining your clients' trust and increasing their dedication to exercise. However, genuine interest, warmth, and enthusiasm are not sufficient in and of

themselves. Strong communication and leadership skills also are central to your effectiveness. In their review of optimal leader qualifications, Lewis and Campanelli (1990) concluded that leaders of exercise and health-education programs for older adults should be:

✓ trained in the areas of physical activity and aging
✓ able to offer a mixture of fun, purposeful activities
✓ able to relate meaningfully to older adults
✓ willing, interested, and empathetic
✓ patient with themselves and others
✓ organized in their methods and directions
✓ firm but not authoritarian
✓ trained in group dynamics
✓ trained in CPR and able to recognize signs of overexertion

Continually strive to improve your professional abilities, just as you expect clients to continue working to improve their fitness levels or general health. As with the behavioral strategies, thinking about how you will apply these communication and leadership skills with clients will help you prepare to use them. After you have read this section, challenge yourself to improve at least one leadership or communication skill. As you make gains in that skill area, try using a new skill. Committing to a process of ongoing professional growth will help you better appreciate a fundamental truth of teaching and leadership: The best instructors learn from their students, even as they are teaching them.

### Tips for Communicating with Older Adults

Most of us are familiar with the saying "communication is a two-way street." It is true that the most effective communication requires two willing parties, but the parties must do more than merely speak. They must be able and willing to listen carefully and respond in respectful, constructive ways. Fitness instructors need to be particularly responsive to the communication needs of their older adult clients. Because older adults often are stereotyped or patronized by others, they may be especially appreciative of attentive listening and understanding. The better the communication between you and your clients, the more likely it is that you will hear about problems that could interfere with their program success.

Unfortunately, younger people who have not spent much time around older adults may feel intimidated about communicating with these individuals, and rely upon familiar stereotypes to guide interactions. Hummert, Nussbaum, and Wiemann (1992), note that language beliefs and attitudes toward the elderly tend to be negatively biased. These negative stereotypes actually can contribute to communication problems and misunderstandings between generations.

One especially common stereotype is that all older adults have problems communicating based on hearing loss, poor memory, or other factors. The reality, though, is that some older clients may have hearing impairments, comprehension problems, or difficulties in finding the right words to express themselves, while others may have excellent communication skills (Hummert, Nussbaum, & Wiemann, 1992).

Younger adults often fail to adjust for individual differences, erring on the side of using what is known as "patronizing speech" or "elderspeak" when addressing older adults (Hummert, Nussbaum, & Wiemann, 1992). This speech style is characterized by simplification strategies (speaking more slowly, using very simple grammar) and clarification strategies (speaking loudly, articulating very carefully) in addition to basing content upon stereotypes of aging. While adjustments in speech pat-

terns may be well-intentioned, older adults may feel they are being "talked down to."

According to Willis and Campbell (1992), the major keys to effective communication are **attending,** listening, and **empathetic responding.** These are useful tools for communicating with any clients, but are even more important if clients are different from you. Attending refers to focusing your attention on another person rather than on yourself or things going on around you. Listening requires actively focusing on both the spoken content and feelings or other messages that are only alluded to.

Empathetic responding can be more challenging. Empathy refers to understanding a person's experience from their perspective. Asking yourself, "How would I feel in their situation?" is a good way to understand your client's point of view. Next, your response should accurately acknowledge their experience. Ideally, empathetic responses slightly increase the client's awareness of their experiences. Consider the case of Vivian, a 68-year-old client who said to Fitness Instructor Joe, "These weight machines are so complicated. I still get confused about how to use them and have to ask for help, even after three weeks in the program!" Joe simply agreed that some of the machines are complicated and then immediately proceeded with reviewing their proper use. While his technical review may have been helpful to Vivian in some ways, Joe's focus upon only technical issues probably left her feeling somewhat misunderstood and unsupported.

Imagine now that Vivian made the same statements to Fitness Instructor Tim. Before responding, Tim asked himself how he would feel in her situation. Tim decided that he would probably feel embarrassed and/or discouraged. Tim then acknowledged these feelings in the empathetic response, "The weight machines can take quite a while to get used to, especially if you haven't used them before. It sounds like you feel badly about having to ask for help after three weeks, but it's great that you ask questions. You are doing a good job of learning the machines—you'll probably find that it will get easier with practice."

Tim's understanding of Vivian's feelings, his reassurance that she was not a failure, and praise for asking questions increased her confidence in being able to master the machines. Once she indicated that she was ready, Tim reviewed the use of the problematic machines. This technical review was important to Vivian's safety and success, and it was of even greater value because it followed an empathetic response, which motivated her to continue her efforts.

Table 2.1 lists other important communication tips for working with older adults, and their application.

---

Table 2.1

## Communication Tips for Working with Older Adults

---

*1. Listen without interruption to your clients' questions and statements before responding.*

Instructors often think they must have all of the answers—and FAST—to look competent. But fitness instructors sometimes miss part of what a client is saying because they are busy thinking about how they will answer. To avoid this problem, hear all of what your client has to say before commenting. If needed, remind yourself to take your time and think about what is being said. If you are at a loss for a response, tell your client that you need to think about the question for a moment, then formulate your answer. If you are "stumped," assure the client that you will consider the question and get back to him or her. If you do this, be sure to follow up with an answer as soon as you have researched one.

*2. Tune out distractions.*

Distractions can occur in the environment (things we see or hear around us), within ourselves (our state of mind or physical condition), or from the speaker (mannerisms or a communication style that make it difficult to pay attention). Because your clients should be the focus of your attention, eliminate or minimize distractions that make it hard for you to listen. Move to a quiet location if surrounding noise or activity is disruptive. If your mind keeps wandering to a personal issue, silently repeat to yourself everything the speaker says. If the speaker's style makes it hard to listen, respectfully work with the speaker to solve the problem (e.g., ask a soft speaker to speak more loudly).

*3. Avoid overuse of filler words.*

Sometimes, instructors feel uncomfortable with brief silences and attempt to fill pauses with words. While it often is helpful to acknowledge that you are listening with an occasional "uh-hum," overuse of filler words can become annoying and should be avoided. If you find yourself using too many filler words, take a deep breath and remind yourself that some pauses and brief silences are natural and productive. Smiling and nodding in a supportive manner can show your interest without being disruptive.

*4. Avoid patronizing language.*

Too often, older adults are spoken to as if they are children, with little regard for their dignity. For example, if a small-framed elderly female fits the "little old lady" stereotype, some adults may unthinkingly address this woman as "dear" or "honey." While the speaker may consider these terms of affection, others may find this approach condescending and offensive. Address older adults as you would any other adults—with respect—in the manner they request. It is not uncommon for older persons to prefer being addressed in a more formal manner (e.g., Mr. Smith, rather than Bill.) If in doubt about addressing an older client by first or last name, ask their preference.

---

5. *Avoid using slang.*

Remember that slang often is age-, gender-, and/or culturally specific. For instance, it might be appropriate for a 25-year-old woman to use the phrase "you guys" to address her close friends, both male and female. Older women, however, might find such a phrase to be disrespectful. It is best to use mainstream English (or whatever primary language your instruction is in). If you are working with an individual or with group members who are from a similar age group and background as yourself, the use of some slang may be acceptable. Be careful, however, not to patronize clients by attempting to use slang terms you would not otherwise use.

6. *Make eye contact.*

This demonstrates your interest in each client. A steady gaze can be threatening, but among most American cultures frequently making brief eye contact with clients shows concern and interest. If you are leading a group or class, be sure to make eye contact with each participant.

7. *Speak at an appropriate volume and pace.*

Nervous and/or enthusiastic leaders tend to speak quite rapidly, often not allowing time for listeners to ask about what was said. If you are a rapid speaker, be conscious of slowing your pace. Additionally, the volume of speech must be loud enough for clients to hear, especially if there is background noise. (Remember that hearing aids amplify all noise—not just your voice—so any background music must be low.)

Ask your clients about volume and pace until you become familiar with their needs. Inquire whether the volume of your voice is OK. Likewise, you can ask clients, "Am I talking too fast?" and adjust accordingly. For hearing-impaired clients, it often is beneficial to slow down the rate of your speech, use some gestures or demonstrations to emphasize points, and look at clients so they can pick up visual cues about what you are saying.

8. *Teach new material at an appropriate pace.*

It has been noted that although the ability to learn new information remains relatively stable over time, the speed of learning may slow with aging (Spotts & Schewe, 1989). There may be tremendous variation from one client to another, but a good rule of thumb is to allow older adults (and, ideally, all of your clients) to learn at their own pace.

Allow clients to tell you when they are comfortable with what you have taught them and when they are ready to move on. Periodically ask individuals to demonstrate new moves or explain what you have just said. Inquire whether additional practice is desired. If the majority of a class is ready to move on, reassure those who want more practice that you will review the information again, making sure to let them know when. In groups, give clients the option of using a familiar move until they become comfortable with the new one. Provide frequent opportunities for older clients to meet with you or peers to work on new steps or exercises.

9. *Visual communication aids should be easy to read.*

Older adults' vision will vary widely. To meet the needs of those with vision difficulties, it is best to make writing on chalk boards, signs, flyers, and instruction sheets easy to read. Keep visual material uncluttered and brief. Color combinations that give maximum contrast should be used, while varying shades of the same colors (like grays) should be avoided. Pictures or diagrams can enhance some messages, but they should be simple and clear.

---

*Remember that the best way to determine if you are meeting clients' needs is simply to ask. Most clients will appreciate your concern and will attempt to tell you how to help them. An old adage about teaching applies well to fitness instructors working with older adults: It is less important to know all the answers than to ask the right questions.*

## Leadership Skills for Fitness Professionals

Communication with clients does not occur in a vacuum. It takes place within the context of a relationship in which you hold a special position. You may alternate among acting as a consultant, instructor, counselor, coach, mentor, or other roles, depending on the nature of your work and your client's needs. In all of these roles, however, you remain the leader, the person who has primary responsibility for defining how clients can best approach their health and fitness goals.

There are many talents that contribute to a leader's effectiveness. You already may naturally possess many of these abilities, but may need to work on developing some of them. Understanding how groups and individuals may relate to you over time can be helpful. Skilled fitness instructors are good at using feedback for educational and motivational purposes, while also making clients feel emotionally safe. In addition to these general leadership skills, an appreciation of gender and cultural differences, and creativity in making exercise sessions fun, can encourage clients to get hooked on their exercise program.

Each of these skills is important to successful work with older clients, whether in individual or group formats. But there is an almost endless list of other positive leadership characteristics as varied as the number of fitness professionals. Therefore, in addition to developing these skills, recognize your own special strengths as a leader, and use them for the benefit of your clients.

## Evolution of Instructor-Client Relationships

Human relationships evolve over time. Understanding the basic stages of relationship development will help you pinpoint and address common client needs, so that your rapport will continue to grow. Table 2.2, which was adapted from a group development model by Ward and Preziosi (1994), summarizes the stages of relationship development, as well as specific tips for instructor behaviors at each stage. These same stages also occur within the context of one-on-one work with clients, so they are as relevant to fitness professionals seeing clients individually as they are for leaders of structured exercise classes and facilitators of exercise-related educational programs. Look to your clients' behaviors and concerns for clues about the current stage of your relationship.

Use this information to improve your skills as a fitness instructor. An isolated comment might not require action on your part, but the validity of suggestions or criticisms that come from two or three people always should be seriously considered. When appropriate to do so, modify your behaviors and programs to address these issues.

Your work with older adults will not be limited to conveying information. These relationships will grow and change over time, and the stage of your relationship may influence the kind of information you choose to share or how you communicate it. This insight and flexibility can help you nurture the development of your working relationships.

## Instructor Responsibilities During Individual and Group Sessions

Just as relationships with individuals and groups grow over time, there is a natural progression of events that should occur each time you meet with clients or lead classes. It is your responsibility to smoothly guide clients through each of these steps, making your time with them productive and focused. For the sake of efficiency, the term "session" here refers to both individual work and group activities.

*Step 1: Beginning the session.* Introduce yourself and let clients know that it is time to begin. Explain what you will be doing that day and how you expect them to participate. This is especially important when working with new clients or class members. Reassure clients that they can participate at their own pace, and that they will not be expected to engage in movements that they are unable to perform or are uncomfortable doing.

Concentrate on:
- ✓ setting a positive tone (I'm glad to see each of you here today!)
- ✓ focusing clients' attention on exercise (Now it's time to get our workout going.)
- ✓ explaining what to expect (Today we'll talk about how your routine is going, and I'll teach you a new exercise for your hamstrings.)
- ✓ reviewing prior performance, if applicable (Last class we learned a new move and all of you started to get it. Is everyone comfortable with that move?)

---

Table 2.2

**Stages of Instructor-Client Relationship Development**

---

1. *Preparation Stage*
   This refers to fitness instructors' preparation prior to meeting with a client. Be comfortable with the information to be covered; appearing scattered and disorganized can damage your credibility, while a calm and organized approach can instill confidence.

   You will need to:
   - ✓ Do your homework. Review fitness assessment or exercise tracking information, if applicable. If you are leading group exercise or offering educational programs, be thoroughly familiar with the information you will be teaching.
   - ✓ Come psychologically prepared [calm, enthusiastic, and focused on the client(s) and your job].
   - ✓ Finalize content to be covered and presentation methods for structured or semi-structured classes or presentations.

2. *Initial Stage*
   Trust issues are central to your clients, since they are figuring out what your sessions will be like, and how they are expected to behave. In this initial stage, older adults in particular may be reluctant to question your authority, to disagree with you or other group members, or to challenge your recommendations. Remember that this is probably not due to unwillingness to cooperate or a lack of interest. For some older adults, you are an expert or authority figure. Initial reluctance to critique your suggestions or to report problems may be based upon long-standing beliefs that one should not question authority. It may take some time and patience to help some of your older clients feel comfortable being candid with you.

   You will need to:
   - ✓ Help clients get acquainted with you (and other group members).
   - ✓ Set the norm for participation by explaining that client input is respected and essential to success.
   - ✓ Provide accepting and constructive responses to both concerns and positive comments.
   - ✓ Point out similarities among your ideas and viewpoints, and those of your clients.
   - ✓ Provide structure and direction.

3. *Transition Stage*
   After you and your clients have worked together for a while, they may begin to ask more questions or offer challenges. Personal agendas and power issues may surface in groups and classes.

You will need to:

✓ Continue identifying perspectives and experiences that are shared by you and clients.
✓ Respond to differences of opinion in a positive manner.
✓ Keep meetings and classes on track.
✓ Respond to challenges to your expertise in an open, non-defensive manner.
✓ With groups or classes, get as many people as possible involved in discussing problems and giving feedback.

4. *Working Stage*

Relationships are characterized by increased open and supportive communication. In groups or classes, interactions become less instructor-focused, and more exchanges occur between group members. In both group and one-to-one situations, feedback is more readily solicited by clients, and empathy among clients and fitness instructors often is high.

One danger that may arise during this stage is that clients' or instructors' desires for approval or acceptance may take priority over exercise goals. For instance, Richard states that he has missed the last three power-walking classes because he has been busy planning a social event for his condo community. In an attempt to maintain a warm and positive relationship with Richard, his fitness instructor may refrain from reminding Richard that walking remains vitally important to his health and well-being, even when he is busy. Similarly, clients who have bonded well with their fitness professional may be reluctant to report when strategies proposed by the instructor are not working well for them.

You will need to:

✓ Encourage members to honestly report what does and does not work for them on a continual basis.
✓ Encourage clients to turn ideas into action.
✓ Remember that your primary role is to provide expert guidance. Tactfulness always is required, but don't hesitate to gently challenge clients or constructively critique their performance when needed. Your main role is not to be a friend, but rather a coach.
✓ Interpret individual or group behavior when it will help clients. (Example: *"I notice that fewer people are coming to class during this holiday season. I know this is a very busy time for some of you, but making time for exercise can help you to stay healthy and reduce tension if you are dealing with a lot of holiday stress. Congratulations for being here today! Please encourage your friends to keep coming, too!"*)

5. *Final Stage*

This is the time to terminate work with an individual or group. Emphasize what your clients have accomplished, and challenge them to carry on with skills they have learned. This also is the time for the fitness instructor to summarize what has been learned and to establish a sense of pride and closure. Many clients naturally will begin to emotionally distance themselves; increased absences for individual sessions or groups is not uncommon.

You will need to:

✓ Address any remaining questions or concerns.
✓ Acknowledge the ending of the current relationship and emotions related to the change (e.g., apprehension, sadness).
✓ Summarize the accomplishments of individual clients, classes, or exercise groups.
✓ Reinforce your clients' exercise-related changes and insights.
✓ Ensure that your clients know how to get more information and support as needed.
✓ Ensure that clients have the knowledge to maintain healthy physical activity behavior changes.
✓ Confirm each client's future exercise commitment(s).

6. *Evaluation Stage*

Focus on assessing your performance as a fitness instructor and your clients' experiences working with you or attending your class or group.

You will need to:

✓ Follow up with your clients regarding their experiences and suggestions, in person and/or through evaluation surveys.

*Step 2: Leading the session.* This is the body of your session, when the bulk of the exercise, education, and/or discussion will occur (* indicates leader behaviors that are especially important for older adults).

Concentrate on:

✓ providing clear instructions (First, let's review your exercise chart. How many times did you swim last week?)

✓ allowing adequate time for questions* (Do you have any questions about where you should feel this stretch?)

✓ presenting options for modifying types of movements, intensity, etc.* [If you aren't comfortable with this new move, you can march in place, like this (demonstrating).]

✓ giving plenty of genuine, positive feedback (You are showing some great endurance.)

✓ actively engaging clients' participation (Who can tell me the purpose of this exercise?)

*Step 3: Closing the session.* This sets the tone for the feelings clients carry away from the session, so be sure to close on a positive note! Review what has been accomplished and what clients should be doing until you meet again.

Concentrate on:

✓ summarizing your clients' achievements (Everyone's form looked terrific today.)

✓ restating clients' "homework," if applicable (So this week you'll buy a new pair of aerobics shoes and will walk three times.)

✓ expressing the expectation of seeing them again (I'll look forward to our next appointment on Thursday morning.)

By carefully performing each of your duties as a fitness leader, you will confirm that you are well-prepared and that your clients' time with you is well spent.

## Creating a Safe Environment for Older Adults

To facilitate the success of your older clients in meeting exercise goals, you must create a safe environment for them. We commonly think of safety for exercise program participants in terms of physical safety issues (Is the floor dry and the surface smooth? Are participants properly warmed up before doing strenuous exercises?) In a review of the challenges of physical education of older adults, Cousins and Burgess (1992) reported that chronic conditions may indeed put some older adults at increased risk of aggravation or pain, or require physical activity modifications. Research has suggested, however, that older adults generally are not more injury-prone than younger adults (Clarkson & Dedrick, 1988), although fears of injury increase significantly with age (Stephens & Craig, 1990). For example, in a study of women over age 70, Cousins (2000) found that her participants generally recognized benefits of physical activity, especially moderate walking. But they often held exaggerated concerns over risks. She concluded that, "Many older women feel physically vulnerable, are unsure about their actual risks and benefits in exercise settings, and in the face of that uncertainty, report medical reasons why they should be excused from fitness-promoting exercise" (Cousins, 2000).

Why might even healthy older adults at low risk for injury be overly fearful of exercise? The answer rests in a frequently overlooked aspect of client safety: the concern for psychological safety. Perceived risk of injury or bad health outcomes is subjective. As a result, you may encounter clients with realistic concerns, while other clients may possess exaggerated risk beliefs that unnecessarily prevent them from exercising or limit their exercise options (Cousins,

2000). Most older clients will not engage in physical activities they perceive to be dangerous, no matter how adamantly you insist that they should.

Increased psychological comfort with exercise programs can dramatically improve program adherence. Help older adults safely exercise at or near their physical ability by accurately identifying and minimizing both physical and psychological risks of exercise. Subsequent chapters suggest specific components of program design intended to minimize the risk of physical injury to your older clients. Table 2.3 presents a few common psychological risks of exercise for older adults. Some of these are based upon the work of researchers (Cousins, 2000;

---

Table 2.3

**Common Psychological Risks of Exercise for Older Adults**

---

*1. Risk of Embarrassment or Ridicule.* This risk may be especially serious for older adults who never have been physically active or who are attempting to engage in exercise after an extended break. All clients may be susceptible to the risk of embarrassment, but remember that older adults are attempting to engage in an exercise plan despite societal messages that exercise is most appropriate for younger adults, and that older adults may be too frail for exercise or too old to develop new skills. (Hence the term, "You can't teach an old dog new tricks.") It is no wonder that some older adults fear criticism.

*To Help Your Older Clients:* Acknowledge your client's wisdom and courage in committing to their health or physical fitness by exercising. Reassure them that the vast majority of individuals in exercise programs are preoccupied with their own performance, leaving little time to worry about what others are doing. Predictions of failure from family members or others, if they occur, can be used as a motivator to succeed and to prove skeptics wrong.

*2. Risk of Facing Diminished Physical Abilities.* This problem can be especially difficult for former athletes or former regular exercisers who have not been active in a long time. Some older adults may compare their current performance to what they could do when they were younger or prior to a medical problem. Finding out that they can do less than expected can be a demotivating blow to self-esteem. Older clients who note declines in their abilities may be reluctant to continue exercise activities that painfully remind them of these changes.

*To Help Your Older Clients:* Encourage them to measure progress from their present starting point. We would never expect a person of any age who has not exercised for a while to be able to automatically perform as they did when they were exercising regularly. Additionally, remind clients that individuals of any age have plenty of room for substantial gains in physical abilities. With time and consistent participation in their exercise routine, they may be pleasantly surprised at how much they can improve.

*3. Risk of Confronting Ageist Stereotypes of Physical Beauty.* Given society's obsession with youth, older women may feel acutely self-conscious while exercising, particularly if the setting is a facility where slim, well-toned young women work out. Males, too, can suffer from damaged self-esteem when comparing their own physiques to those of well-conditioned young men who exercise at the same facility.

*To Help Your Older Clients:* Remind your clients that the only people they need to please are themselves. Suggest they concentrate on the benefits from participating in an exercise program regardless of how they fit into the visual profile of others attending a facility. Point out, too, that by actively taking steps to improve their health, appearance, and self-esteem by exercising, they are improving their own physical attractiveness.

---

*These are just a few of a wide variety of psychological risks your clients may associate with physical activity programs. By supportively encouraging them to come to terms with these and other risks, you will free your clients of restrictive barriers to exercise and fears that may impact many aspects of their lives.*

Caserta & Gillett, 1998; Cousins and Burgess, 1992), and others are based upon fitness professionals' experiences. Suggested strategies for helping older clients to overcome each of these risks are also given in Table 2.3.

## Types and Uses of Feedback to Clients

A primary task of fitness instructors is to provide clients with helpful feedback. Different types of feedback serve different functions. Feedback may be technical, as when you comment on a client's form as they use a piece of equipment or perform an exercise. It also may take the form of counseling, as when you work with clients to set new physical-activity goals or problem-solve their barriers to exercise. Another intent of feedback may be to reassure clients about their performance, or to enhance their motivation.

Positive feedback is a response that tells a person or group what they are doing right. Telling an exercise class, "I see that everyone is moving their weights slowly and with control; that's great!" is an example of positive feedback. In contrast, negative feedback is a response that tells a person or group what they are doing wrong. For example, "I see some people getting into the pool to swim laps without doing any initial stretching or warm-up. That's not good for your body, which needs time to prepare for exercise." Negative feedback is necessary to teach clients to avoid errors that could put them at risk for injury.

It is not helpful for clients to hear that they are doing something wrong if they are not informed about how to correct the problem. Therefore, negative feedback should be immediately followed by corrective information. Corrective feedback is a response to observed behavior that provides specific instruction on how to improve the technique or performance.

Even if clients are not in danger of injuring themselves, corrective feedback that can lead to improved health or fitness benefits should be given. This type of feedback also can be used to correct client misconceptions about their exercise program, the use of behavior-change skills, or fitness in general. In the case of teaching physical movements, it often is helpful to supplement corrective feedback by modeling (demonstrating) the proper form.

Prevent clients from jumping to the conclusion that they are doing everything wrong by giving negative and corrective feedback in conjunction with positive feedback. Researchers and leadership specialists have suggested the "sandwich technique," which simply refers to placing negative and corrective feedback between two instances of positive feedback (Hughes, Ginnet, & Curphy, 1993). When commenting on client performance, start on a positive note and end on a positive note. For example: "Frank, you are doing a great job of keeping your back against the mat as you start your sit-ups. Try not to pull your head forward; that puts strain on your neck. Keep your neck and elbows back like this (while demonstrating proper form). Your form on these floor exercises is really improving."

Remember to give positive feedback as soon as clients improve their form or correct mistakes. Do not wait to give encouragement until they have perfect form because it may take many attempts for them to succeed. To keep clients motivated, give positive feedback about each successive step toward the desired outcome, in conjunction with corrective instructions. "That is much better, Frank! Now see if you can extend your arms even further. Good work."

Redirective feedback attempts to switch the subject under discussion by keeping conversations on target. For example, a personal trainer might have to change the subject from a client's extended discussion of his vacation to strength-training goals. Redirection can also be used to alter the way a process is being handled. For instance, if an experienced step aerobics participant is commenting on a new class member's performance in a hurtful way, the instructor could use redirection to guide how feedback should be given. The instructor might say, "Rose, I'm sure you remember how hard it was trying to learn the steps we use in our classes. It seems like an awful lot to remember at once. Would you be willing to demonstrate just one of the steps?" Redirection can be relatively painless for the redirected clients if it is done with respect and sensitivity.

Keep in mind the tasks to be accomplished during your meetings with individual clients or in groups or classes. Discussions that trail into extended tangents quickly get boring or seem chaotic, leaving clients questioning the value of participating. Therefore, try to stay on track with what you planned to accomplish, using redirection when needed.

This does not mean, however, that fitness professionals should become tyrants, never tolerating the slightest bit of non-exercise commentary. Some older adults may want to use their exercise program for social connection, as well as health benefits. They may want to share information about themselves to help you and others get to know them, and may ask you details about yourself and your life.

Other older clients may feel a natural and compelling need to make sense of new information by relating it to their past experiences. In such cases, older clients need room to share information that may not be directly related to their health or fitness programs. Accept and welcome this type of communication if it helps your clients to bond with you or others in a fitness program, or to generally feel understood and cared about. Think of redirection as a tool to help you maintain a comfortable balance between accomplish-

ing exercise-related tasks and your clients' needs for individual expression.

If you find yourself using redirection techniques often, try to examine why. The need for frequent redirection might be expected if you are dealing with older adults who suffer from cognitive impairments that lead to disorientation, short-term memory problems, or difficulty paying attention. But with clients without cognitive difficulties, the need for frequent redirection might signal problems with the information you are presenting. Is the material interesting to your clients? Is it clearly relevant to their lives? Distractions also can make it harder for clients to stay on task; is there activity or noise in the background that makes it hard for clients to focus or hear what you are saying? Are your questions and instructions clear so clients understand the desired response? A client's response may seem off-target simply because they don't understand what kind of response you want. Lastly, difficulties staying on track almost always suggest a client's need for more consistent positive feedback when they are on track.

No matter what type of feedback you are giving, following certain rules will increase the chance that it will be beneficial. Hughes and colleagues (1993) suggest a number of tips for improving feedback skills. Among others, they suggest that feedback should always:

✓ Be helpful. (Emphasize behaviors that are under the client's control.)

✓ Be specific. (Give a clear understanding of what behaviors need to be changed and how to change them.)

✓ Be timely. (Give feedback as soon as possible after the behavior is observed.) If the immediate situation is not a good time for your client to hear feedback (for example, they are surrounded by people and you know that they would be embarrassed by receiving corrective feedback in front of others), offer the feedback at the earliest appropriate opportunity.

✓ Include positive and corrective feedback. A mix of recognition for what is right, plus ongoing suggestions for improvement, can optimize your clients' ability to develop the skills you are teaching.

A final note: Feedback may elicit different feelings in different listeners. Something that you said for the sake of simple redirection may be interpreted as negative by one client and positive by another. Remember that the overall goal of feedback is to help your clients. Carefully observe the effects of your feedback on each person. Over time, you will learn how particular clients receive your comments, allowing you to tailor your feedback so that it has the intended effect.

## Sensitivity to Gender and Ethnic/Cultural Differences

At first glance, the differences between a fitness professional and a client may seem to far outweigh the similarities. Fitness instructors are called upon to work with clients from different age groups, genders, ethnicities, cultures, economic situations, life experiences, and personalities. Don't become overwhelmed by the diversity; successful fitness instructors approach differences as interesting aspects of clients that deserve both consideration and appreciation. Each client's beliefs, perspectives, and lifestyle will impact their health and fitness goals and the ways in which they will want to meet them. Exercise programs must take into account the individuals for whom they are designed, and must work with that person's values. Appreciating differences will help you consistently demonstrate respect and acceptance. Always remember that if all clients were clones, your job would be pretty dull!

Clients' exercise interests may be highly influenced by cultural messages about appropriate male and female behavior. Much of older adults' life experiences occurred during times that were more restrictive in terms of gender-appropriate behavior. Although most older clients may have revised their perspectives many times over the years, and some may always have been progressive in their thinking about sex roles, some older adults may be influenced by historic notions of "acceptable" male and female behavior. For example, some older females may be concerned with issues of modesty, finding the scanty workout clothes worn by some people at a fitness facility offensive. A few older male and female clients may feel strongly that women have no business in the weight room. Older males may think participating in traditional aerobics, yoga, or flexibility classes is not masculine. Older women and men may prefer exercise groups of the same gender over co-educational instruction.

As a fitness professional, your main task is to help your clients engage in exercise activities that best serve their health and fitness needs and interests. As much as possible, recommend activities that are a good match for client perspectives, as well as the desired outcomes. That is not to say that you should never challenge a client to broaden their thinking. It may be extremely helpful for an older woman who is experiencing difficulty with daily household tasks that require upper-body strength to try some strength exercises using weight-training equipment. Similarly, an older man who attends a stretching class might benefit from increases in flexibility and be pleasantly surprised to see other males in the room.

Remember to be sensitive to clients' feelings. Provide gentle encouragement and occasional challenges to clients' thinking without attacking entire perspectives. As your relationship develops and you patiently encourage new activities, your older clients may become willing to branch out into some new exercise behaviors. If this does not happen, continue working within the parameters of their current attitudes to meet the primary objective of keeping them actively engaged in their exercise program.

Cultural and ethnic differences also can impact your work and effectiveness in communication with clients (Li, 1999). In a discussion on communicating with older adults of different ethnic and cultural backgrounds, Joan Wood (1989) noted that most research and health-related programs have been developed from white, urban, middle-class models that ignore variations. She also noted that health professionals are more likely to come from upper-class non-minority backgrounds, and that there is a great need to develop effective cross-cultural communication skills to better serve all older adults. Some important points from her discussion and suggestions for improving cross-cultural communication skills follow.

Culture refers to socially transmitted beliefs, institutions, and norms for behavior, while ethnicity refers to a shared history, culture, and sense of peoplehood. Culture and ethnicity are inseparable from other components of an individual's identity. Lifelong patterns of socialization within an ethnic group play a major role in shaping personality, so sensitivity to culture is crucial to individualizing the services you provide to older adults.

One example of how ethnic differences may impact your work is the variation in the social status of older adults in many minority cultures vs. white, middle-, and upper-class American cultures. Although older adults from minority groups may be isolated or segregated from the mainstream white culture, remember that they may be fully integrated within their own cultural group. Unlike white older adults, who often experience decreases in respect and power with age, older adults from some ethnic minority groups occupy positions of great honor, respect, and authority. In some minority cultures, older adults frequently provide a home for younger children and grandchildren, use their own homes as the gathering place for culturally important events, and preside over important community and family decision-making processes. In economically disadvantaged situations, older adults may provide the most stable income (from retirement or benefits programs) and take on substantial parenting responsibilities for grandchildren whose parents work.

While the roles of older adults vary dramatically even among the same culture, this example highlights several important implications. First, failure to treat older adults with sufficient respect may impair your ability to build a trusting and positive relationship with them. The best approach is to consistently show in your actions and words that they are valued. This will increase the likelihood that your client will share important information with you and continue to invest in working with you to meet their health or fitness goals.

It can be dangerous to make generalizations about clients' lifestyles. For instance, you cannot assume that all retired men sit home most of the day, and have no obligations other than addressing their physical-activity goals. Take the case of an African-American older adult who holds a position of authority in his church, does extensive volunteer work with agencies in his community, and frequently chairs committees that organize and implement important cultural events. This client may be too busy for an exercise program that demands two hours in the fitness facility four times a week. Inquire about the lifestyle of each client, rather than make assumptions about what the client should be willing and able to do.

Here are some suggestions to increase sensitivity to the needs of older adult clients from varied cultures:

✓ Treat all older adults with respect. Do not minimize the importance of their other activities, and do not patronize them.

✓ Understand that cultural beliefs may have a large impact on ideas about health and fitness. Some cultural beliefs actually may suggest that physical activity is an undesirable or unattractive behavior, or that health outcomes are mostly determined by factors other than personal exercise habits (such as spiritual or religious forces, or emotional states). Beliefs about exercise or physical activity will influence clients' compliance with their exercise programs, as well as their motivation. As you develop program goals and assess progress, strive to understand the beliefs that may be influencing your client. You do not have to agree with all of their beliefs, but show respect for them, and make exercise recommendations that fit their belief system.

✓ Seek out expertise when needed. Read about, or attend training on, cross-cultural communication. Enlist the help of cultural mediators from various ethnic groups, either on a formal basis (working with ethnic minority staff) or informal basis (receiving advice from friends, co-workers, or other members of ethnic groups).

✓ Be empathetic. As much as possible, listen to your client's experience and attempt to see their perspective. Preferring our own way is not the only barrier to empathy. Automatic assumptions that clients' values, viewpoints, and reactions will be the same as ours also should be avoided.

Currently, minority elderly populations are growing more rapidly than the white elderly population. According to the Centers for Disease Control and Prevention (2003), from 2000 to 2030, the proportion of racial minority persons age 65 or older is expected to increase from 11.3% to 16.5%. The proportion of Hispanic elders, for example, is expected to rise from 5.6% to 10.9%. This implies that the already vital need for exercise programs designed and offered to minority elders will only increase.

Working with clients who are different from you need not be intimidating. It can be one of the most enjoyable and exciting challenges of your work as a fitness professional. If you approach all of your clients with respect and a willingness to learn about their perspectives, your working relationships will be productive and rewarding.

## The Fun Factor: Leadership Strategies for Making Exercise Enjoyable for Older Adults

As previously discussed, enjoyment is a valuable asset for exercise adherence. Here are a few strategies to make exercise more enjoyable for your older clients.

### HUMOR

You can take your work seriously without always taking yourself seriously. Human resource research has determined that leaders who use humor often are perceived as both more likable and effective. Environments where humor is welcome result in benefits ranging from increased motivation, creativity, satisfaction, and productivity to decreased stress. Humor is a wonderful tool for capturing your clients' attention and having fun as you lead exercise classes or work individually. According to Dean (1993), humor:

✓ shows people that you are approachable and "down to earth"

✓ conveys confidence in your relationship with clients

✓ decreases tension or anxiety if clients are nervous

✓ puts issues into perspective in a non-threatening way

✓ demonstrates that you value and encourage spontaneity

Here are a few tips for appropriate uses of humor, adapted from the work of Ozzie Dean (1993):

✓ Making fun of yourself from time to time is OK, but do not make fun of others.

✓ Laugh with others, not at them. Do not tell a funny story about someone in the group or known to the group unless you have first obtained their permission to do so.

✓ Avoid any sort of age-related, ethnic, or sexist jokes or insults.

✓ Show clients that it is OK to laugh. If you are able to relax and laugh from time to time, you have given them permission to do so as well.

Try to be open to using humor to make the exercise skills you are teaching or the activity you are leading more interesting. Humor should not detract from your exercise goals for the group or person, but should contribute to clients' motivation.

## MUSIC

Although there may be tremendous variation, appropriate use of music can greatly enhance exercise experiences, especially in structured exercise classes. Frequently, Big Band music, show tunes, or instrumental music is enjoyable to the greatest proportion of older clients. However, avoid making assumptions about the types of music that older adults should or will like. The best way to learn about their music preferences is to ask for specific suggestions.

No matter what the type of music, volume should be kept low. High volumes may interfere with an older client's ability to hear your instructions and can be especially problematic if they wear hearing aids. The rhythm should be easy to follow and the tempo appropriate for clients' physical abilities and skill levels. By listening to older adults' input, you can determine the degree to which music can enhance their exercise activities.

## OTHER WAYS TO ADD NOVELTY AND VARIETY

People naturally enjoy activities that are interesting and fresh, which usually requires adding variety, such as occasional changes in exercise routines. Remember that some older adults may require more time to learn new movements or skills. Experts in programming for older adults frequently warn fitness instructors to avoid overwhelming older clients with sudden changes to established routines.

Whether you are leading fitness classes or working with clients on a one-to-one basis, the rate of change should be physically safe, and comfortable for the client. New steps or equipment should be introduced gradually, with plenty of time for practice. Remember that successful experiences are good motivators, whereas feeling lost or unable to perform new movements can be embarrassing and frustrating. Ensure success with new movements by keeping them simple at first. In the case of fitness classes, offer frequent demonstrations of movements for different ability levels and encourage modification of movements as needed. Frequently returning to familiar basic movements such as marching in place will enable even new participants to be successful. When working with older clients, provide plenty of positive feedback as they try new exercises or activities and make sure that plenty of time is spent on tasks they perform well.

## Tips for Handling Nervousness or Anxiety

No matter how knowledgeable you are about providing fitness instruction, leading new kinds of classes or working with new kinds of clients can sometimes make even seasoned fitness professionals nervous. If you do find yourself feeling anxious, the following tips may help.

Before the session:

✓ Be sure you are at ease with the material by rehearsing your role.

✓ Visualize yourself as a confident and successful fitness instructor. Picture the best-case scenario of how you would like your appointment or class to go.

✓ If needed, enlist the help of an experienced co-leader the first few times you do a new type of class or training session.

During the session:

✓ Focus on the value of what you are teaching, and how it will help your clients. (This takes your focus off yourself and places it back on your clients.)

✓ Practice empathy. Focusing on your clients' perspectives not only helps you to serve them better, but also takes attention away from your own anxiety.

## CONCLUSION

An older client's exercise-program satisfaction and participation is often directly related to their relationship with you. Your knowledge and application of behavior-change principles can help clients develop and sustain new exercise habits. Showing interest and frequently giving sincere praise are especially motivating to older adults. Because they may not have recent exercise experiences or physically active peers to help them understand what to expect, your support becomes even more important when older adults are just beginning to exercise.

Invest time and energy into getting to know your clients. Nurture your relationships with them by showing acceptance and interest in their well-being. Make an ongoing effort to improve your own communication and leadership skills. In addition to enhancing your own professional abilities, the uplifting effect you will have on many of your older adult clients may become its own reward.

# REFERENCES AND SUGGESTED READING

Ajzen, I. (1991). The theory of planned behavior. *Organizational Behavior and Human Decision Processes, 50,* 179–211.

Arias, E. & Smith, B.L. (2003). Deaths: Preliminary data for 2001. *National Vital Statistics Reports, 51,* 5, 1–44.

Barke, C.R. & Nicholas, D.R. (1990). Physical activity in older adults: The stages of change. *Journal of Applied Gerontology, 9,* 2, 216–223.

Barone, D.F., Maddux, J.E., & Snyder, C.R. (1997). *Social Cognitive Psychology: History and Current Domains.* Fort Lauderdale, Fla: Plenum.

Becker, M.H. & Maiman, B.A. (1975). Sociobehavioral determinants of compliance with health and medical care recommendations. *Medical Care, 13,* 1, 10–24.

Belisle, M., Roskies, E., & Levesque, J.M. (1987). Improving adherence to physical activity. *Health Psychology, 6,* 2, 159–172.

Blumenthal, J. et al. (1999). Effects of exercise training on older patients with major depression. *Archives of Internal Medicine, 159,* 2349–2356.

Brawley, L.R., Rejeski, W.J., & King, A.C. (2003). Promoting physical activity for older adults: the challenges for changing behavior. *American Journal of Preventive Medicine, 25,* 172–183.

Brown, D.R. (1992). Physical activity, aging, and psychological well-being: An overview of the research. *Canadian Journal of Sports Science, 17,* 3, 185–193.

Brown, D.R. (1990). Exercise fitness and mental health. In C. Bouchard et al. (Eds.) *Exercise, Fitness and Health: A Consensus of Current Knowledge,* (607–626). Champaign, Ill.: Human Kinetics.

Brownell, K.D. et al. (1986). Understanding and preventing relapse. *American Psychologist, 41,* 765–782.

Buckworth, J. & Dishman, R.K. (2002). *Exercise Psychology.* Champaign, Ill: Human Kinetics.

Burlew, L.D., Jones, J., & Emerson, P. (1991). Exercise and the elderly: A group counseling approach. *Journal for Specialists in Group Work, 16,* 3, 152–158.

Butler, R.N. et al. (2000). Anti-aging medicine: What makes it different from geriatrics? *Geriatrics, 55,* 6, 36–43.

Cantor, M. (1991). Family and community: Changing roles in an aging society. *The Gerontologist, 31,* 3, 337–346.

Carstensen, L. & Turk-Charles, S. (1994). The salience of emotion across the adult life span. *Psychology and Aging, 9,* 2, 259–264.

Caserta, M.S. & Gillett, P.A. (1998). Older women's feelings about exercise and their adherence to an aerobic regimen over time. *The Gerontologist, 38,* 5, 602.

Center for Disease Control and Prevention (2003). Trends in aging: United States and worldwide. *Morbidity and Mortality Weekly Report, 52,* 6, 101–106.

Clark, D.O. (1999). Identifying psychological, physiological, and environmental barriers and facilitators to exercise among older low-income adults. *Journal of Clinical Geropsychology, 5,* 51–62.

Clarkson, P.M. & Dedrick, M.E. (1988). Exercise-induced muscle damage, repair and adaptation in old and young subjects. *Journal of Gerontology: Medical Sciences, 43,* 4, M91–96.

Cousins, S.O. (2000). "My heart couldn't take it:" Older women's beliefs about exercise benefits and risks. *Journal of Gerontology: Psychological Sciences, 55B,* 5, 283–294.

Cousins, S.O. & Burgess, A. (1992). Perspectives on older adults in physical activity and sports. (Special Issue: Educational Gerontology in Canada). *Educational Gerontology, 18,* 5, 164–481.

Culos-Reed, S.N., Gyurcsik, N.C., & Brawley, L.R. (2001). Using theories of motivated behavior to understand physical activity: Perspectives on their influence. In Singer, R.N., Hausenblas, H.A., Janelle, C.M. (Eds.) *Handbook of Sport*

*Psychology* (2nd ed.). (695–717). New York: John Wiley & Sons.

Davis, K. (1986). Paying the healthcare bills of an aging population. In A. Pifer & L. Bronte (Eds.) *Our Aging Society: Paradox and Promise*. New York: W.W. Norton & Co.

Dean, O. (1993). The effective use of humor in human resource development. In J.W. Pfeiffer (Ed.) *The 1993 Annual Developing Human Resources*. San Diego: Pfeiffer and Company.

Deci, E.L. (1977). Intrinsic motivation: Theory and application. In D.M. Landers & R.W. Christina (Eds.) *Psychology of Motor Behavior and Sport* (388–396). Champaign Ill.: Human Kinetics.

Deci, E.L. & Ryan, R.M. (1985). The general causality orientations scale: Self-determination in personality. *Journal of Research in Personality*, 19, 109–134.

Dishman, R.K. (1991). Increasing and maintaining exercise and physical activity. *Behavior Therapy*, 22, 345–378.

Dishman, R.K. (1988). Overview (1–9). In R.K. Dishman (Ed.) *Exercise Adherence: Its Impact on Public Health*. Champaign, Ill.: Human Kinetics.

Dychtwald, K. (1989). *Age Wave: The Challenges and Opportunities of an Aging America*. Los Angeles: Jeremy Tarcher, Inc.

Epstein, L.H. (1998). Integrating theoretical approaches to promote physical activity. *American Journal of Preventive Medicine*, 15, 257–265.

Ferrini, A.F., & Ferrini, R.L. (1993). *Health in the Later Years* (2nd ed.). Dubuque, Iowa: William C. Brown.

Hagger, M.S., Chatzisarantis, N.L., & Biddle, S.J. (2002). The influence of autonomous and controlling motives on physical activity intentions within the theory of planned behavior. *British Journal of Health Psychology*, 7, 283–297.

Hausenblas, H.A., Carron, A.V., & Mack, D.E. (1997). Application of the theories of reasoned action and planned behavior to exercise behavior: A meta-analysis. *Journal of Sport and Exercise Psychology*, 19, 1, 36–51.

Himes, C. (1992). Social demography of contemporary families and aging. *Generations*, 3, 13–16.

Hughes, R.L., Ginnet, R.C., & Curphy, G.J. (1993). *Leadership: Enhancing the Lessons of Experience*. Homewood, Ill.: Irwin.

Hummert, M.L., Nussbaum, J.F., & Wiemann, J.M. (1992). Communication and the elderly: Cognition, language, and relationships. (Special Issue: Communication and aging: Cognition, language, and relationships). *Communication Research*, 19, 4, 413–422.

Kane, R., Oslander, J., & Abrass, I. (1989). *Essentials of Clinical Geriatrics* (2nd ed.). New York: McGraw-Hill, Information Services Co.

Kaplan, M.S. et al. (2001). Demographic and psychosocial correlates of physical activity in late life. *American Journal of Preventive Medicine*, 21, 306–312.

Kaplan, R.M., Sallis, J.F., & Patterson, T. L. (1993). *Health and Human Behavior*. New York: McGraw-Hill, Inc.

Keysor, J.J. (2003). Does late-life physical activity or exercise prevent or minimize disablement? A critical review of the scientific evidence. *American Journal of Preventive Medicine*, 25, 129–136.

King, A.C. et al. (2000). Personal and environmental factors associated with physical inactivity among different racial-ethnic groups of U.S. middle-aged and older-aged women. *Health Psychology*, 19, 354–364.

King, A.C. et al. (1992). Determinants of physical activity and interventions in adults. *Medicine and Science in Sports and Exercise*, 24, 6, S221–S235.

Kogan, N. (1990). Personality in aging. In J.E. Birren & K.W. Schaie (Eds.) *Handbook of the Psychology of Aging* (3rd ed.). San Diego: Academic Press.

Lavie, C. et al. (1999). Effects of cardiac rehabilitation and exercise training programs in women with depression. *American Journal of Cardiology*, 83, 1480–1483.

Lee, C. (1993). Factors related to the adoption of exercise among older women. *Journal of Behavioral Medicine*, 16, 323–334.

Levy, et al. (2000). Reducing cardiovascular stress with positive self-stereotypes of aging. *Journal of Gerontology, 55,* 4, 205–213.

Lewis, C.B. & Campanelli, L.C. (1990). *Health Promotion & Exercise for Older Adults: An Instructor's Guide.* Rockville, Md.: Aspen Publishers.

Li, H.Z. (1999). Communicating information in conversations: A cross-cultural comparison. *International Journal of Intercultural Relations, 23,* 3, 387–409.

Maddux J.E. (1993). Social cognitive models of health and exercise behavior: An introduction and review of conceptual issues. *Journal of Applied Sport Psychology, 5,* 116–140.

Marcus, B.H. & Forsyth, L.H. (2003). *Motivating People to be Physically Active.* Champaign, Ill.: Human Kinetics.

Marcus, B.H. & Owen, N. (1992). Motivational readiness, self-efficacy and decision-making for exercise. *Journal of Applied Social Psychology, 22,* 3–16.

Marcus, B.H., Rakowski, W., & Rossi, J.S. (1992). Assessing motivational readiness and decision-making for exercise. *Health Psychology, 11,* 4, 257–261.

Marcus, B.H. & Stanton, A.L. (1993). Evaluation of relapse prevention and reinforcement interventions to promote exercise adherence in sedentary females. *Research Quarterly for Exercise and Sport, 64,* 447–452.

Marlatt, G.A. & Gordon, J.R. (1985). *Relapse Prevention: Maintenance Strategies in Addictive Behavior Change.* New York: Guilford Press.

Marlatt, G.A. & Gordon, J.R. (1980). Determinants of relapse: Implications for the maintenance of behavior change. In P.O. Davidson & S.M. Davidson (Eds.) *Behavioral Medicine: Changing Health Lifestyles* (410–452). New York: Guilford Press.

Mook, D.G. (1996). *Motivation: The Organization of Action* (2nd ed.). New York: W.W. Norton & Company.

Morgan, W.P. (1997). *Physical Activity and Mental Health.* Washington, D.C.: Taylor & Francis.

Myers, G.C. (1990). Demography of aging. In R.H. Binstock & L. K. George (Eds.) *Handbook of Aging and the Social Sciences* (3rd ed.). San Diego: Academic Press.

Ostrow, A.C. (1984). *Physical Activity and the Older Adult: Psychological Perspectives.* Princeton, N.J.: Princeton Book Co.

Prochaska, J.O. & DiClemente, C.C. (1983). Stages and processes of self-change of smoking: Toward an integrative model. *Journal of Consulting and Clinical Psychology, 51,* 390–395.

Prochaska, J.O. & DiClemente, C.C. (1982). Transtheoretical therapy: Toward a more integrative model of change. *Psychotherapy: Theory, Research, and Practice, 20,* 161–173.

Rebok, G.W. & Plude, D.J. (2001). Relation of physical activity to memory functioning in older adults: The memory workout program. *Educational Gerontology, 27,* 241–259.

Rosenstock, I.M. (1966). Why people use health services. *Milbank Memorial Fund Quarterly, 44,* 94–124.

Rowe, J.W. & Kahn, R.L. (1998). *Successful Aging.* New York: Parthenon Books.

Ryan, R. M. et al. (1997). Intrinsic motivation and exercise adherence. International *Journal of Sport Psychology, 28,* 335–354.

Sallis, J.F. & Owen, N. (1999). *Physical Activity and Behavioral Medicine.* Thousand Oaks, Calif.: Sage.

Salthouse, T. (1990). *Theoretical Perspectives on Cognitive Aging.* Hillsdale, N.J.: Lawrence Erlbaum Associates.

Seguin, R. & Nelson, M.E. (2003). The benefits of strength training for older adults. *American Journal of Preventive Medicine, 25,* 141–149.

Sonstroem, R.J. & Morgan, W.P. (1989). Exercise and self-esteem: Rationale and model. *Medicine and Science in Sports and Exercise, 21,* 329–337.

Spirduso, W. & MacRae, P.G. (1990). Motor performance and aging. In J. Birren et al. (Eds.) *Handbook of the Psychology of Aging* (3rd ed.). San Diego: Academic Press.

Spotts, H.E., Jr. & Schewe, C.D. (1989). Communicating with the elderly consumer: The growing health care challenge. *Journal of Health Care Marketing, 9,* 3, 36–44.

Stephens, T. & Craig, C. (1990). *The Well-being of Canadians.* Ottawa, Ontario: Canadian Fitness and Lifestyle Research Institute.

Steuart, G.W. (1993). Social and behavioral change strategies. *Health Education Quarterly,* (Supplement 1), 113–135.

U.S. Department of Health and Human Services (1996). *Physical Activity and Health: A Report of the Surgeon General.* Atlanta, Ga.: U.S. Department of Health and Human Services, Centers for Disease Control and Prevention, National Center for Chronic Disease Prevention and Health Promotion, and The President's Council on Physical Fitness and Sports.

Viney, L.L., Benjamin, I.Y.N., & Preston, C.A. (1988). Promoting independence in the elderly: The role of psychological, social and physical constraints. *Clinical Gerontologist, 8,* 3–17.

Wankel, L.M. (1987). Enhancing motivation for involvement in voluntary exercise programs. In M.L. Maehr (Ed.) *Advances in Motivation and Achievement: Enhancing Motivation* (vol. 5). Greenwich, Conn.: JAI Press.

Ward, P.J. & Preziosi, R.C. (1994). Fostering the effectiveness of groups at work. In J.W. Pfeiffer (Ed.) *The 1994 Annual Developing Human Resources.* San Diego: Pfeiffer and Company.

Williams, D.M., Anderson, E.S., & Winett, R.A. (2005). A review of the outcome expectancy in physical activity research. *Annals of Behavioral Medicine, 29,* 1.

Willis, J.D. & Campbell, L.F. (1992). *Exercise Psychology.* Champaign, Ill.: Human Kinetics.

Wood, J.B. (1989). Communicating with older adults in health care settings: Cultural and ethnic considerations. (Special Issue: Developing Leadership in Geriatric Education.). *Educational Gerontology, 15,* 4, 351–362.

# Common Health Challenges Faced

## BY OLDER ADULTS

## James H. Rimmer

*James H. Rimmer, Ph.D., is a professor in the Department of Disability and Human Development at the University of Illinois at Chicago. For the past 25 years, Dr. Rimmer has been developing and directing health promotion programs for people with disabilities. He has published more than 70 peer-reviewed journal articles and book chapters on various topics related to physical activity,*

*health promotion, and disability. He is director of two federally funded centers, the National Center on Physical Activity and Disability and the Rehabilitation Engineering Research Center on Recreational Technologies and Exercise Physiology. Dr. Rimmer is a member of the Scientific and Medical Advisory Board for Life Fitness Academy.*

The fastest growing segment of adults older than 65 is composed of those older than 85 (Centers for Disease Control and Prevention, 2003). This remarkable extension of life brings with it the reality that most older adults will have to live for years, maybe even decades, with one or more chronic conditions. However, though these conditions limit the ability of older adults to exercise, they should not be a deterrent to physical activity. Adults now entering their seventh and eighth decades of life have heard for the last quarter century that exercise is one of the most important aspects of a healthy lifestyle. As a result, many are continuing to participate in physical activity well into their 70s, 80s, and 90s.

Clearly, despite the number of chronic health problems that an elderly person may acquire in later life, exercise can and should be an integral part of maintaining and, in some cases, improving functional mobility.

Research demonstrates that persons with chronic conditions such as arthritis or diabetes can improve their physical function by engaging in regular physical activity (Jette & Keysor, 2003; Rimmer et al., 2002).

Older adults with heart disease or osteoporosis also can improve their health by choosing to remain physically active (Lewis & Bottomley, 1994), and regular physical activity can positively impact many other chronic conditions (Rimmer, 1994).

Given this demographic shift toward an older, more frail population, fitness professionals must understand the major types of chronic conditions that affect the elderly, and be able to develop safe and effective exercise programs for this clientele. This chapter presents the chronic conditions most commonly experienced by older adults, and discusses guidelines for developing exercise programs that address them.

## THE DEVELOPMENT OF HEALTH PROBLEMS IN THE ELDERLY

Lawrence and Jette (1996) developed a model to describe what they refer to as the disablement process. According to their model, disability and health problems among the elderly occur with several rapid changes in an individual's life.

During the first stage, **pathology**, a person develops a disorder such as rheumatoid arthritis or osteoporosis that causes an **impairment**. Impairments can be classified as both anatomical (e.g., bone loss) and structural (e.g., muscle atrophy) in nature, and often lead to a **functional limitation** that causes a restriction in certain physical or mental tasks (e.g., difficulty walking). If the individual does not reverse this process through exercise and rehabilitation, the functional limitation usually worsens, resulting in a **disability.** During this final stage, the individual is

unable to perform certain essential movements, such as dressing, walking, getting in and out of a bathtub or shower, and climbing steps, and depends more on others for care. The loss of physical mobility often sets off a spiral of depression and failing health.

Your role as a fitness professional is to prevent older adults with chronic health conditions from entering the impairment or functional limitation stages by helping them to incorporate exercise into their lifestyles. Exercise can slow the decline in physical function by preventing further deterioration and, in some instances, by improving the individual's functional mobility.

The goal of an exercise program for older persons with chronic health conditions is not to eliminate the disorder, but to increase the person's fitness level so they are able to maintain as much physical independence as possible. For example, an exercise program for a person with rheumatoid arthritis is not aimed at eliminating the condition, but rather at improving their ability to perform basic and instrumental activities of daily living, giving them greater control over their environment.

## MAJOR CHRONIC HEALTH PROBLEMS EXPERIENCED BY OLDER ADULTS

Age-related medical conditions that affect the elderly can be divided into six categories: cardiovascular, respiratory, musculoskeletal, metabolic, neurological, and sensory (Table 3.1).

### Cardiovascular Disorders

Heart disease is the number one killer of Americans and the most common cause of death among the elderly (Abrams, Beers, & Berkow, 2000). While nearly every older adult has an

Table 3.1

**Chronic Conditions Often Experienced by Older Adults**

| Cardiovascular | Respiratory | Musculoskeletal |
|---|---|---|
| Heart disease | Asthma | Osteoarthritis |
| Hypertension | Chronic Obstructive Pulmonary Disease (COPD) | Rheumatoid arthritis |
| | | Low-back pain |

| Metabolic | Neurological | Sensory |
|---|---|---|
| Diabetes | Alzheimer's disease | Visual disorders |
| Obesity | Parkinson's disease | Auditory disorders |
| Osteoporosis | | |

element of heart disease, recent medical advances allow more and more individuals with advanced coronary heart disease to live longer.

## CORONARY ARTERY DISEASE

Coronary artery disease (CAD) is the primary type of heart disease experienced by older adults. As a person ages, fatty plaque forms inside the arterial walls and causes the arteries to become narrow or blocked. Consequently, blood flow to the myocardium (heart muscle) is reduced. This process is known as **atherosclerosis,** a condition that causes the artery walls to become narrow and brittle. When the arteries become almost completely blocked, the person may experience a heart attack (myocardial infarction), irregular heart rhythm, or **congestive heart failure.**

Other cardiovascular complications include hypertension (high blood pressure), pump failure, valvular problems, and peripheral vascular disease (atherosclerosis in the legs). Any of these conditions make the heart less effective in pumping blood to the working muscles, and should be considered when developing exercise programs for older clients.

### Symptoms

An early symptom of coronary artery disease is **angina pectoris** (chest pain or discomfort), but it is less common in older adults than in younger persons.

More common symptoms of coronary artery disease in older individuals include **dyspnea** (difficulty breathing), diminished exercise tolerance, chronic fatigue, and disorders of the heart rhythm, which may cause **syncope** (faintness), **paresthesia** (tingling sensation), and confusion. Electrocardiographic findings are similar to those found in younger persons with CAD (Abrams, Beers, & Berkow, 2000).

### Developing a Safe Exercise Program

A cardiac rehabilitation program administered under the guidance of a physician, nurse, and/or exercise specialist is the safest exercise environment for a person with known coronary artery disease. However, there may come a point when both the client and physician decide that a fitness center is an acceptable place to exercise. If an older adult with coronary artery disease wants to exercise under your guidance, it is imperative to make certain that the exercise regimen is safe for them. Request a specific **exercise prescription** from the client's physician, and do not alter the program without written approval. Adhere to the following safety concerns when working with clients with coronary artery disease:

**Reduce physical exertion.** Be aware of the signs of heart distress (chest pain, irregular pulse, difficulty breathing, dizziness), and make sure the client does not exhibit any of these symptoms while exercising. If these symptoms do appear, stop the exercise immediately and notify the client's doctor. Always keep emergency telephone numbers on file in case a client needs immediate medical attention. Clients who are symptomatic during exercise should move into a **Phase II** or **Phase III cardiac rehabilitation program** where they will be closely monitored and supervised.

**Avoid exposure to extreme heat or cold.** As a person ages, their body becomes more sensitive to heat and cold, and it is more difficult to retain or dissipate heat. Maintain a comfortable temperature and humidity level inside the exercise room, and avoid extreme hot or cold temperatures. Frequent water breaks and adequate ventilation are two ways to avoid temperature-induced problems.

**Mitigate emotional stress.** Emotional stress is a marker for heart problems. If your client exhibits early signs of depression, or you notice a personality change, there may be new sources of stress in their life. This could exacerbate a heart condition or predispose them to new problems. The loss of a spouse or close friend, for example, can be a tremendous hardship. If your client is experiencing more stress than usual, reduce exercise intensity and spend a few extra minutes with them. Weekly three- or four-minute phone calls during these difficult times may enhance your relationship with your client.

**Discourage consumption of large meals before exercise.** Older adults should never exercise after eating a large meal. Consumption of a large meal could trigger a heart attack in an older client with advanced coronary artery disease. If combined with exercise, large meal consumption may put clients at an even higher risk. Always check to make sure your older clients do not exercise sooner than one hour (ideally closer to two hours) after a meal.

## Exercise Guidelines

1. Because it may be impractical to have every older adult with heart disease perform a stress test before beginning an exercise program, a physician's written consent should be in each older client's file. The consent should indicate that the client's heart condition will not complicate the exercise regimen you develop. Adhere to the exercise prescription and do not alter it in any way unless written approval is given by the physician.

2. Make sure that the client has taken their heart medication before each exercise session and always check their heart rate and blood pressure before beginning activity. If the client's blood pressure is significantly higher than normal, do not allow them to exercise that day. Take blood pressure readings before, during, and after exercise to ensure that there are no major cardiovascular changes occurring during the session.

3. Use the Rating of Perceived Exertion (RPE) scale to gauge exercise intensity in clients who are taking beta blockers, a heart medication that blunts the heart-rate response to exercise. You may have to teach the client how to measure RPE to ensure accuracy.

4. Individualized exercise programs are recommended for persons with severe cardiovascular disease, because group activities usually do not allow the attention that is required to monitor a client's vital signs (i.e., blood pressure, heart rate, respiration, skin color, RPE, general feelings). Though a physician-prescribed program is the safest method, your client may prefer group exercise. Their physician must give written approval for a program that includes group exercise, and may recommend activities that can be performed within a specified intensity level.

## HYPERTENSION

Hypertension is a cardiovascular problem for more than 50% of

Americans over age 65 (Abrams, Beers, & Berkow, 2000). It has been coined the silent killer because half the people who have hypertension are unaware of it. There is a strong relationship between hypertension and coronary artery disease, stroke, congestive heart failure, and peripheral vascular disease (Lueckenotte, 2000).

According to the *Seventh Report of the Joint National Committee on Detection, Evaluation and Treatment of High Blood Pressure,* hypertension is defined as a systolic blood pressure greater than 140 mmHg or a diastolic pressure greater than 90 mmHg (National Institutes of Health, 2003). One of the more common hypertension conditions among older persons is isolated systolic hypertension, which is defined as a systolic pressure of greater than 160 mmHg and a diastolic pressure less than 90 mmHg. Several clinical studies have shown that an elevated systolic blood pressure is a better predictor of cardiovascular complications than an elevated diastolic blood pressure. Moreover, people with isolated systolic hypertension are much more likely to die of heart failure or stroke (Abrams, Beers, & Berkow, 2000).

### Symptoms

Most people with mild to moderate hypertension do not exhibit any symptoms, but those with severe hypertension may experience headaches, fatigue, dizziness, and heart palpitations.

### Exercise Guidelines

1. The American College of Sports Medicine (2000) recommends a pre-exercise screening and assessment before developing an exercise program for persons with hypertension. Since there are other factors to consider in older clients with hypertension (e.g., age, number of chronic conditions, medication), their physician should provide specific guidelines for exercise intensity, frequency, and duration.

2. Persons with an elevated blood pressure should not begin an exercise program until drug therapy has been initiated (Goldberg & Elliot, 1994). Participation in an exercise program should only begin once the medication has controlled the hypertension and the person does not experience any side effects.

3. Use RPE to monitor exercise intensity in clients taking beta-blocking drugs. Consult with their physicians to determine the RPE value that should be targeted.

4. Always take the client's pre-exercise blood pressure to ensure they have taken their medication (older persons who have forgotten to take their medication will have an elevated blood pressure). To avoid potential problems, clients should not exercise on days when they have not taken their medication.

5. Do not include isometric exercises in programs for clients with hypertension, since such exercises can induce an exaggerated rise in blood pressure.

6. Instruct all hypertensive individuals to maintain normal breathing patterns while resistance training, since breath holding can induce a Valsalva effect, causing an excessive, transient rise in blood pressure.

7. Hypertensive individuals should avoid high-intensity exercise (American College of Sports Medicine, 2000). This is especially true for older clients with hypertension since heart disease progresses significantly faster in seniors than in younger individuals.

8. A weight-training program for clients with limited strength should emphasize a high number of repetitions at a low resistance (American College of Sports Medicine, 2000).

9. Along with the exercise program, encourage clients with hypertension to lose weight (if obese); limit daily alcohol intake to less than 24 ounces of beer, 8 ounces of wine, or 2 ounces of spirits; reduce sodium intake; stop

smoking; and reduce dietary saturated fat and cholesterol (American College of Sports Medicine, 2000).

## Respiratory Problems

The three most common respiratory problems in older adults are asthma, bronchitis, and emphysema. As a group, these conditions are called **chronic obstructive pulmonary disease (COPD),** a functional diagnosis given to any pathologic process that decreases the ability of the lungs and bronchi to get air into and out of the lungs (Warden-Tamparo & Lewis, 2000). Respiratory disorders are ranked among the top 10 leading causes of death among older persons.

### ASTHMA

Asthma, which comes from the Greek word meaning to pant, is defined as a reversible-obstructive-airway disease in which the airways become narrow, resulting in labored breathing. Three pathological changes simultaneously occur during an asthma attack, making it extremely difficult for the person to breathe:

1. The smooth muscles around the bronchioles, which are the small airway tubes in the lungs, go into spasm, contracting and squeezing the bronchial tubes and making it difficult for air to enter.

2. Thick secretions of mucus accumulate inside the bronchial tubes, further deteriorating the lungs' ability to get oxygen into the blood.

3. The lining of the bronchial tubes thickens and becomes engorged with blood.

### Causes of Asthma

The causes of asthma include everything from allergens (substances to which one can acquire a sensitivity) to stress. If a person's asthma is related to a specific allergen, it is called **extrinsic asthma;** if it is not related to a specific allergen, it is called **intrinsic asthma** (Pauls & Reed, 1996). Most people with asthma suffer from a combination of the two.

**Allergens.** Common **allergens** include pollen; animal dander; certain types of foods, such as strawberries, nuts and chocolates; food additives, such as monosodium glutamate; feathers; certain medications, such as aspirin and penicillin; and dusts and molds.

**Chemical Irritants.** These include dust, paint, deodorants, perfumes, and cigarette smoke. For some, the chlorine found in swimming pools also may be a chemical irritant, and new carpeting may precipitate an asthma episode in others. Identify which clients have asthma and alert them to any changes in the exercise facility that may cause an attack.

**Temperature.** Cold air is a primary trigger of asthma attacks. Many older individuals with asthma may not want to venture out of their homes during the cold winter months to get to a fitness center.

**Psychological and Nervous Stimuli.** Emotional outbursts of laughter, crying, or screaming can stimulate the vagus nerve, which causes the muscles in the bronchial lining of the lungs to tighten and trigger an attack (Plaut, 1998).

**Infection.** The increased mucus production caused by sinusitis or influenza further narrows the airways and increases the risk of an attack. Pay close attention to a client with asthma who is recovering from a respiratory infection.

**Exercise.** Researchers speculate that asthma attacks occur during exercise because the temperature in the respiratory passages is lowered and water vapor is removed. This causes a cooling and drying effect in the lungs, which may trigger an asthma attack.

### Symptoms of Asthma

**Shortness of Breath.** The major symptom of asthma is shortness of breath. This uncomfortable feeling has been described as trying to breathe through a pinched straw, and can be an extremely fearful experience for older adults.

**Coughing.** Persons with asthma may experience a great deal of coughing, particularly during the winter months when cold air exacerbates their condition. The coughing sometimes is associated with an upper respiratory infection, which also can trigger an asthma attack.

**Wheezing.** When the coughing sounds as if it originates in the lungs, and audible vibrations can be heard within the chest, the person is wheezing. The wisping noise that is heard when a person is wheezing is related to air being forced through the mucus-filled air passages in the lungs.

## Medications Used to Treat Asthma

Familiarize yourself with the drugs most often used to treat asthma and their common side effects. The following medications are listed by their generic name and are sold by various pharmaceutical companies under different trade names.

**Theophylline.** One of the most commonly prescribed medicines for asthma, theophylline can be taken in pill or liquid form, and should be ingested with a light snack since it can irritate the lining of the stomach. The most common side effects are nervousness, hyperactivity, stomach upset, nausea, vomiting, loss of appetite, and headache (Rund, 1990).

**Beta-adrenergic Agents.** These are sometimes referred to as beta-agonists. Common types include albuterol, isoproterenol, bitolterol, pirbuterol, metaproterenol, and terbutaline sulfate. These medications are usually administered with inhalers, and are prescribed to prevent or control exercise-induced asthma.

**Cromolyn Sodium.** Persons with asthma often use cromolyn sodium as a daily medication, or in place of theophylline if that drug is not well-tolerated. It is usually administered through an inhaler. Cromolyn sodium will pre-

vent an asthma attack from occurring, but will not reverse an attack once symptoms, such as wheezing, have already started. At that point, a beta-agonist must be inhaled to prevent the attack from getting worse.

**Corticosteroids.** A newer class of drugs called corticosteroids are used to treat many conditions, but are particularly helpful for controlling severe asthma. Effective in reducing airflow obstruction by stopping the inflammatory reaction, corticosteroids can be administered as tablets or pills, by injection in emergency situations, or with an inhaler for everyday management. Popular corticosteroids include beclomethasone diproprionate, flunisolide, and triamcinolone acetonide.

## Exercise Guidelines

1. Older adults with asthma need to be involved in a safe, structured exercise program. It is important to pay close attention to the client, particularly during the early stages of the program when the risk of an asthma episode is higher.

2. Some older clients with asthma have difficulty exercising for extended periods of time; short, intermittent bouts of exercise may be more effective than one long bout. The exercise program should consist of five or six one- to two-minute exercise routines, with a one-minute rest between each. Once the client becomes conditioned to the program and is able to tolerate longer periods of activity, progressively increase the duration of exercise.

3. Clients with asthma should rest as often as necessary, particularly during group activities. If the client exhibits any shortness of breath, they should stop the activity and rest until they feel comfortable returning to the group. If the client prefers to do something while they are waiting to rejoin the group, have them perform the breathing exercises described in Tables 3.2 and 3.3.

Table 3.2

**How to Perform Diaphragmatic Breathing**

✓ Lie supine on a mat.

✓ Place one hand on the chest and the other hand on the stomach.

✓ Inhale slowly through the nose.

✓ The aim is to inhale so that only the hand on the stomach moves (elevates); the hand on the chest should remain still. This is an indication that the diaphragm is being used to breathe.

✓ Exhale slowly through pursed lips. The stomach muscles should contract.

✓ Rest and repeat several times.

4. Older persons with asthma should always begin exercising at a very low intensity. Watch for shortness of breath during the initial stages of the program. Once the client increases their conditioning level, gradually increase the intensity as long as there are no asthma symptoms. Some older clients with asthma may not have any trouble exercising at 60 to 75% of their age-adjusted maximum heart rate, provided they take their medication before the activity. Other clients with a more severe form of asthma will have difficulty exercising at this intensity.

5. The frequency of exercise can range from three to seven days per week, depending on the client's interest and the severity of the asthma.

6. Much of the research on exercise and asthma indicates that swimming is one of the best exercise modalities for this clientele. The temperature and humidity just above the water's surface allow airways to remain warm and moist, thus preventing an asthma episode. For older persons who do not like to swim, short bouts of exercise using a stair stepper, stationary cycle, or rowing machine should be relatively safe. Jogging appears to be one of the biggest triggers for exercise-induced asthma and is only recommended for the person who prefers no other modality. Low-impact aerobic dance may be safe if it is not too strenuous.

7. You must make sure that older adults with asthma take their medication before exercising to prevent the onset of an attack. In addition, clients should always carry their inhalers with them. If asthma symptoms arise during the early stages of the program, reduce the activity to a level that will not excessively elevate the client's heart or breathing rates.

8. Warm-ups and cool-downs are especially important for persons with asthma. Research demonstrates that a 15-minute low-intensity warm-up (e.g., brisk walking, riding a stationary bike) can reduce the incidence of asthma

Table 3.3

**How to Perform Pursed-lips Breathing**

✓ Can be done with diaphragmatic breathing or separately.

✓ Inhale slowly through the nose, keeping the mouth closed.

✓ Pucker the lips as if trying to whistle.

✓ Exhale slowly, blowing the air through the pursed lips.

✓ Exhalation should be at least twice as long as inhalation. Begin with a two-second inhalation and a four-second exhalation.

✓ Rest and repeat several times.

episodes during activity in younger athletes. How this translates into an exercise program for older adults is not known at this time, but it does appear that a sufficient warm-up allows the respiratory system to slowly adapt to the activity and helps prevent an asthma episode.

9. Any person with asthma who enters a fitness center *must* carry a bronchodilator at all times. Always check to make sure your client has their inhaler (e.g., Proventil, Ventolin) with them before they begin exercising, as using it is the only way to reverse an attack.

10. A small plastic device, called a peak flow meter, measures how quickly a person expires air from their lungs and is a reliable instrument for determining airflow obstruction before an asthma attack occurs. You should have access to a peak flow meter at the exercise site.

Measuring peak flow rate (Table 3.4) before a class or exercise session informs you whether the client can safely exercise on that day. A general guideline is that the exercise program should be modified to avoid an asthma episode if peak flow is less than 15% of the normal values for the client (which should be established on good days when the client is free of obstruction). It is a good idea also to measure peak flow after exercise, so that both pre-exercise and post-exercise values may be compared.

11. It is crucial to know what to do when an older client has an asthma attack. Refer to Table 3.5 for specific recommendations.

## BRONCHITIS AND EMPHYSEMA

Two other types of COPD commonly seen in the elderly are chronic bronchitis and emphysema. Chronic bronchitis is an inflammation of the bronchi, the larger airway tubes in the lungs. This condition causes an irritating and productive cough that lasts up to three months and recurs for at least two consecutive years (Pauls & Reed, 1996). It is often linked to heavy cigarette smoking.

Emphysema usually occurs in people between the ages of 60 and 70 years, and is characterized by progressive destruction of the alveoli, the spongelike tissues in the lungs where the exchange of oxygen and carbon dioxide takes place. It also is linked to heavy cigarette smoking.

### Symptoms

The symptoms of these two chronic obstructive pulmonary diseases are similar, and include dyspnea (difficulty breathing), coughing, and increased mucus production that can be heard in the chest when coughing and wheezing.

### Exercise Guidelines

Before developing an exercise program for a client with COPD, classify the client at one of four levels (Rimmer, 1994). Descriptions of these levels are given in Table 3.6. Since it is highly unlikely that a fitness instructor in a community-based setting will work with clients in levels 3 or 4, these guidelines focus on clients in levels 1 and 2.

Table 3.4

**How to Measure Peak Flow Rate**

1. Have the client stand, take a deep breath, and place their lips around the cardboard mouthpiece that slides into the peak flow meter.

2. The client should blow as fast and as hard as possible into the peak flow meter.

3. Perform peak flow three times and record the highest score.

4. Perform peak flow during the early stages of the program to obtain baseline values on your client.

Table 3.5

**What to do if a Client is Having an Asthma Attack**

1. Remove the person from the class or room and bring them to a quiet area of the facility.

2. Place the client in a comfortable position (usually sitting down with the arms placed over a table or chair to "open" up the chest).

3. Encourage the person to breathe deeply and slowly (diaphragmatic breathing).

4. If necessary, use a beta-agonist inhaler (this should be left up to the client).

5. A warm drink may help loosen mucus secretions. Do not allow the client to drink cold beverages since this may cause further tightening of the chest.

6. Seek medical attention if symptoms do not improve in a few minutes.

1. Always consult with the client's physician and/or a respiratory therapist for ideas and tips on preventing dyspnea during exercise. There is a good possibility that the client may already have undergone some kind of a rehabilitation program, and that there are written reports on the client's physical status that may help you develop a safe and effective program.

2. Measure peak expiratory flow rate (see Table 3.4) before and after exercise to determine the effects of the activity on breathing capacity. Some activities may produce better airflow readings than others. Those that cause the lowest amount of dyspnea should be used in the program.

3. The American College of Sports Medicine (2000) recommends that a rating of dyspnea be used to gauge the intensity of exercise in persons with COPD. The dyspnea rating scale goes from 0 to 10 (similar to the Borg RPE scale), and a score of 3 is an indication that the person is exercising at an intensity of approximately 50% of $\dot{V}O_2$ peak. The scores for the dyspnea scale are:

0.5 - very, very slight

1 - very slight

2 - slight

3 - moderate

4 - somewhat severe

5 - severe

7 - very severe

10 - very, very severe

Record heart rate along with the dyspnea rating to determine the relationship between the two measures.

4. Emphasize interval training techniques for clients exhibiting a high degree of dyspnea during exercise. Providing short periods of rest (one to two minutes) between exercise bouts (one to five minutes in duration) should reduce dyspnea.

Table 3.6

**Functional Classification of Persons with COPD**

| | |
|---|---|
| Level 1 | No basic limitations need be observed. The client is in the early stages of the disease. |
| Level 2 | A moderate impairment exists. Duration of exercise may have to be severely restricted. |
| Level 3 | A severe impairment exists. While exercising, the client may need to be carefully monitored by a medical doctor in a controlled setting, such as a laboratory or hospital where oxygen is available as needed. |
| Level 4 | The client may be in chronic respiratory and cardiac failure and may need constant oxygen to survive. |

5. Exercises that do not produce huge fluctuations in oxygen cost are safer and more effective for this clientele. High-impact exercises or activities that result in dramatic increases in oxygen cost (e.g., running or walking briskly up a flight of stairs) may cause dyspnea.

6. Each exercise session should be preceded by a 10- to 15-minute warm-up that gradually elevates the client's heart rate. Walking outdoors or on a treadmill at a pace that allows the individual to carry on a conversation is a good warm-up activity.

7. End each exercise session with cool-down activities that include flexibility exercises, relaxation techniques, and breathing exercises. **Diaphragmatic breathing** and **pursed-lips breathing** are recommended for persons with COPD. These techniques, described in Tables 3.2 and 3.3, have been shown to increase the amount of air taken in through the damaged tissues of the lungs and reduce the incidence of dyspnea.

8. Some clients with COPD have a tendency to hyperventilate during exercise. This causes further dyspnea since shallow breathing does not allow oxygen to reach the deepest layers of the lungs where gases are exchanged. If a client has a tendency to hyperventilate, teach them how to breathe correctly using diaphragmatic and pursed-lips breathing while walking, riding a stationary cycle, or using an upper-arm ergometer.

9. For muscular endurance activities, incorporate high repetitions at a low resistance to avoid dyspnea. Emphasize smooth, coordinated movements that do not require tremendous variations in breathing rate, as would occur while doing push-ups or pull-ups.

10. Exercise programs may need to be modified during the winter months. Respiratory infections and cold temperatures often worsen COPD, and many clients will have to severely curtail their activity levels during illness or when temperatures drop below freezing. Suggest that clients wear a scarf or surgical mask while traveling to the facility during the winter months. Breathing in cold air before exercise can precipitate dyspnea.

11. Some clients with COPD (or their spouses) continue to smoke, even though they have been diagnosed with a serious disease. Provide as much information as possible about smoking-cessation techniques, and remind these clients that even second-hand smoke can exacerbate their condition.

12. Be familiar with the warning signs for the cardiorespiratory complications that are listed in Table 3.7. If any of these signs appear during exercise, stop the activity and contact the client's physician for further advice.

13. Consider using an oximeter to record oxygen saturation when working with clients with COPD. This device ensures that the exercise program is not causing an oxygen saturation level that is too low, which could lead to respiratory complications. Most respiratory therapists recommend that oxygen saturation remain above 85% during exercise (at rest, oxygen saturation is around 97 to 98%). If oxygen saturation drops below 85%, exercise should be stopped and the client should rest and perform

Table 3.7

**Warning Signs of Cardiorespiratory Complications in Clients Who Have COPD**

✓ Dyspnea that gradually worsens

✓ Swollen ankles

✓ Sudden weight gain

✓ High resting heart rate (over 100 bpm)

diaphragmatic and pursed-lips breathing before resuming the activity.

# Musculoskeletal Conditions

It is rare to find an older person in their 70s or 80s who does not experience joint pain. The most common cause is arthritis. Although there are many different types of arthritis (called a **rheumatic disease**) the two most common types affecting approximately 30 to 40 million Americans are osteoarthritis and rheumatoid arthritis.

## OSTEOARTHRITIS

**Osteoarthritis** is sometimes referred to as **degenerative joint disease** or **osteoarthrosis.** Osteoarthrosis means an abnormal condition of the joint, which some experts say is a more accurate term than arthritis, which means an inflammation of the joint. There is usually little joint inflammation with osteoarthritis. Most of the pain is due to the progressive deterioration of **articular cartilage,** which covers the ends of the bones inside diarthrodial joints.

### Pathology

Osteoarthritis usually is divided into two types: **primary osteoarthritis** and **secondary osteoarthritis.** Primary osteoarthiritis, which is of unknown origin, is the most common. Secondary osteoarthritis results from an injury or a mechanical derangement of the joint (Mongan, 1990). The joints most often affected by osteoarthritis are the cervical and lumbar spine, hip, knee, and distal joints of the hand (the joints closest to the ends of the fingers).

Osteoarthritis is caused by a deterioration in articular cartilage, normally smooth tissue that allows the ends of the bones to glide without friction. The water content of this cartilage increases, indicating that the collagen that provides its structure is breaking up. The cartilage loses its ability to withstand compressive forces, and starts to fray and develop fissures (clefts) that extend into the bone. These bone fragments are called **osteophytes,** or bone spurs. The deteriorating articular cartilage and the accompanying osteophytes create a great deal of pain for millions of older adults.

## RHEUMATOID ARTHRITIS

Although rheumatoid arthritis can occur at any time during a person's life, it most often occurs between the ages of 25 and 60. In most instances, rheumatoid arthritis is more disabling than osteoarthritis, and causes greater joint deformity, typically in the hands (particularly the middle joints of the fingers and the knuckles), wrists, and feet.

### Pathology

Although much has been learned about rheumatoid arthritis, its exact cause is still unknown. It is classified as an **autoimmune disease,** which means that the person's immune system attacks healthy tissue and damages the joint (Rimmer, 1994).

Rheumatoid arthritis manifests itself in the synovial tissue that lines the outside of the joint, and progresses to an erosion of articular cartilage and bone. In severe cases, the tendons and occasionally the muscles that surround the joint also may become inflamed.

### Symptoms

Many of the symptoms and treatment strategies for osteoarthritis and rheumatoid arthritis are similar.

**Pain.** Many people equate the pain of arthritis to a nagging, dull toothache. Pain caused by rheumatoid arthritis is symmetrical, or bilateral, meaning that both joints are affected. The pain of osteoarthritis is often asymmetrical, meaning that only one joint is affected, although it is not uncommon to feel pain in both joints. Clients who have a high tolerance for pain are able to participate in more activity.

**Decreased Range of Motion.** Another common symptom of arthritis is decreased range of motion. Sometimes this occurs because of a shortening of muscle fibers associated with inactivity; other times it is due to joint destruction. A client may try to protect the joint by becoming inactive, causing further shortening of the muscle fibers.

**Joint Instability.** The affected joint often becomes unstable as a result of overstretching the supportive ligaments that protect it. This occurs more often with rheumatoid arthritis than osteoarthritis.

**Muscle Weakness.** Muscle weakness is common in older adults with arthritis because they often think that they protect the joint by not exercising. On the contrary, a lack of physical activity leads to other physical problems and can worsen the symptoms of arthritis.

**Diminished Endurance.** Just as muscle weakness occurs as a result of inactivity, cardiovascular endurance is lower in sedentary persons with arthritis. Many individuals with arthritis do not understand the value of maintaining good cardiovascular endurance, and think that exercise will do more harm than good.

## CLASSIFYING PEOPLE WITH ARTHRITIS

People with arthritis represent a diverse group. The classification criteria shown in Table 3.8 is a useful guide in determining what type of exercise program best meets the needs of your clients. You will be able to develop a more challenging program for clients in Classes 1 and 2, but may have to work closely with a physical therapist to develop a safe program for clients in Classes 3 and 4.

## Exercise Guidelines

Hochberg et al. (1995) note that exercise is a cornerstone of therapy for persons with arthritis. No matter how severe the condition, it is extremely important for older clients with arthritis to participate in physical-activity programs because a deterioration in fitness will clearly worsen their condition. People with arthritis who are deconditioned lose strength, flexibility, and endurance, all of which are needed to overcome the pain and physical limitations associated with this disease.

### Flexibility

People reluctant to move a painful joint experience extreme tightness in the muscles, ligaments, and tendons that surround it. Although protecting the joint from further injury is important, immobilizing the joint may do more harm than good by increasing the tightness/stiffness in and around it. Therefore, flexibility exercises are an essential component of the exercise program for an older-adult client with arthritis.

Follow these general guidelines when developing a flexibility program:

✓ Discontinue flexibility exercises that cause immediate pain, or pain that

---

Table 3.8

**Classifying Clients with Arthritis Based on Severity of the Condition**

| | |
|---|---|
| *Class 1* | Complete ability to carry on all usual duties without a high level of pain or discomfort |
| *Class 2* | Adequate ability for normal activities despite the handicap, discomfort, or limited motion at one or more joints |
| *Class 3* | Ability limited to little or none of the duties of usual occupation or self-care |
| *Class 4* | Totally incapacitated, bedridden, or confined to a wheelchair; little or no self-care |

develops within 24 to 48 hours after exercise.

✓ Teach clients to distinguish between soreness and pain. Soreness, which occurs when sedentary people begin an exercise program, is usually located in the muscle. Pain originates in the joint and indicates that the client may have exercised that joint too strenuously. Soreness will ease after the first few weeks of the program, but pain will last longer than a few weeks and may result in further joint damage.

✓ Warming the tissues that surround the affected joint may make the exercise feel more tolerable. Try using hydrocollator pads, which come in different sizes and shapes to fit different joints (e.g., shoulder, knee, ankle), to warm the tissue. Some clients prefer having the joint warmed before starting the exercise program, while others do not. Hayes (1996) also notes that some clients may prefer ice to decrease joint pain.

✓ Each of your clients has an individual threshold for holding a static stretch. Some will be able to hold a stretch for six to eight seconds, others longer.

✓ Make sure flexibility exercises are executed correctly, and do not allow the client to bounce during the stretch.

### Strength Exercises

It is a misconception that strength exercises will do more harm than good for clients with arthritis. Several studies have documented that strength exercises help people to better cope with their arthritis by improving muscle function and reducing the load on the joint (Feldmann, 1996). Furthermore, strength training arthritic joints improves functional mobility.

Follow these general strength-training guidelines for older adults with arthritis:

✓ Excessive weight training can cause an inflammatory response that results in pain and reduced mobility. Therefore, make sure the client experiences no pain (discomfort or soreness is acceptable, but there should be no pain) during the activity.

✓ If the joints are severely damaged, isometric exercise may be the preferred method of conditioning. Several researchers have noted that isometric activity does not cause inflammation or pain (Basmajian, 1987). Contractions should last approximately six to eight seconds and be performed two to three times for each muscle group. Isometric exercises can be done with or without weights, depending on the client's initial levels of strength.

### Cardiovascular Endurance

Clearly, the best cardiovascular exercise for a client with arthritis is one that does not cause pain. People who have arthritis have successfully used water exercise for years. Some fitness facilities, including the YMCA, even have their own arthritis swim programs. The pool temperature is elevated and participants perform different exercises in the water. (Note: The pool also can be used to develop flexibility and strength.)

Cardiovascular equipment that can be used by most clients with arthritis without causing high levels of pain includes the arm ergometer (particularly for clients who have knee or hip arthritis), stationary or recumbent bike, and recumbent stepper. These machines do not excessively overload the joints and can usually be used for several minutes without pain. Combination arm-leg devices such as the Schwinn Air-Dyne cycle ergometer or the NuStep recumbent stepper may be popular choices because clients can use their arms and legs to propel them. This reduces the load on their hip and knee joints.

Follow these general guidelines for improving the cardiovascular endurance of older clients with arthritis:

✓ Use smooth, repetitive motions, such as those used in swimming, cycling, and walking.

✓ Jogging or other jarring activities, such as high-impact aerobics, are contraindicated for this clientele.

✓ Use interval training or circuit training routines with clients who are unable to tolerate continuous activity. For example, a client might spend one minute on the bicycle ergometer, followed by a 30-second rest, and then complete another minute on the ergometer. The client may do this for five or 10 minutes and then move to a new machine that uses different joints, such as the arm ergometer.

✓ Keep the intensity level within the client's comfort zone. The duration and frequency of exercise is more important than the intensity. Encourage 60-minute exercise sessions that allow the client to take periodic breaks. They may be actually exercising for only 30 minutes, but still need a full 60 minutes to incorporate rest periods.

✓ A client with rheumatoid arthritis may occasionally have an acute flare-up. This is called an exacerbation, which means that the arthritis has worsened. This has nothing to do with the exercise program, but is part of the disease's progression. The client will probably not be able to exercise during an exacerbation and may have to rest until the symptoms subside.

✓ Clients with arthritis will often fatigue easily. This may be due to a number of problems, including a low fitness level, side effects from certain medications, and not sleeping well at night. Make sure that you do not cause excessive fatigue during the early stages of the program when the client is at high risk for dropping out.

## LOW-BACK PAIN

Low-back pain is a common complaint among individuals of all ages, but may become a chronic problem for older persons who also have arthritis. In fact, some low-back pain in older persons may be a direct consequence of osteoarthritis in the spine or another type of rheumatic condition, such as fibromyalgia (Pauls & Reed, 1996).

Low-back pain usually is classified as either acute or chronic. Acute back pain is present less than three months and is frequently associated with sciatica or back-related leg pain (Oldridge & Stoll, 1997). Symptoms often clear within three days to six weeks when treated with rest and anti-inflammatory drugs (Plowman, 1992). Chronic back pain lasts longer than three months and treatment includes exercise. However, it is important to consider secondary conditions (e.g., arthritis, fibromyalgia, coronary heart disease) when designing an exercise program.

### Exercise Guidelines

Exercises for acute low-back pain should be developed by the client's physician or possibly a physical therapist. However, once the client is cleared to return to full physical activity, you can play an important role in preventing another occurrence of low-back pain.

1. A major goal of an exercise program for persons with chronic low-back pain is to prevent deconditioning. The person may avoid movement for fear of re-injuring the back; in the interim, the muscles weaken and the low back loses some of its extensibility.

2. The exercise program must remain within the client's pain threshold and should not exacerbate any underlying

conditions. Sharp pain may be an indication that the exercise is harmful to the condition.

3. Aerobic exercise that puts minimal stress on the back may help to maintain cardiorespiratory endurance. A recumbent bike may be a good modality for mitigating low-back pain in some clients. Check with each client to determine which type of exercise produces the least amount of pain or discomfort.

4. Strength and flexibility exercises may be helpful for some clients with low-back pain. Their physician or physical therapist may be able to provide you with an established regimen of strength and flexibility exercise for the low back.

## Metabolic Disorders

The three most common metabolic conditions seen in elderly adults are **diabetes, obesity,** and **osteoporosis.** In 2001, the prevalence of obesity (i.e., BMI >30) in the United States was 20.9% and the prevalence of diabetes was 7.9% (Mokdad, 2003).

When you consider the millions of older Americans who suffer from osteoporosis, it becomes clear that metabolic disorders are the most prevalent and costly conditions in our society. Obesity and diabetes often are seen in the same individual, since 80% of people who have type 2 diabetes also are overweight (Franz & Norstrom, 1994).

### DIABETES

Diabetes is characterized by reduced insulin secretion by the pancreatic beta cells and/or reduced sensitivity to insulin. Diabetes causes abnormalities in the metabolism of carbohydrates, protein, and fat and, if left untreated, can be deadly. This is of particular concern since the symptoms of diabetes are not always evident in the early stages.

People with diabetes are at greater risk for numerous health problems, including kidney failure, nerve disorders, eye problems, and heart disease, and are two to four times more likely to develop cardiovascular disease. Prolonged and frequent elevation of blood sugar can damage the capillaries, a condition called microangiopathy that leads to poor circulation. In addition, people with diabetes are at greater risk for permanent nerve damage.

There are two main types of diabetes. **Type 1 diabetes** is caused by the destruction of the insulin-producing beta cells in the pancreas, which leads to little or no insulin secretion. Type 1 diabetes generally occurs in childhood and regular insulin injections are required to regulate blood glucose levels.

The typical symptoms of type 1 diabetes are excessive thirst and hunger, frequent urination, weight loss, blurred vision, and recurrent infections. During periods of insulin deficiency, a higher-than-normal level of glucose remains in the blood because of reduced uptake and storage. A portion of the excess glucose is excreted in the urine, which leads to increased thirst and appetite and weight loss. Chronically elevated blood glucose levels is a condition known as **hyperglycemia.**

**Type 2 diabetes** is the most common form of diabetes, affecting 90% of all diabetic patients. It typically occurs in adults who are overweight and is characterized by a reduced sensitivity of insulin target cells to available insulin, called insulin resistance. Insulin resistance, a condition in which the body is unable to use its own insulin efficiently, affects approximately 60 million people in the United States, one in four of whom will develop type 2 diabetes. Unfortunately, increasing numbers of children are being diagnosed with type 2 diabetes, making the term "adult-onset diabetes" obsolete. Some people with type 2 diabetes never exhibit any of the classic symptoms of diabetes. Treatment usually includes diet modification, medication, and exercise.

## Table 3.9

### Symptoms of an Insulin Reaction (Hypoglycemia)

✓ Anxiety, uneasiness

✓ Insomnia

✓ Irritability

✓ Nausea

✓ Extreme hunger

✓ Confusion

✓ Double vision

✓ Sweating, palpitations

✓ Headache

✓ Loss of motor coordination

✓ Pale, moist skin

✓ Strong, rapid pulse

Type 2 diabetes also is characterized by frequent states of hyperglycemia, but without the increased catabolism of fats and protein. Because 75% of individuals with type 2 diabetes are obese or have a history of obesity, it is important to note that this condition is often reversible with permanent weight loss.

## Effective Diabetes Control

Long-term regulation of blood glucose levels is necessary to effectively control diabetes. In type 1 diabetes, glucose regulation is achieved through regular glucose assessment, proper diet, exercise, and appropriate insulin medication. For type 2 diabetes, it is achieved through lifestyle changes centered around proper diet, weight management, exercise, and insulin or oral agents if needed. A well-designed diet and exercise regimen can result in weight loss and weight control, improved circulation and cardiorespiratory fitness, a reduced need for insulin, improved self-image, and a better ability to deal with stress.

## Exercise Guidelines

1. The intensity, frequency, and duration of exercise will depend to a large extent on the severity of the diabetes and the client's initial fitness level. In general, emphasize frequency and duration over intensity.

2. If a client has type 2 diabetes and is overweight, follow these guidelines along with the guidelines recommended for obesity on pages 87–88.

3. A common side effect of type 1 diabetes is foot ulcers. Diabetes causes deterioration in the small blood vessels in the feet, diminishing blood flow to these tissues and resulting in foot ulcers. Foot ulcers can last several months or longer, and are exacerbated by high-impact exercise, such as jogging or aerobics. Discourage clients with foot problems from participating in weightbearing, jarring exercises such as jogging or racquet sports.

4. Be aware that clients with type 1 diabetes must coordinate insulin shots and food intake with their exercise program. Too much exercise, too much insulin, or too little food can cause glucose levels to drop to a dangerously low level. Exercise should not be initiated when glucose levels are under 100 mg/dL.

5. Your major concern when working with older clients with type 1 diabetes should be a condition known as hypoglycemia, or what some experts call an insulin reaction. This is defined as a blood glucose level less than 60 mg/dL. An extremely dangerous situation could develop when blood glucose levels drop below this value. Table 3.9 describes the signs and symptoms of an insulin reaction. Exercising under these conditions is a serious hazard and should be avoided until food is consumed and glucose levels rise above 100 mg/dL. Refer to Table 3.10 for guidelines on what to do if a client is having an insulin reaction.

6. Become familiar with a small, pocket-size device called a glucometer that measures blood glucose levels with the prick of a finger and a drop of blood. Clients who have trouble regulating their glucose levels should bring a glucometer to the exercise session so that blood glucose levels can be checked before, during, and after the activity. In general, blood glucose levels should remain between 100 mg/dL and 250 mg/dL during an exercise session. If blood glucose levels drop below 100 mg/dL, a small snack (e.g., soft drink, orange juice, Gatorade) should be consumed before the exercise session. Have the client wait 10 to 15 minutes and then check their blood glucose level again to make sure that it is in the suggested range. If blood glucose levels rise above 250 mg/dL, discourage the

Table 3.10

**What to Do If a Client Is Having an Insulin Reaction**

1. Stop the activity immediately.

2. Have the client consume a quickly absorbing carbohydrate, such as fruit juice, jelly beans, or soda (do not use diet soda).

3. Have the person sit down and check their blood glucose level with a glucometer.

4. Allow the client to rest and return to normal function.

5. When the client feels better, recheck their blood glucose level.

6. If the blood glucose level is above 100 mg/dL, and the client feels better, resume activity.

client from exercising, since activity could cause the blood glucose level to go even higher.

7. Clients who have type 1 diabetes and are taking beta blockers for a heart condition have a higher risk for developing hypoglycemia because the drugs mask the symptoms of an insulin reaction.

## OBESITY

Obesity is a common problem among older populations because older adults often think they need not be as concerned with their weight as younger people. People over age 65 rarely follow diet and exercise programs for weight loss. On the contrary, weight should be a greater concern for older populations because of the higher occurrence of secondary conditions (e.g., hypertension, arthritis, heart disease). In addition, as a person grows older and experiences a decline in strength, balance, and cardiovascular endurance, any excess weight makes performing activities of daily living (ADL) more difficult. For these reasons, weight reduction always should be a goal for any older individual who has been classified as overweight or obese.

### Exercise Guidelines

1. Exercising three days per week is a good start for obese clients over the age of 65. As the client adjusts to the program, progressively work up to five days per week, varying the program on alternating days to prevent boredom.

2. The higher the level of obesity, the more difficult it will be to exercise. Start with three 10-minute bouts of exercise that consist of 10 minutes of cardiovascular activity (e.g., stationary cycling), 10 minutes of strength training (e.g., biceps curls and triceps extensions using 5-pound dumbbells), and 10 minutes of flexibility exercises. Add minutes to each area of fitness as the client becomes more capable and comfortable with the program. Provide as much rest as is necessary to prevent premature fatigue.

3. The major objective of exercise for obese clients is to keep them moving, so intensity should not be a focus of the program. Use RPE to gauge exercise intensity if you would like a general index.

4. Utilize structured exercise programs with obese individuals who have never exercised before.

5. Because many obese adults are self-conscious about their weight, it may be beneficial to hold separate classes for males and females.

6. Exercises that compress the chest cavity may impair breathing in the severely obese. Be sure that chest exercises, such as the bench press, do not cause breathing problems.

7. Weightbearing activities may be difficult for the novice exerciser who also is obese. Try to incorporate nonweightbearing activities, such as aquatic exercise, and arm and leg cycling.

8. Obese clients will be more susceptible to injury, fatigue, and dehydration because of their excess weight. Because

these conditions make them more likely to drop out of the program, do not exercise this clientele too strenuously.

9. If the client is interested in an aerobics program, make sure it is low-impact, low-intensity, and performed on a type of flooring that will not excessively load the joints.

10. Do not be too concerned about the client's weight during the early stages of the program. The goal is to keep them in the program. Teach the client that even a 10% loss in weight will result in tremendous health benefits.

11. Obese people generally have very low self-esteem, so be generous with praise and encouragement, and never place the client in an uncomfortable situation.

12. Develop mini-lectures on dietary guidelines for this clientele. Without a reduction in calories, an exercise program aimed at weight reduction will probably fail.

## OSTEOPOROSIS

Osteoporosis is a metabolic bone disease that affects about 10 million older adults according to the National Osteoporosis Foundation (2003). It is characterized by a gradual reduction in bone mass, which leads to pain, especially in the back and in weightbearing bones. Like hypertension, osteoporosis has been referred to as a silent killer because there are frequently no clinical symptoms until a fracture occurs.

Fractures associated with osteoporosis are often seen in the thoracic vertebra (dowager's hump or **kyphosis**), the neck of the femur, and the wrist. Fractures can occur through routine bending, lifting, and even coughing. Sometimes the affected bones are so thin that lightly tapping a wrist against a hard surface or sitting down too quickly can cause a fracture (Kane, Ouslander, & Abrass, 1994).

### Exercise Guidelines

1. The key to managing osteoporosis is prevention through smoking-cessation classes, adequate calcium intake, estrogen replacement, and exercise.

2. Weightbearing activities increase bone mass. Simply standing for several minutes at a time has been shown to slightly increase bone mass in people with severe osteoporosis.

3. Resistance training within the client's tolerance level must be a major cornerstone of the exercise program. Begin with light weights and progressively add more resistance, provided no pain is experienced.

4. Avoid quick, jarring movements that may precipitate a fall or fracture. Twisting movements and increases in intra-abdominal pressure could cause pain.

5. If a dowager's hump is present, avoid excessive overload of the back.

6. Unsupported flexion at the spine could cause excessive loading of the lower vertebrae. Be careful when performing any back exercises, and if the client complains of pain, stop the activity.

7. No weightbearing activities should be performed prior to six to eight weeks after a hip fracture.

## Neurological Disorders

### DEMENTIA OR ALZHEIMER'S DISEASE

As you become more accustomed to working with older clients, you will be exposed to a number of older adults who have memory loss and several different types of **cognitive** impairments. When a person loses memory and other intellectual capacities (e.g., orientation, attention, calculation, language, motor skills), it is called **dementia.** Alzheimer's disease is the most common cause of dementia in older adults.

## Exercise Guidelines

### Early Stages of Dementia

1. During the early stages of dementia, the client may forget to come to an exercise session or how to do certain exercises. Be patient, understanding, and sensitive to the mental anguish that the person is experiencing. Memory loss is one of the most devastating conditions that older adults may experience during their lifetime. Provide moral support and make regular phone calls to remind them of their exercise class.

2. Depression is common in this clientele and may lead to a higher dropout rate. To prevent clients from dropping out of the program, contact them regularly and make sure their caregivers understand the importance of the exercise program.

3. Replace complex exercise routines with simpler activities, such as walking, stationary cycling, and basic stretches. Free weights, treadmills, and other pieces of equipment that require steady control of the body could be dangerous to clients with cognitive disorders.

4. Part of the focus of an exercise program for clients with dementia is keeping them interested. Provide lots of verbal praise and positive reinforcement (e.g., birthday card, phone calls, short letters, client-of-the-week award) to encourage adherence.

5. The intensity of the exercise program is not as important as the frequency and duration. The preferred frequency is five days per week, preferably at the same time each day, so that the client develops a structured exercise routine. Mornings are typically better than afternoons since the client will be rested in the morning and may experience more agitation and fatigue as the day progresses.

### Later Stages of Dementia

1. Clients with Alzheimer's disease may sometimes exhibit extreme outbursts of anger and physical aggression. Be aware that this behavior has nothing to do with you or the exercise program. These acts of aggression occur randomly and often will last only a few minutes. If the client disrupts a class, remove them from the group until they calm down. Understand that these outbursts are a symptom of the disease and the client often does not understand what they are saying.

2. Memory loss will become more pronounced during the later stages of a progressive cognitive disorder. When this occurs, the client may have to switch from a group exercise class to individual training sessions.

3. The client's caregiver may need to be present during the exercise program. A person with severe dementia often will not want to be left alone with anyone but the caregiver they are most familiar with.

4. It is important to provide a structured exercise routine with little variation for a client in the later stages of a cognitive disorder. An introduction to new activities may confuse them.

5. Never leave a client with Alzheimer's disease alone because they will often wander to other parts of the facility.

6. Playing music from the client's generation during the exercise session will occasionally bring back memories and may be a good way to keep them interested in the program.

## PARKINSON'S DISEASE

Although Parkinson's disease can occur in younger populations, it is most often seen in individuals older than 50 (Abrams, Beers, & Berkow, 2000). Characterized as a chronic, progressive disease that causes movement and postural problems, the condition is caused by a shortage of a chemical produced by the brain called **dopamine,** which is responsible for transmitting messages across nerve pathways in the brain. When there is not enough dopamine available for the brain to send these messages, voluntary muscle movement and coordination are affected. Tremor (shaking), muscle rigidity, and the loss of postural reflexes also characterize the condition. During the early stages of Parkinson's disease, shaking is isolated to the hands. Other symptoms include slowness in ambulation and dressing; difficulty getting out of a chair; shuffling gait; stooped-over posture; and difficulty in starting movements.

### Exercise Guidelines

1. Relaxation techniques appear to be very helpful in reducing tremors (Lewis & Bottomley, 1994). Begin a relaxation class in the supine position and gradually progress to sitting and standing.

2. Flexibility exercises also are an important part of the exercise program. Clients with Parkinson's disease will exhibit a great deal of muscle tightness and may need some assistance with flexibility routines.

3. Since balance is a major problem for people with Parkinson's disease, take every precaution to assure that the exercise environment is safe and that there is a minimal risk of the client falling. You should always be in close contact with the client in case they lose their balance. If the client is participating in group exercise classes, recommend that they hold on to a railing or chair, or sit down during the exercise routine.

4. Clients with Parkinson's disease usually have a delay when starting a movement, so allow more time to initiate movements.

5. Balance exercises must be an integral part of the exercise program. Both static and dynamic balance exercises should be incorporated into the routine while sitting and standing.

6. Breathing exercises also are important for persons with Parkinson's disease. Teach the client to use diaphragmatic and pursed-lips breathing, and have them practice expiring air (e.g., blowing out candles) to strengthen respiratory muscles.

7. Encourage participation in cardiovascular and strength exercises to prevent secondary conditions, such as osteoporosis and muscle atrophy. Be sure that the machines and equipment selected are safe for a clientele with a high risk of falling.

8. Aquatic exercises are extremely beneficial to this clientele, and help eliminate the risk of a serious fall while performing strength and balance exercises. However, keep in mind that clients with Parkinson's disease may have difficulty dressing and undressing, and may not want to go through this burden in order to swim. Be sure the pool temperature is at least 86° F (30° C).

The instructional strategies listed in Table 3.11 will help you design a program that will lower the frustration level of clients with neurological disorders, as well as your own.

## Visual and Auditory Disorders

When working with clients who have visual and auditory problems, remember that the environment must be safe.

### SUGGESTIONS FOR WORKING WITH OLDER ADULTS WITH VISUAL PROBLEMS

1. Use brightly colored tape (e.g., hot pink or yellow, depending on the background color) to mark objects above and below eye level. Because many older clients will not have a good vertical range of vision, machines that contain parts higher than the client's head or lower than their knees may be bumped into. Objects left in the middle of the floor have the potential to cause a fall.

2. The display panel on some pieces of exercise equipment may be difficult

Table 3.11

**Instructional Strategies for Working with Clients Who Have a Neurological Cognitive Disorder**

1. *Make the Exercises Simple and Straightforward.* Don't change the exercise routines on a regular basis because it may frustrate a client with memory loss.

2. *Explain Each Movement Clearly and Frequently.* Many clients with neurological impairments will need a frequent explanation of the activity. They will often forget how to perform certain movements and will need to be reminded regularly. Repetition is very important with this group. It may seem boring to you, but will make the client more successful.

3. *Keep the Exercise Routine Structured.* For some clients with dementia, a structured exercise routine (i.e., same room, same equipment, same music, same professional) may need to be established. New activities or surroundings can be frightening for some clients and will agitate others.

4. *Slow Down All Activities.* Everything will have to be slowed down (i.e., speech, tempo, activity) for some clients with dementia. This is especially true for clients with Parkinson's disease.

5. *Touching Is a Double-edged Sword.* Some clients will like to be touched; others will become agitated. You may try to show a client a correct movement and they may become offended by your touch. Keep track of which clients you can and cannot touch. As a client gets to know you, they may become more willing to be touched by you.

6. *Avoid Talking Down to the Client.* Many fitness professionals talk to older clients with a neurological disorder as if they are a child, since some of the behaviors are similar to what may be observed in children. This may offend the client or their caregiver. Always treat them like adults.

7. *Always Listen and Be Responsive.* Occasionally, clients with dementia will say something that does not make sense. Instead of laughing or becoming agitated, understand that this is part of the disease process and respond to the client in an appropriate manner.

8. *Do Not Tolerate Verbal or Physical Abuse.* If a client is verbally or physically abusive to you or other members of a class, understand that although this is part of the disorder, it should not be permitted in your class. Remove the client from the group until they calm down.

for clients with visual problems to see. Use brightly colored tape to mark the dials, or make arrows that show the client which button to press to increase or decrease time or intensity.

3. Certain types of exercise machines, such as a treadmill, may be hazardous for clients with poor eyesight. To increase safety, use equipment that requires a sitting position, such as a stationary cycle or a recumbent stepper.

4. Because clients with visual impairments may not be able to clearly see your movements, verbal instructions must be precise. Physically guide the client through the correct movement to make the verbal instructions more clear.

5. Clients with visual impairments often use certain pieces of equipment as markers for where they are located in a room. Inform them if any equipment is moved or rearranged.

## SUGGESTIONS FOR WORKING WITH OLDER ADULTS WITH AUDITORY PROBLEMS

1. Always face the client when you speak. Some older adults may be able to read lips, and when this is combined with the little hearing they have, they will be better able to follow your instructions.

2. Never eat or chew gum while working with the client, as this will make it difficult to understand your speech.

3. Reduce background noise or move to a quiet area while talking to the client.

4. Keep your hands away from your face. If you block your mouth, a client

who can read lips will be unable to understand.

5. Do not shout at the client, but speak with a normal, clear tone. Shouting will distort the sound of your voice.

6. Use visual cues as often as possible and combine them with your verbal instructions. Clients with hearing impairments respond well to visual cues (e.g., pictures of the exercises, demonstrations).

# MEDICATIONS AND EXERCISE

Almost every adult older than 65 is taking one or more medications. Despite the benefits that these drugs provide, there are many side-effects that could compromise the client's ability to exercise. Although it is beyond the scope of this chapter to review the hundreds of medications that older adults may be taking, it is important that you become familiar with the most common drugs used by this clientele, and that you understand some of the concerns related to exercise and medication.

## Beta Blockers

Beta blockers are drugs used to treat cardiovascular disease, including angina pectoris, hypertension, and cardiac arrhythmias. They slow down the heart rate and decrease blood pressure by blocking the catecholamine released from the autonomic nervous system. Common brands include Propranolol (Inderal), Nadolol (Corgard), Atenolol (Tenormin), and Metoprolol (Lopressor).

### EXERCISE CONCERNS

Beta blockers often cause depression, fatigue, and dizziness, thus forcing the client to cut down on exercise. Because the function of a beta blocker is to decrease heart rate, heart rate measures are not a good indicator of exercise intensity. It is recommended that rating of perceived exertion (RPE) be used to monitor the intensity of exercise for clients taking beta blockers.

## Diuretics

Diuretics are used to treat hypertension and congestive heart failure. They increase the excretion of sodium and chloride in the urine, producing diuresis. Blood pressure is decreased through the loss of fluid. Common brands include Furosemide (Lasix), Spironolactone (Aldactone), and Hydrochlorothiazide (Esidrix, Hydrodiuril, Oretic, Thiuretic).

### EXERCISE CONCERNS

Some older adults who are taking diuretics can also occasionally get **postural hypotension.** Postural hypotension causes a drop in systolic and/or diastolic blood pressure, which could lead to dizziness, lightheadedness, or a loss of consciousness that could result in a fall. Since clients who are taking diuretics are removing higher levels of fluid from their body, they may need to go to the bathroom more often. This loss of fluid, combined with exercise, could lead to dehydration. Make sure the client is adequately hydrated after the exercise class by having them drink a couple of glasses of water before they leave the fitness center.

Diuretics also can cause weakness and fatigue by depleting the body of its potassium stores. This condition is called **hypokalemia.** If a client complains of weakness or fatigue and is taking a diuretic, ask them to check with their physician to make sure that they do not have this condition.

## Hypnotics and Tranquilizers

Hypnotics and tranquilizers are powerful drugs used to calm or quiet an anxious person. The mechanism of action is not completely known. Common brands include Diazepam (Valium), Chlordiazepoxide (Librium), Oxazepam (Serax), Prazepam (Centrax), and Lorazepam (Ativan).

## EXERCISE CONCERNS

Hypnotics and tranquilizers calm a person, but also increase drowsiness and make it difficult for the client to exercise. It is probably not a good idea for the client to exercise too soon after taking this type of medication. Some hypnotics and tranquilizers also block sweating, thus increasing body core temperature and the risk of hyperthermia (overheating). Make sure that the client has adequate fluid intake before exercise and does not overheat during or after the exercise session. Intensity and duration of exercise may need to be lowered in clients who overheat too quickly.

## Antidepressants

Antidepressants are used to treat depression, a condition that afflicts millions of older Americans. The function of an antidepressant is to block the reuptake of **neurotransmitters** in the brain so that there is an increase in their concentration. Common brands include Imipramine (Tofranil), Amitriptyline (Amitril, Elavil, Endep), Nortriptyline (Pamelor), Desipramine (Norpramin, Pertofrane), and Doxepin (Adapin, Sinequan). A newer class of antidepressants include Fluoxetine (Prozac), Sertraline (Zoloft), Paroxetene (Paxil), and Venlafaxine (Effexor).

## EXERCISE CONCERNS

Antidepressants can cause dizziness, weakness, and lightheadedness. Therefore, pay close attention to the client to avoid a fall. Antidepressants also may cause the client to have a dry mouth, which exercise could exacerbate.

It is important to encourage your client to consume small amounts of water before, during, and after the exercise session. The newer class of antidepressants (e.g., Prozac, Zoloft) appears to have fewer side effects than the older medications.

## Analgesics

Analgesics are widely used by millions of older adults to relieve some form of joint pain. The function of an analgesic is to block the pain receptors that lead from the brain to the joint. Many of these drugs are over-the-counter medicines, while others require a prescription. Common analgesics are aspirin, acetaminophen (Tylenol), ibuprofen (Advil, Motrin), naproxen (Naprosyn), and Fenprofen (Feldene). Aside from aspirin and acetaminophen, the other drugs are classified as nonsteroidal anti-inflammatory drugs (NSAIDs).

## EXERCISE CONCERNS

The side effects of NSAIDs in older adults include indigestion, stomach ulcers, kidney problems, and, occasionally, gastrointestinal bleeding. Because exercise causes a shifting in blood distribution from the gastrointestinal tract to the working muscles, you must make sure that indigestion or stomach pain is not worsened by exercise. NSAIDS are relatively safe drugs provided they are not taken in high dosages.

## CONCLUSION

Older adults constitute the fastest growing segment of the population. More and more older persons with chronic conditions are electing to remain physically active. Despite their physical limitations, older adults are interested in quality exercise programs delivered by competent fitness professionals. As a result of these demographic shifts, fitness professionals will emerge as major players in health promotion among older adults in this new century.

For more information on fitness programming for older adults with chronic conditions, contact your local heart association, lung association, diabetes association, and arthritis association, or log onto the National Center on Physical Activity and Disability Web site at www.ncpad.org.

# REFERENCES AND SUGGESTED READING

Abrams, W.B., Beers, M.H., & Berkow, R. (Eds.) (2000). *Merck Manual of Geriatrics* (3rd ed.). Whitehouse Station, N.J.: Merck Research Laboratories.

American College of Sports Medicine (2003). *ACSM's Exercise Management for Persons with Chronic Diseases and Disabilities.* Champaign, Ill.: Human Kinetics.

America College of Sports Medicine (2002). *ACSM's Resource for Clinical Exercise Physiology: Musculoskeletal, Neuromuscular, Neoplastic, Immunologic, and Hemotologic Conditions.* Philadelphia: Lippincott Williams & Wilkins.

American College of Sports Medicine (2000). *ACSM's Guidelines for Exercise Testing and Prescription* (6th ed.). Baltimore: Lippincott Williams & Wilkins.

Basmajian, J.V. (1987). Therapeutic exercise in the management of rheumatic diseases. *Journal of Rheumatology,* 15(suppl. 15), 22–25.

Centers for Disease Control and Prevention (2003). Trends in aging: United States and worldwide. *Morbidity & Mortality Weekly Report,* 52, 101–106.

Feldmann, S. (1996). Exercise for the person with rheumatoid arthritis. In R. W. Chang (Ed.) *Rehabilitation of Persons with Rheumatoid Arthritis* (91–102). Gaithersburg, Md.: Aspen.

Franz, M.J. & Norstrom, J. (1994). *Diabetes Actively Staying Healthy (DASH).* Minneapolis, Minn.: DCI Publishing.

Goldberg, L. & Elliot, D.L. (1994). *Exercise for Prevention and Treatment of Illness.* Philadelphia: F.A. Davis.

Hayes, K.W. (1996). Heat and cold in the management of rheumatoid arthritis. In R.W. Chang (Ed.) *Rehabilitation of Persons with Rheumatoid Arthritis* (77–89). Gaithersburg, Md.: Aspen.

Hochberg, M.C. et al. (1995). Guidelines for the medical management of osteoarthritis. *Arthritis and Rheumatism,* 38, 1541–1546.

Huang, Y. et al. (1998). Physical fitness, physical activity, and functional limitation in adults aged 40 and older. *Medicine and Science in Sports and Exercise,* 30, 9, 1430–1435.

Jette, A.M. & Keysor, J.J. (2003). Disability models: Implications for arthritis exercise and physical activity interventions. *Arthritis and Rheumatism: Arthritis Care and Research,* 49, 114–120.

Kane, R.L., Ouslander, J.G., & Abrass, I.B. (1994). *Essentials of Clinical Geriatrics.* New York: McGraw-Hill.

Lawrence, R.H. & Jette, A.M. (1996). Disentangling the disablement process. *Journals of Gerontology,* 51B, S173–S182.

Lewis, C.B. & Bottomley, J.M. (1994). *Geriatric Physical Therapy.* Norwalk, Conn.: Appleton & Lange.

Lueckenotte, A.G. (2000). *Gerontologic Nursing* (2nd ed.). St. Louis: Mosby.

Mokdad, A.H. (2003). Prevalence of obesity, diabetes, and obesity-related health risk factors, 2001. *Journal of the American Medical Association,* 289, 76–79.

Mongan, E. (1990). Arthritis and osteoporosis. In B. Kemp, K. Brummel-Smith, & J.W. Ramsdell (Eds.), *Geriatric Rehabilitation* (91–105). Boston: Little Brown.

National Institutes of Health (2003). The Seventh Report of the Joint National Committee on Prevention, Detection, Evaluation, and Treatment of High Blood Pressure: The JNC 7 Report. *Journal of the American Medical Association,* 298, 2560–2571.

National Osteoporosis Foundation (Oct. 2003). www.nof.org/osteoporosis/stats.htm.

Oldridge, N.B. & Stoll, J.E. (1997). Low back pain syndrome. In J.L. Durstine (Ed.) *ACSM's Exercise Management for Persons with Chronic Diseases and Disabilities* (155–160). Champaign, Ill.: Human Kinetics.

Pauls, J.A. & Reed, K.L. (1996). *Quick Reference to Physical Therapy.* Gaithersburg, Md.: Aspen.

Plaut, T. (1998). *Children with Asthma: A Manual for Parents* (2nd ed.). Amherst, Mass.: Pedipress.

Plowman, S.A. (1992). Physical activity, physical fitness, and low back pain. In J.O. Holloszy (Ed.) *Exercise and Sport Science Reviews,* vol. 20, (221–242). Baltimore, Md.: Williams & Wilkins.

Rimmer, J.H. (2003). Alzheimer's disease. In J.L. Durstine (Ed.). *ACSM's Exercise Management for Persons with Chronic Diseases and Disabilities* (311–315). Champaign, Ill.: Human Kinetics.

Rimmer, J.H. (2002). Health promotion for people with disabilities: A new era for managing medical costs and improving quality of life. *Disease Management and Health Outcomes,* 10, 337–343.

Rimmer, J.H. (1994). *Fitness and Rehabilitation Programs for Special Populations.* Dubuque, Iowa: Brown & Benchmark.

Rimmer, J.H. et al. (2002). Feasibility of a health promotion intervention for a predominantly African-American group of women with type 2 diabetes. *The Diabetes Educator,* 28, 571–580.

Rimmer, J.H., Braddock, D., & Pitetti, K.H. (1996). Research on physical activity and disability: An emerging national priority. *Medicine and Science in Sports and Exercise,* 28, 1366–1372.

Rund, D.A. (1990). Asthma. *The Physician and Sportsmedicine,* 18, 143–146.

Volicer, L. et al. (1988). *Clinical Management of Alzheimer's Disease.* Gaithersburg, Md.: Aspen.

Warden-Tamparo, C. & Lewis, M.A. (2000). *Diseases of the Human Body* (3rd ed.). Philadelphia: F.A. Davis.

PRE-EXERCISE

# Screening and Fitness Assessment

## Gregory L. Welch

*Gregory L. Welch, M.S., is an exercise physiologist and president of SpeciFit,™ a Seal Beach, Calif.–based non-profit entity established to further the progression of wellness for women. Welch specializes in exercise programming for special-needs populations, has published several articles on exercise for older adults, and is a nationally recognized presenter.*

More and more, older adults are urged to get some exercise. Virtually all healthcare professionals advocate some form of physical activity for this special population. But what does a recommendation to get some exercise mean? How does an exercise program begin and what determines if it is adequate and appropriate? It all starts with the development of an exercise program, which is the successful integration of exercise science and behavioral techniques that leads to long-term program compliance and attainment of the individual's goals (American College of Sports Medicine, 2000). The FITT principle (Frequency, Intensity, Time, and Type) is a clever acronym identifying the components of an exercise program. But how are the questions "How often?" (frequency), "How hard?" (intensity), "How long?" (time/duration), and "Which exercise?" (type) answered? Will an exercise program for an 80-year-old cardiac patient be the same as that for a 60-year-old person with diabetes who has not exercised a day in his life?

The answers to these questions lie in exercise screening and fitness assessment. Though the exercise program is a vital link to improving the quality of older adults' lives, it may not have a chance to succeed without some form of measurement to determine the individual's current fitness and/or functional status. For this reason, a complete assessment of the older adult is essential for developing adequate and appropriate exercise programming. This chapter provides a comprehensive rationale for determining a prudent assessment protocol and details a wide range of measurement and monitoring methods and tools.

## THE BEGINNING

The pre-exercise screening and fitness assessment of any individual, regardless of age, involves the gathering of pertinent information. Preventing or reducing the loss of function as a person grows older is dependent, in part, on the detection and treatment of any physical declines that may be precursors to more serious functional losses (Rikli & Jones, 1997). Anthony (2003) states that the screening process allows you to:

1. Identify health conditions and/or risk factors that may necessitate referral or place the client at risk when participating in certain activities.

2. Identify possible contraindicated activities.

3. Design an appropriate exercise program.

4. Adhere to the legal and ethical requirements of the fitness industry.

5. Open lines of communication between you and any appropriate healthcare professionals.

Once this information is acquired, the assessment can proceed to the evaluation of the client's functional capabilities. Cotton (2003) suggests using a sound fitness testing battery to evaluate the function of the heart, blood vessels, lungs, and muscles according to the physical demands of an individually defined optimal lifestyle. The key to this phrase lies in its latter half. An exercise program should be specific to the physical endeavors of the individual. Similarly, particularly with older adult clients, physical assessments should be specific to each client's needs, abilities, and objectives. The benefits of exercise can be measured to the degree that individual limitations are accommodated within exercise training methodology (Williams & Sketch, 1988). This becomes clearer as we attempt to categorize the older adult before beginning the testing process.

## IDENTIFYING THE OLDER ADULT

Chapter 1 of this manual provides excellent information about the physiological effects of aging. Because the aging process is complex, physiology must be the first consideration when working with an older adult client; this consideration is vital to proceed with the assessment protocol. Likewise, it is imperative to ascertain both the general characteristics and the specific needs of the elderly (Skinner, 1993).

### Chronological Age

No existing single model or paradigm clearly defines the older adult population; rather, a variety of approaches is blended according to individual differences. Because of the relationship between time and the aging process, chronological age is used as an initial identification. The following examples are offered by Spirduso, Francis, and MacRae (2005) as simple ways to describe aging: (1) the "young-old" (65–74 years), the "old" (75–84 years), the "old-old" (85–99 years), and the "oldest-old" (>100 years); and (2) sexagenarians (60–69), septuagenarians (70–79), octogenarians (80–89), nonagenarians (90–99), and centenarians (100+). The span of this population is greater than in any other age group, and to label a person as an older adult based solely on age does not give many clues to their fitness level (Evans & Rosenberg, 1992).

## Biological Age

Scientists have theorized that **biological age** is a better tool than chronology when identifying the older adult. Biological aging is the process or group of processes that causes the eventual breakdown of mammalian homeostasis with the passage of time (Spirduso, Francis, & MacRae, 2005). It is common to hear someone refer to a person as "young for their age," suggesting that the person apparently has not suffered the decremental effects of biological aging that often accompany **chronological age.** However, simple observation of a person's appearance does not provide much more information about a person's functional capacity than chronology.

Because identifying age by outward appearance seems of minimal value, researchers are investigating a biological measurement called a biomarker that is independent of chronological age. This type of measurement has been the focus of gerontologic research for many decades (Mooradian, 1990). Evans and Rosenberg (1992) formulated a list of 10 measurable, modifiable, and "vitality-influencing" biomarkers based on a philosophy of maintaining good health for the longest period of time:

1. muscle mass
2. strength
3. basal metabolic rate
4. body-fat percentage
5. aerobic capacity
6. blood-sugar tolerance
7. cholesterol/HDL ratio
8. blood pressure
9. bone density
10. ability to regulate internal body temperature

For assessment purposes, Evans and Rosenberg (1992) suggest that biological age is best calculated on an individual basis. There is, however, a fundamental problem with the biological measurement. Spirduso, Francis, and MacRae (2005) states that theories suggesting the existence of a single biological age score assume the existence of a uniform rate of aging across different systems. This criticism is the foundation for the growing interest in biomarkers of aging, including how they are influenced and their potential use for exploring why aging occurs at different rates (Hochschild, 1990). Mooradian (1990) agrees that the rate of aging within a species is quite variable. Furthermore, he states that the availability of biomarkers allows aging rates to be determined on an individual basis, and also allows the impact of various interventions—such as food restriction or exercise—on the aging process to be monitored. By comparing the rates of performance declines in master athletes, Bortz (1996) has suggested that the rate of decline in $\dot{V}O_2$max of 0.5% per year may be a basic biomarker of the aging process.

## The Rate of Aging

The rate of aging is the change in function of organs and systems per unit of time. Under normal circumstances, these changes roughly follow a linear pattern over the life span (Spirduso, Francis, & MacRae, 2005). There are, however, a number of factors that confuse what is regarded as normal. Spirduso, Francis, and MacRae cite disease, trauma, genetics, nutrition, theories of damage and gradual imbalance, and even gender as factors that affect the rate of deterioration and aging.

There is convincing evidence that physiologic aging advances more rapidly with an accumulation of years of inactivity:

✓ Sedentary individuals have nearly a two-fold faster rate of decline in VO$_2$max as they age as compared to active individuals (Bruce, 1984).

✓ Muscle mass reduction is primarily responsible for the age-associated loss of strength, which reflects a loss of total muscle protein caused by inactivity, aging, or both (Imamura et al., 1983).

✓ The major cause of declining flexibility is a lack of movement in joints not usually used in daily activities (Heath, 2001).

✓ The relative risk of fatal coronary heart disease among the sedentary is about twice that of active individuals (Powell et al., 1987).

✓ Movement times for active people, both young and old, are faster than those in corresponding age groups who are less active (Spirduso, 1975).

✓ Reaction times of older men who have remained active for 20 or more years are equal to or faster than those of inactive men in their 20s (Spirduso, 1975).

✓ Athletes over age 60 have consistently larger-than-expected values for vital capacity, total lung capacity, residual volume, maximum voluntary ventilation, and forced expiratory volume based on their body size. The values also are significantly larger than those of sedentary, age-matched, healthy counterparts (Hagberg et al., 1988).

✓ Sedentary living may result in functional capacity losses that are as great as the effects of aging itself (McArdle, Katch, & Katch, 2001).

✓ Physical inactivity is an independent determinant of hip fracture in the elderly (Coupland, Wood, & Cooper, 1993).

✓ Sarcopenia, the loss of muscle mass and strength with age, is a part of normal aging. However, it is clearly accelerated by physical inactivity (Roubenoff, 2000).

✓ Declining muscle function through a loss of muscular strength may decrease functional independence and mobility and increase the risk for falls and injuries, physical frailty, and **disability.** Two major contributors to the decline in muscle function as a person ages are disuse and physical inactivity (Brill et al., 1999).

✓ At all age levels, and especially in the elderly population, a sedentary lifestyle and low fitness levels are independent risk factors for all causes of mortality, including cardiovascular mortality (Keller & Lemberg, 2002).

✓ Physical inactivity is an important determinant of disability and mortality risk. Even a recent increase in activity level can have an important effect, although the benefits are also easily lost when the activity level is again reduced (Westerterp, 2000).

The pre-exercise screening assessment can identify lifestyle behaviors and patterns that are integral to the development of an exercise program.

## Activities of Daily Living

Activities of Daily Living (ADL) are the basic tasks of everyday life and independent living, such as eating, bathing, and going to the bathroom (Wiener et al., 1990). General measures of health status (e.g., diagnoses or medical conditions) are limited indicators of an individual's independence and functional capabilities (Fillenbaum, 1985). Therefore, researchers have devoted considerable attention to developing health and functional status measures that correspond to practical applications of everyday life as shown in Table 4.1 (Rimmer, 1994). There are more than 43 different published indexes that assess ADL in both patients and populations (Feinstein, Joseph, & Wells, 1986).

ADL are classified into three levels of function by the American Geriatrics Society (1989) as basic (BADL),

Table 4.1

**Classification Schema for Elderly Clientele**

| | |
|---|---|
| *Level I* | Healthy: No major medical problems; in relatively good condition for age; has exercised for the past several years. |
| *Level II* | Ambulatory/nonactive: No major medical problems; has never participated in a structured exercise program. |
| *Level III* | Ambulatory/disease failure: Diagnosed as having severe coronary artery disease, arthritis, diabetes, or chronic obstructive pulmonary disease. |
| *Level IV* | Frail elderly: Relies on partial assistance from professional staff for ADL; can stand or walk short distances (usually less than 100 feet) with an assistive device; spends most of the day sitting. |
| *Level V* | Wheelchair-dependent: Relies on total assistance from professional staff for ADL; cannot stand or walk. |

Rimmer, J.H. (1994). Fitness and Rehabilitation Programs for Special Populations. *Madison, Wis.: Brown and Benchmark.* Reprinted with permission.

intermediate (IADL), and advanced (AADL). BADL include the elemental items of self-care (Katz et al., 1970). IADL also are referred to as independent ADL and include tasks essential to maintaining independence (Fillenbaum, 1985). AADL are functions well beyond the status necessary for living alone, and tend to be specific to each individual. These include recreational, occupational, and community-service functions (American Geriatrics Society, 1989). ADL measurements are often used to determine whether an older adult is capable of living independently (Table 4.2). ADL are simple or complex, depending on the lifestyle history of the individual. For example, stair climbing may or may not be considered a lifestyle activity, depending on the person's need to negotiate stairs. Ultimately, as a matter of lifestyle normalcy, it would be beneficial to train individuals to climb stairs. However, in terms of assessment, determining the person's immediate needs and abilities is the primary objective. Measurement of the activities of daily living is a tremendous tool for answering the question, "What can the older adult actually do?" (Spirduso, Francis, & MacRae, 2005).

# THE PROCEDURE

The main purposes of exercise testing for the elderly are the same as those for all adults: to define the degree of risk associated with varying work loads, and to establish appropriate intensities for an exercise program (Skinner, 1993). An exercise program should only be developed and used if it is based on sound information obtained from a reliable screening and assessment protocol. Many tests exist to ascertain the information needed to develop an exercise program; you must determine which is most applicable to each client. Skinner (1993) states that not all older people can or should be given exercise tests to determine their fitness level. This is why you must conduct a pre-exercise screening.

## Pre-exercise Screening

The pre-exercise screening is the best way to begin gathering information about the older adult's individual needs. A self-reported medical history and an interview enable you to discern the most appropriate exercise-testing protocol.

Table 4.2

**Hierarchy of Physical Function of the Old (75–85 Years) and Oldest-Old (86–120 Years)**

_Physically elite_
Sports competition; Senior Olympics
High-risk and power sports (e.g., hang-gliding, weightlifting)

_Physically fit_
Moderate physical work;
All endurance sports and games; Most hobbies

_Physically independent_
Very light physical work; Hobbies (e.g., walking, gardening)
Low physical-demand activities (e.g., golf, social dance,
handcrafts, traveling, automobile driving)
Can pass some AADL, all IADL

_Physically frail_
Light housekeeping; Food preparation; Grocery shopping
Can pass some IADL, all BADL; May be homebound

_Physically dependent_
Walking; Bathing; Dressing; Eating; Transferring
Needs home or institutional care

_Disability_

_From W.W. Spirduso, Physical Dimensions of Aging, 2nd ed., Figure 11.1 (in press). © 2005 by Waneen W. Spirduso. Reprinted with permission from Human Kinetics (Champaign, Ill.)._

## MEDICAL HISTORY AND CLEARANCE

Lifestyle behavior, rate of aging, and individual differences produce many health issues to consider. Each older adult client should provide a medical history and waiver form prior to beginning any physical assessment procedure. At this time you should completely disclose the risks of an exercise program to your client.

It also is beneficial to acquire a client's physician's consent once an exercise program has been developed. This not only informs the client's physician of the type of exercise the individual will be participating in, but also confirms the validity of the program you have developed and allows the physician to make modifications.

### Medication

Be knowledgeable about the various medications that are prescribed for older adults (Tables 4.3 & 4.4). The use and misuse of medication can lead to adverse physical side effects, such as headache, drowsiness, loss of coordination, fatigue, impaired vision and hearing, nausea, irregular heartbeat, orthostatic hypotension, constipation, urinary incontinence, irritability, depression, an inability to concentrate, and confusion (Jones, 1986). Older adults are more vulnerable to adverse reactions to medication because of the aging process, lifestyle behaviors,

Table 4.3
## Cardiac Medications: Their Use, Side Effects, and Effects on Exercise Response

| Type/Trade Name | Use | Side Effects | Effects on Exercise Response |
|---|---|---|---|
| **I. Antianginal Agents** | | | |
| A. Nitroglycerin compounds [*Amyl nitrate; Isordil; Nitrostat*] | Smooth muscle relaxation; decrease cardiac output | Headache, dizziness, hypotension | Hypotension; increase exercise capacity |
| B. Beta blockers [*Inderal; Propranolol; Lopressor; Corgard; Biocadren*] | Block beta receptors; decrease sympathetic tone; decrease HR, contractility, BP | Bradycardia, heart block, insomnia, nausea, fatigue, weakness, increased cholesterol and blood sugar | Decrease HR; hypotension; decrease cardiac contractility |
| C. Calcium antagonists [*Verapamil; Nifedipine; Procardia*] | Block influx of calcium; dilate coronary arteries; suppress dysrhythmias | Dizziness, syncope, flushing, hypotension headache, fluid retention | Hypotension |
| **II. Antihypertensive Agents** | | | |
| A. Diuretics [*Thiazides, Lasix, Aldactone*] | Inhibit $NA^+$ and $Cl^-$ in kidney; increase excretion of sodium and water, and control high BP and fluid retention | Drowsiness, dehydration, electrolyte imbalance, gout, nausea, pain, hearing loss, elevated cholesterol, and lipoproteins | Hypotension |
| B. Vasodilators [*Hydralazine, Captopril, Apresoline, Loniten, Minoxidil*] | Dilate peripheral blood vessels; used in conjunction with diuretics; decrease BP | Increase HR and contractility; headache, drowsiness, nausea, vomiting, diarrhea | Hypotension |
| C. Drugs interfering with sympathetic nervous system [*Reserprine, Propranolol, Aldomet, Catapres, Minipress*] | Decrease BP, HR, and cardiac output by dilating blood vessels | Drowsiness, depression, sexual dysfunction, fatigue, dry mouth, stuffy nose, fever, upset stomach, fluid retention, weight gain | Increase exercise capacity; increase myocardial contractility |
| **III. Digitalis Glycosides, Derivatives** [*Digoxin, Lonoxin, Digitoxin*] | Strengthen heart's pumping force and decrease electrical conduction | Arrhythmias, heart block, altered ECG, fatigue, weakness, headache, nausea, vomiting | |
| **IV. Anticoagulant Agents** [*Coumadin, Sodium Heparin, Aspirin, Persantine*] | Prevent blood clot formation | Easy bruising, stomach irritation, joint or abdominal pain, difficulty in swallowing, unexplained swelling, uncontrolled bleeding | |
| **V. Antilipidemic Agents** [*Cholestyramine, Lopid, Niacin, Atromid-S, Mevacor, Questran Zocor*] | Interfere with lipid metabolism and lower cholesterol and low-density lipoproteins | Nausea, vomiting, diarrhea, constipation, flatulence, abdominal discomfort, glucose intolerance | |
| **VI. Antiarrhythmic Agents** [*Cardioquin, Procaine, Quinidine, Lidocaine, Dilantin, Propranolol, Bretylium tosylate, Verapamil*] | Alter conduction patterns throughout the myocardium | Nausea, palpitations, vomiting, rash, insomnia, dizziness, shortness of breath, swollen ankles, coughing up blood, fever, psychosis, impotence | Hypotension; decrease HR; decrease cardiac contractility |

*McArdle, W.D., Katch, F.I. & Katch, V.L. (2001). Exercise Physiology. (5th ed.) Baltimore: Lippincott Williams & Wilkins. Reprinted with permission.*

Table 4.4

**Medications and Substances
Affecting Balance**

*Medications that reduce alertness*

- narcotics

- hypnotics

- sedatives

- tranquilizers

- alcohol

*Medications that retard central conduction*

- narcotics

- hypnotics

- sedatives

- tranquilizers

- analgesics

*Medications that impair cerebral perfusion*

- vasodilators

- antihypertensives

- some antidepressants

*Medications that affect postural control*

- diuretics

- digitalis

- some beta blockers

- some antihypertensives

*Source: Modified from Professor Bernard Isaacs as cited in appendix A: "A glossary on falls" in Danish Medical Bulletin, Gerontology Special Supplement Series, No. 4: The Prevention of Falls in Later Life: A Report of the Kellogg International Work Group on the Prevention of Falls by the Elderly, 1987.*

acute and chronic diseases, the mixing of drugs, and diet.

Numerous drug regimens are prescribed for a variety of reasons. According to Jones (1986), the most common prescriptive and over-the-counter medications with the greatest risk of adverse effects are:

**Prescriptive:**

antihypertensive drugs (beta blockers, diuretics)

antiparkinsonism drugs (antidepressants)

psychotropic drugs (sedatives, antianxiety, anticonvulsants, hypnotics, antipsychotics)

**Over-the-counter:**

aspirin

multivitamins

laxatives

calcium

antacids

antihistamines

For additional information about medications for older adults, refer to Chapter 3 of this book, *ACSM's Guidelines for Exercise Testing and Prescription* (6th ed.), and the *ACE Personal Trainer Manual* (3rd ed.).

## The Aging Process and Pharmacokinetics

Pharmacokinetics involve the absorption, distribution, metabolism, and excretion of drugs in the human body. Following are five physiological changes that affect the pharmacokinetics of medications in older adults:

**Decrease in lean body mass as body fat increases.** A decrease in lean body tissue and an increase in body fat are due not only to the aging process, but also are partially dependent upon lifestyle behaviors. Body weight rises between the ages of 40 and 60 due to an increase in fat tissue, then declines between the ages of 60 and 80 as lean muscle mass is lost. These changes profoundly affect the distribution and elimination of drugs outside the circulatory system. If a drug must bind to protein tissues, such as acid-organic drugs (diazoxide, digitoxin, penicillin), its distribution is adversely affected by the decrease in muscle mass. When body fat increases, liposoluble drugs, such as barbiturates and psychotropic agents, accumulate in fat tissue and increase the chance of prolonged and toxic effects.

**Reduction in total body water.** The body consists of about 80% water at birth. This figure decreases gradually with age, and it is generally agreed that total body water drops by 10 to 15% between the ages of 30 and 80. Since body water helps dilute water-soluble medications (i.e., diuretics), this decrease in the amount of water in the body lessens the distribution and increases the concentration of these drugs, causing a higher susceptibility to the drugs' toxic effects in older adults.

**Decreased efficiency of the gastrointestinal tract.** As people age, the efficiency of the gastrointestinal tract diminishes. Enzyme and glandular secretion, blood flow, gastric motility, and sphincter activity decrease, and the effective surface area available for drug absorption is reduced. Thus, the absorption of oral medications in the gastrointestinal tract is slow and less complete. Differences in drug absorption are due to gastrointestinal diseases associated with the aging process, mixing various medications, drug/nutrient interactions, and the effects of exercise.

**Decreased cardiac output.** Reductions in **cardiac output** decrease blood flow to various body parts. Reduced blood flow to major body organs, such as the liver and kidneys, can result in less efficient drug distribution, metabolism, and elimination from the body and, consequently, accumulation and toxicity of drugs taken over an extended period of time.

**Decreased efficiency of the liver and kidneys.** The liver is the most predominant organ in drug metabolism. As humans age, liver mass diminishes, hepatic blood flow decreases, and fat tends to accumulate in the liver. Combined with other lifestyle abuses, these conditions cause a decline in liver function and a slower, less complete metabolism of drugs. This slower metabolism of drugs—particularly cardiac medications—increases an older adult's vulnerability to adverse effects.

Aging also induces changes in the structure and function of the kidneys. Research has shown that by age 85, kidney mass is about 25% less than that of a younger person and renal plasma flow is less than half. These and other changes, such as the build-up of fatty tissue, decrease the filtration rate and secretion in the kidneys by about 35% over a lifetime and account for a slower removal of drugs.

## THE INTERVIEW

The interview process often is the most comfortable way to begin gathering information and establishing a relationship. A seemingly casual conversation can reveal philosophical and attitudinal biases toward exercise. By having your client describe their past and present experiences with physical activity, whether it be play, sport, or occupation, you can gain an overall appreciation of their health status.

## PHYSICAL SCREENING

The purpose of a physical evaluation is to identify possible unknown conditions and to establish initial baseline data.

## Blood Pressure

The American College of Sports Medicine (2000) considers blood pressure measurement an integral component of the pretest evaluation. Blood pressure is defined as the force of blood distending the arteries and is measured in millimeters of mercury (mmHg). It is determined by cardiac output (CO) and **total peripheral resistance (TPR)** and, therefore, can be elevated by an increase in either or both (American College of Sports Medicine, 2000).

Blood pressure readings are divided into a top (systolic) and bottom (diastolic) number. The systolic blood pressure represents the maximum pressure created by the heart during ventricular contraction. The diastolic value is the minimum pressure that remains in the arteries during the filling phase of the cardiac cycle, which occurs when the heart relaxes.

A sphygmomanometer and a stethoscope are the tools of blood pressure measurement. The sphygmomanometer consists of a rubber bladder enclosed in a nylon cuff and connected to an inflatable bulb and manometer from which the pressure is read. The stethoscope is used in conjunction with the sphygmomanometer to listen to the sounds made by the vibrations of the vascular walls. These sounds, referred to as Korotkoff sounds, were named after their discoverer in 1905.

Blood pressure assessment can be influenced by client anxiety over unfamiliar surroundings and other stressors, so it may be helpful to let the individual relax quietly for several minutes prior to taking the measurement. With the client seated, place the cuff of the sphygmomanometer around the upper portion of their bare arm, about 1 inch above the crease of the elbow joint. The middle of the bladder should be over the brachial artery on the inner part of the upper arm. Have the client rest their arm comfortably on a table or arm of a chair at heart level. Place the bell of the stethoscope firmly on the brachial artery. You can locate the brachial artery by feeling for a pulse at the inner portion of the elbow joint. Interfering noise, called artifact, can occur if the stethoscope comes in contact with anything during the reading.

While listening to the pulse through the stethoscope, pump the cuff until the pulse disappears. Release the pressure from the cuff at a rate that will cause the pressure to fall about 2 to 3 mmHg per second. If the pressure is released too fast, it will be difficult to obtain an accurate reading. If released too slowly, pressure builds within the arm and causes discomfort and an inaccurate reading. The blood pressure assessment must be performed within 60 seconds to avoid the likelihood of falsely elevated readings. (See Table 4.5 for other potential sources of error in blood pressure assessment.)

As the pressure falls, the Korotkoff sounds can be heard in four or five phases. The first sound represents the systolic blood pressure reading. As the mercury continues to fall, the sound becomes louder and changes to a sharp tapping. This marks the second and third phases, which are not significant. At rest, the fourth and fifth phases usually coincide and involve the disappearance of sound.

Table 4.5

**Potential Sources of Error in Blood Pressure Assessment**

1. Inaccurate sphygmomanometer
2. Improper cuff size
3. Auditory acuity of technician
4. Rate of inflation or deflation of cuff pressure
5. Experience of technician
6. Reaction time of technician
7. Improper stethoscope placement or pressure
8. Background noise
9. Allowing patient to hold treadmill handrails
10. Certain physiological abnormalities (e.g., damaged brachial artery, subclavian steal syndrome, a-v fistula)

The point at which the sound disappears is the diastolic reading. During exercise, there may be an audible muffling of the fourth phase; this is the diastolic reading. Because it is not unusual for the vibrations to be heard near zero levels, the fifth phase is not a valid indicator of diastolic pressure (Table 4.6).

Table 4.6

**Classification of Blood Pressure for Adults Age 18 and Older***

| Category | Systolic (mmHg) | | Diastolic (mmHg) |
|---|---|---|---|
| Normal† | <120 | and | <80 |
| Prehypertension | 120–139 | or | 80–89 |
| Hypertension‡ | | | |
| Stage 1 | 140–159 | or | 90–99 |
| Stage 2 | ≥160 | or | ≥100 |

* Not taking antihypertensive drugs and not acutely ill. When systolic and diastolic blood pressures fall into different categories, the higher category should be selected to classify the individual's blood pressure status. For example, 140/82 mmHg should be classified as stage 1 hypertension, and 154/102 mmHg should be classified as stage 2 hypertension. In addition to classifying stages of hypertension on the basis of average blood pressure levels, clinicians should specify presence or absence of target organ disease and additional risk factors. This specificity is important for risk classification and treatment.

† Normal blood pressure with respect to cardiovascular risk is below 120/80 mmHg. However, unusually low readings should be evaluated for clinical significance.

‡ Based on the average of two or more readings taken at each of two or more visits after an initial screening.

Source: National Institutes of Health (2003). *The Seventh Report of the Joint Committee on Prevention, Detection, Evaluation, and Treatment of High Blood Pressure.* NIH Publication No. 03-5233.

## EXERCISE RESPONSE

Systolic blood pressure increases at the onset of exercise due to a rise in cardiac output (Wilmore & Costill, 1999). As exercise intensity increases, the systolic pressure increases linearly (McArdle, Katch, & Katch, 2001). Williams (1994) states that a systolic reading above a maximal range of 220 to 240 mmHg is considered a hypertensive response to exercise. A drop in systolic blood pressure (or failure of systolic pressure to increase) that occurs with increased exercise intensity should be viewed as an abnormal test response (American College of Sports Medicine, 2000).

Contrary to the normal rise in systolic blood pressure that occurs during dynamic exercise, diastolic blood pressure should remain constant or decrease by 10 to 20 mmHg as a result of the dilation of the peripheral arterioles of exercising muscle (Williams, 1994). Figure 4.1 illustrates the generalized response for systolic and diastolic blood pressure during continuous, graded treadmill exercise testing.

The ACSM criteria for contraindicative resting blood pressure for older adults are systolic pressure >200 mmHg or diastolic pressure >110 mmHg (American College of Sports Medicine, 2000).

## Body Composition

Body composition refers to the overall make-up of the body's total mass. Body composition assessment determines the relative percentages of lean body mass and fat mass.

Sedentary people often boast that their weight is at, or close to, what it was many years before. However, ideal weight, as determined by the bathroom scale, is a well-rooted misconception that does not consider the relationship between lean body mass and fat mass. In reality, though increases in body weight begin to level off at about age 50 and even begin to decline in the seventh decade, body fat continues to increase

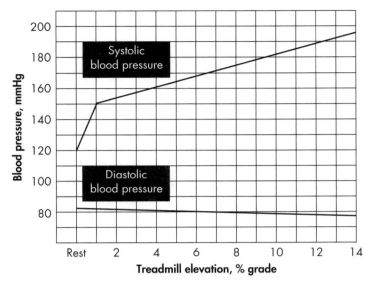

FIGURE 4.1
Generalized response for systolic and diastolic blood pressure during continuous, graded treadmill exercise testing.

McArdle, W.D., Katch, F.I., & Katch, V.L. (2001). Exercise Physiology (5th ed.). Baltimore: Lippincott Williams & Wilkins. Reprinted with permission.

(Spirduso, Francis, & MacRae, 2005) and lean muscle mass decreases (Stamford, 1988; Muritani, 1981). The loss of lean muscle mass results in an accumulation of body fat (Bemben, Kuchera, & Bemben, 1989) and connective tissue (Lexel, 1993). It is clear that a person who maintains their weight without participating in an exercise program to preserve lean muscle tissue is not the picture of health. In fact, excess body fat has been associated with a number of health risks, including heart disease, diabetes, hypertension, arthritis, gall bladder disease, cirrhosis of the liver, hernia, intestinal obstruction, and sleep disorders (Cotton, 2003).

There are a variety of methods used to measure body composition. Hydrostatic weighing and skinfold thickness are commonly used with younger populations, but there are notable disadvantages to using these methods with older adults. Hydrostatic (underwater) weighing may make an older individual uneasy as they must be completely submerged in water while the reading is taken. More importantly, while the individual is underwater, they must exhale all the air from their lungs and then wait for a signal before surfacing. This is likely to be very uncomfortable for many older adults. In addition, there is a likelihood of gross inaccu-

racy due to the difficulty of performing the **forced expiratory volume** (FEV) procedure. It seems safe to say that only a small portion of the older adult population (e.g., the competitive senior) would fare well with this measurement protocol.

The use of skinfold thickness to measure body composition also is not optimal for older adults. As with hydrostatic weighing, the normative data used to determine the actual percentage of body fat are grouped together in a category listed as 60+ years. This general grouping cannot be considered reliable for a population that is so varied, since, realistically, the senior population potentially spans age 50 and above. Also, the pinching required by this method can create uneasiness and possible pain, and may lead to a negative perception of exercise and cause program dropout. The sensitivities and idiosyncrasies of the older adult population must always be considered when conducting the physical screening.

You can gain appreciable information about a client's body composition without using such abrasive techniques. Two methods that work well together and are easily performed are body mass index (BMI) and waist-to-hip ratio (WHR).

Table 4.7
**Body Mass Index**

| Height (inches) | 19 | 20 | 21 | 22 | 23 | 24 | 25 Weight (pounds) | 26 | 27 | 28 | 29 | 30 | 35 | 40 |
|---|---|---|---|---|---|---|---|---|---|---|---|---|---|---|
| 58 | 91 | 95 | 100 | 105 | 110 | 115 | 119 | 124 | 129 | 134 | 138 | 143 | 167 | 191 |
| 59 | 94 | 99 | 104 | 109 | 114 | 119 | 124 | 128 | 133 | 138 | 143 | 148 | 173 | 198 |
| 60 | 97 | 102 | 107 | 112 | 118 | 123 | 128 | 133 | 138 | 143 | 148 | 153 | 179 | 204 |
| 61 | 100 | 106 | 111 | 116 | 121 | 127 | 132 | 137 | 143 | 148 | 153 | 158 | 185 | 211 |
| 62 | 104 | 109 | 115 | 120 | 125 | 131 | 136 | 142 | 147 | 153 | 158 | 164 | 191 | 218 |
| 63 | 107 | 113 | 118 | 124 | 130 | 135 | 141 | 146 | 152 | 158 | 163 | 169 | 197 | 225 |
| 64 | 110 | 116 | 122 | 128 | 134 | 140 | 145 | 151 | 157 | 163 | 169 | 174 | 203 | 233 |
| 65 | 114 | 120 | 126 | 132 | 138 | 144 | 150 | 156 | 162 | 168 | 174 | 180 | 210 | 240 |
| 66 | 117 | 124 | 130 | 136 | 142 | 148 | 155 | 161 | 167 | 173 | 179 | 185 | 216 | 247 |
| 67 | 121 | 127 | 134 | 140 | 147 | 153 | 159 | 166 | 172 | 178 | 185 | 191 | 223 | 255 |
| 68 | 125 | 131 | 138 | 144 | 151 | 158 | 164 | 171 | 177 | 184 | 190 | 197 | 230 | 263 |
| 69 | 128 | 135 | 142 | 149 | 155 | 162 | 169 | 176 | 182 | 189 | 196 | 203 | 237 | 270 |
| 70 | 132 | 139 | 146 | 153 | 160 | 167 | 174 | 181 | 188 | 195 | 202 | 209 | 243 | 278 |
| 71 | 136 | 143 | 150 | 157 | 165 | 172 | 179 | 186 | 193 | 200 | 207 | 215 | 250 | 286 |
| 72 | 140 | 147 | 155 | 162 | 169 | 177 | 184 | 191 | 199 | 206 | 213 | 221 | 258 | 294 |
| 73 | 144 | 151 | 159 | 166 | 174 | 182 | 189 | 197 | 204 | 212 | 219 | 227 | 265 | 303 |
| 74 | 148 | 155 | 163 | 171 | 179 | 187 | 194 | 202 | 210 | 218 | 225 | 233 | 272 | 311 |
| 75 | 152 | 160 | 168 | 176 | 184 | 192 | 200 | 208 | 216 | 224 | 232 | 240 | 279 | 319 |
| 76 | 156 | 164 | 172 | 180 | 189 | 197 | 205 | 213 | 221 | 230 | 238 | 246 | 287 | 328 |

Note: Find your client's height in the far left column and move across the row to the weight that is closest to the client's weight. Their body mass index will be at the top of that column.

## BODY MASS INDEX (BMI)

The body mass index measures weight in relation to stature, and is calculated by dividing weight (kg) by height squared (m²). A BMI conversion chart is found in Table 4.7.

Evans and Rosenberg (1992) have listed ideal BMI values for men ages 60 to 69 at 26.6, and ages 70 to 79 at 27. The respective index values for women in the same age categories are 27.3 and 27.8. The researchers also state that figures 20% above these ideal values indicate obesity. Spirduso, Francis, and MacRae (2005) adds that critical risk factors are associated with extreme BMI values. Very low values indicate a deficiency in muscle mass, whereas very high BMI values suggest excessive fat.

## WAIST-TO-HIP RATIO

Waist-to-hip (WHR) ratio measurements help determine the distribution of fat storage just above and below the waist. The ratio is a simple calculation of the circumference of the waist measured at the level of the navel, divided by the circumference of the hips at the point of greatest protrusion. Men and women have very different ratios that coincide with their gender characteristics. Table 4.8 illustrates the relative risk ratings for WHR ratios. It should also be noted that waist circumference is a reliable and easily measured indicator of abdominal obesity (National Heart, Lung, and Blood Institute, 1998). Waist circumferences of greater than 40 inches (102 cm) in men and 35 inches (89 cm) in women are considered strong indicators of abdominal obesity.

Table 4.8
**Waist-to-Hip Ratios and Associated Level of Health Risks**

| Classification | Men | Women |
|---|---|---|
| High risk | > 1.0 | > 0.85 |
| Moderately high risk | 0.90–1.0 | 0.80–0.85 |
| Lower risk | < 0.90 | < 0.80 |

Adapted, with permission, from: Van Itallie, T.B. (1988). Topography of Body Fat: Relationship to Risk of Cardiovascular and Other Diseases. In: *Anthropometric Standardization Reference Manual.* Lohman, T.G., Roche, A.F., & Martorell, R. (Eds.). Champaign, Ill.: Human Kinetics.

## Flexibility

Flexibility is defined as the range of motion around a joint, and is associated with the closeness of the articulating bones and the elasticity of the muscles, ligaments, and tendons around the joint (Rimmer, 1994). Normative data for adults over the age of 65 is virtually non-existent and the individual differences are high. Therefore, while standard flexibility exercise assessment protocols are appropriate, measures should only be recorded and periodically checked for progress. Chapter 5 provides a variety of flexibility exercises that you can use in assessing client flexibility.

## TOOLS OF THE TRADE

Baseline data established during the pre-exercise screening and assessment is used to devise the initial exercise program and serves as a standard for the comparison of future results to determine progress. Therefore, continual monitoring of an individual as they exercise is just as important

as assessing them at the beginning of the program. This ongoing assessment allows you to: (1) reduce the intensity or curtail the exercise program, (2) maintain the intensity or vary the exercise program, or (3) advance the exercise program.

The health history questionnaire, physician's release form, and initial interview are important tools to use when beginning the pre-exercise screening portion of the assessment. You should encourage continuous self-reporting to help identify subjective attitudes toward exercise (e.g., enthusiasm, boredom, discomfort, and mental and physical fatigue) and to begin to pinpoint possible precursors to injury.

Many of the measuring and monitoring tools and techniques that you use throughout an exercise program can and should be taught to the older adult. Your role as a facilitator of wellness is to educate the individual so they can continue the exercise program autonomously. This is not always as easy as it sounds because the exercise environment is dynamic; by nature, an exercise program is subject to change. An individual must be able to make intelligent decisions based on quality data when dealing with potential changes. Following are the tools and rationale to support the many decisions to be made when assessing and monitoring older adults for an exercise program.

## Heart Rate

Heart-rate values are an effective assessment tool. Given their relatively linear relationship to $VO_2$max, heart-rate measures are a beneficial guide to exercise intensity (American College of Sports

Why not place the power to control workout intensity with the participant? As in any industry, technological advances eventually win out over traditional methods, and it is surprising that with wireless telemetry, portable heart monitors have not swept the international fitness community. Use of a portable heart monitor together with the Rating of Perceived Exertion (RPE) scale would give each exercise participant the precise information needed to gauge the intensity of their workout.

Medicine, 2000). A great deal of information can be discerned when heart-rate measures are used in conjunction with the rating of perceived exertion (RPE) scale. Heart rate traditionally has been determined by palpating the pulse for 10 seconds and extrapolating that value over a minute by multiplying by six. Although this method is well accepted, it is highly impractical and, according to Dunbar and Balanos (1996), significantly inaccurate.

For example, heart rates taken during an aerobics class do not represent the work done over the entire class period, regardless of what point they are taken during the class. The pace of an aerobics class can change dramatically or remain constant, depending on the instructor. Although the instructor cannot be expected to control the exertion levels of the entire class, most people believe they do because the instructor chooses the pace of the music and the difficulty of the choreography and provides encouragement throughout the session. And while heart rate indicates whether a participant's pulse is above their training zone, by the time the pulse is found and time is started, three to five seconds have passed. Add to that the 10 seconds of counting, plus the varying rate of recovery, and you have an imprecise value. If a person does determine that their heart rate is too high, at what point in the workout should they reduce the intensity? This value does not reflect the intensity of the exercise at any previous point during the session.

During a fitness assessment, many cardiovascular testing protocols measure heart rate only at the end of an exercise bout. However, an older adult may take anywhere from 15 to 40 minutes to complete the one-mile walking test, and a great deal of information can be gathered during this time. A heart-rate measurement taken only at the end of the work eliminates a valuable opportunity to collect revealing data. Additionally, because the normative data for evaluating the older adult during this test is unavailable beyond the seventh decade of life, the information extrapolated from it is of little use. Heart-rate and RPE measurements taken throughout the session could be the only reliable data available. If heart rate is considered an important measurement, then it must be monitored accurately throughout the exercise session with at-a-glance convenience.

## CALCULATING THE TRAINING RANGE

There are two primary methods used to determine heart-rate training range. The first computes the percentage of maximum heart rate (HR max). The second is known as the Karvonen, or heart-

## Maximum Heart Rate: How Useful Is The Prediction Equation?

Two methods exist for determining maximum heart rate (HR max). The most accurate way is to directly measure the HR max with an EKG monitoring device during a graded exercise test. The other way is to estimate HR max by using a simple prediction equation or formula. In 1970, the formula "220 – age" was introduced and was widely accepted by the health and fitness community. Recently, however, the validity of the formula has come under attack for several reasons. The subjects used in the study to determine the formula were not representative of the general population. In addition, even if the prediction equation did represent a reasonable average, a significant percentage of individuals will not fit the average. In fact, standard deviations of plus or minus 10 to 20 beats per minute have been observed. Consequently, basing a client's exercise intensity (i.e., training heart rate) on a potentially flawed estimation of HR max is somewhat dubious. When the training heart rate is based on an estimated HR max, it should be used in combination with the perceived exertion scale (Table 4.9). Modify the intensity of the workout if your client reports a high level of perceived exertion, even if his or her training heart rate has not been achieved.

## Heart Rate Example

**Determine the heart rate range from 40% to 80% for an 85-year-old individual with a resting heart rate of 62 beats per minute.**

| % of HR max | % of HRR |
|---|---|
| 220 − 85 = 135 (estimated HR max) | 220 − 85 = 135 (estimated HR max) |
| 40% x 135 = 54 beats per minute BPM | 135 − 62 = 73 |
| 80% x 135 = 108 BPM | 40% x 73 = 29 |
| 40% to 80% = 54 to 108 BPM | 29 + 73 = 102 BPM |
| | 80% x 73 = 58 |
| | 58 + 73 = 131 BPM |
| | 40% to 80% = 102 to 131 BPM |

rate reserve, method (see Table 5.4, page 136). This technique factors in resting heart rate and reflects the percentage of the maximum volume of oxygen ($VO_2$max). When using the **Karvonen method,** the percent of heart-rate reserve corresponds to approximately the same percentage of the individual's functional capacity, or $VO_2$max (American College of Sports Medicine, 2000).

Because true maximum heart-rate values are acquired by using a maximum exercise tolerance test, the constant of 220-minus-age will have to suffice when working with older adults. Remember, though, that this common method has a minimum variability of 10 beats per minute (Franklin, 2001). The example above illustrates the superiority of the Karvonen method in establishing a training range and clearly illustrates that the training range determined by the **heart-rate reserve** method is more reliable.

The additional data contained in the estimated percent of oxygen consumption is a valuable marker. ACSM recommends that the intensity of exercise be 60 to 90% of HR max, or 50 to 85% of $VO_2$max or HR reserve. Many older adults with low initial fitness levels respond to a low exercise intensity (e.g., 40 to 50% $VO_2$max) (American College of Sports Medicine, 2000).

## Rating of Perceived Exertion (RPE)

In the early 1950s, Gunnar Borg developed the rating of perceived exertion scale to subjectively measure an individual's effort during exercise. The RPE scale has a strong linear relationship to heart rate (Carlton & Rhodes, 1985). Use of this scale can help assess older adult fitness, especially when heart-rate values are not available, such as with cardiac patients taking beta-blockers. Although RPE has been considered an alternative to heart rate, both are uniquely valuable and should be used together when assessing the older adult.

The original scale is a 15-point system that begins at 6 and ends at 20. A more recent, simplified scale begins at 0 and progresses to 10. The terminology used with the revised scale is believed to be better understood by the subject. When using the 15-point scale, values of 12 to 13 (somewhat hard), and 16 (hard) correspond to 50 to 74% (average of 60%), and 85% of heart-rate reserve, respectively (American College of Sports Medicine, 2000). The respective values on the Borg 10-point scale are 4 and 6 (Skinner, 1993). Table 4.9 includes the original and revised RPE scales.

Borg (1982) also believed that the subjective perception carried over to additional aspects of measurement rather than

Table 4.9

**Rating of Perceived Exertion and Other Subjective Perception Scales**

| Original RPE Scale* | | Revised RPE Scale | | Rate of Perceived Breathlessness (RPB) | | Weak Link Index | | Degree of Difficulty | |
|---|---|---|---|---|---|---|---|---|---|
| 6 | No exertion at all | 0 | Nothing at all | 0 | Nothing at all | 0 | Nothing at all | 0 | Nothing at all |
| 7 | Extremely light | .5 | Very, very weak | .5 | Very, very slight | .5 | Very, very slight | .5 | Very, very easy |
| 8 | | 1 | Very weak | 1 | Very slight | 1 | Very slight | 1 | Very easy |
| 9 | Very light | 2 | Weak | 2 | Slight | 2 | Slight | 2 | Easy |
| 10 | | 3 | Moderate | 3 | Moderate | 3 | Moderate | 3 | Moderate |
| 11 | Light | 4 | Somewhat strong | 4 | Somewhat severe | 4 | Somewhat severe | 4 | Somewhat difficult |
| 12 | | 5 | Strong | 5 | Severe | 5 | Severe | 5 | Difficult |
| 13 | Somewhat hard | 6 | | 6 | | 6 | | 6 | |
| 14 | | 7 | Very strong | 7 | Very severe | 7 | Very severe | 7 | Very difficult |
| 15 | Hard (heavy) | 8 | | 8 | | 8 | | 8 | |
| 16 | | 9 | Very, very strong | 9 | Very, very severe | 9 | Very, very severe | 9 | Very, very difficult |
| 17 | Very hard | 10 | Maximal | 10 | Maximal | 10 | Maximal | 10 | Maximal |
| 18 | | | | | | | | | |
| 19 | Extremely hard | | | | | | | | |
| 20 | Maximal exertion | | | | | | | | |

\* To understand the RPE scale and its administration all users should read: Borg, G. (1998). *Borg's Perceived Exertion and Pain Scales*. Champaign, Ill.: Human Kinetics.

just fatigue. For example, Gordon (1993b) has modeled the 0-to-10 scale to reflect the rate of perceived breathlessness (RPB) for patients with breathing disorders. The terminology is similar, but the words "weak" and "strong" on the Borg scale are substituted with "slight" and "severe" (see Table 4.9). In his book on arthritis, Gordon (1993a) details a 100-point scale on which individuals rate their perception of pain in each joint.

The solicitation of information about any discomfort in various parts of the body at discrete points during the evaluation is prudent because it helps prevent possible injury if the problem was ignored. For example, a person who is closely monitored because they are expected to discontinue a walking assessment due to low functional capacity might actually have to quit because of lower leg, hip, or back pain. Conversely, an unmonitored person who experiences discomfort in a quadriceps tendon halfway through the test, for example, but completes the exercise, may have begun to establish tendonitis. Even if the pain never becomes significant, it still may induce a negative mindset about exercise and lead to dropout.

When working with older clients, it may be prudent to follow suit with Borg and Gordon regarding the concept of perception, specifically as it applies to discomfort or pain. It may be directly or indirectly related to the physical assessment and can manifest itself in a variety of ways in the older adult. It is important to realize that any physical activity can continue only as far as the failure of the body's weakest link (Welch, 1996b). Therefore, the Weak Link Index (WLI) was created in which the same terminology used in the RPB scale is used to quantify the rate of perceived pain (RPP) (see Table 4.9).

## DEGREE OF DIFFICULTY

Seeking any form of maximal effort from deconditioned (sedentary) muscle or connective and joint capsular material is imprudent and unnecessary in the establishment of a fitness program. It is wise to break from this tradition in the initial assessment and early conditioning of older adults. Jones (1996) developed a 1–5 point scale to protect the deconditioned individual, stating that controlling the resistance intensity helps to prevent excessive compression and sheer force. An initial test for absolute strength or even an extrapolated maximum test puts the individual at risk of injury and can create a psychological deterrent to exercise. Additionally, the validity of an actual test for strength is questionable due to a lack of consideration of true contractile force vs. lack of neuroexcitation, also known as fiber recruitment.

Fitness professionals can incorporate the Degree of Difficulty, an additional 0–10 point assessment scale, similar to the Weak Link Index, but specific to the effort involved in performing a resistance exercise. It is simply a value of the effort, based on the individual's perception of how difficult it is to perform the exercise (see Table 4.9). Monitoring this perception of effort is equally as sensible as seeking RPE values during cardiovascular work.

## The Talk Test

The talk test is another tool used to evaluate an individual during the physical assessment. The ability to engage in conversation during exercise represents work at or near a steady rate (steady state). When the oxygen supply meets demand, a person is able to breathe rhythmically and comfortably. If the work intensity encroaches upon anaerobic metabolism, respirations increase due to an elevation in **lactic acid** production and the ability to talk diminishes.

Although the talk test is considered somewhat conservative, it is especially useful in assessing the older adult for three reasons:

1. It helps to prevent the individual from working in a potentially at-risk environment.

2. It helps to prevent the psychological deterrent of exhaustion.

3. It helps to ensure the validity of the cardiovascular testing procedure by staving off anaerobic metabolism.

As the client becomes more conditioned, there may be a desire for higher-intensity work, and possibly an interval training protocol (Welch, 1996a). However, during the initial stages of assessment, the talk test maintains a prudent level of work intensity.

## Post-assessment Report

To accurately develop an appropriate exercise program and gain an appreciation for the individual's post-assessment perception, there must be follow-up to the initial test phase. The client may be experiencing some level of discomfort or even pain, which can cause them to discontinue an exercise program.

The fact that an individual accomplished a particular amount of work with apparent success does not mean that the level of intensity is appropriate. It is important to discuss the ramifications of the tests with your client one to three days after they have finished the assessment. The information you collect will allow for adjustments if discomfort is experienced due to arthritis, sciatica, lower leg pain, muscle soreness, etc. It is not out of the ordinary for an individual to experience no specific discomfort, but feel completely exhausted. This extended lack of recovery may be due to other lifestyle activities that collectively add to a client's fatigue. It may appear normal, but there is still a potential risk of over-exhaustion.

The report is completed through another conversation one to three days after the test protocol. Use the interview to differentiate any problems related to the assessment from any that may have occurred from their regular lifestyle activity. Do not try to diagnose a particular problem, but identify any concern that could (1) lead to a greater problem should exercise continue, (2) represent the need to reduce the intensity of the program, or (3) be a necessary cause for referral to an appropriate healthcare professional.

## THE ART OF ASSESSMENT

There is an art to the physical assessment of the older adult and it lies in the understanding of this unique population. Spirduso, Francis, and MacRae (2005) point out that assessment is determining what the older adult can actually do. Taking this concept a step further, it is more important to determine what an individual can do successfully rather than what they can do maximally. Assessment in the field setting not only needs to be feasible, but socially acceptable as well (Rikli & Jones, 1997). Maximal testing of sedentary, deconditioned muscle tissue is certainly not socially acceptable.

Although the pre-exercise screening is often taken for granted in younger individuals, it begins the true identification process when working with older adults. As mentioned at the start of this chapter, for every individual who desires to begin an exercise program, there is a myriad of potential roadblocks that must first be identified. Remember, the very reason we are performing an assessment is to establish a rational and calculated training program. It does not make sense to test a person and not be able to intelligently determine from the results where their training program should begin. In other words, the results from the assessment should directly transfer to the sets, repetitions, and load of each exercise recommended.

## The Pre-exercise Interview

Begin the pre-exercise interview by addressing your client's present level of daily activity. Use questions of frequency, duration, and perceived intensity to identify activities of daily living and the extent to which they are carried out. Remember, one person's ceiling is another person's floor; everyone is at some level of activity. You must discover each person's true level before proceeding with further investigation.

Begin with a simple statement that can open a treasure chest of information about the individual's ADL: *Tell me about a typical week in your life.* Ask them to be specific: *Are you still working, or are you retired? If you're working, is any part of your work physical? Do you consistently face stairs, ladders, lifting, or walking? Do you participate in consistent business activities, such as travel and entertaining, that extend the hours of your work day or week? How do you spend your time away from work? Do you participate in any regular physical activity, recreational travel, or physical play? Do you experience any pain during movement?*

If the person is retired, ask what their occupation was. Depending on the answer, the same line of questioning detailed above may be appropriate. Based on how long ago the individual was employed, they may maintain a certain level of fitness due to on-the-job physical training. The contrary also is true regarding a deconditioning level if the individual spent most of their time behind a desk. Ask if they retired by choice or disability. Further questioning after an answer of disability may lead to relevant information specific to the physical assessment: *Have you ever fallen? If so, what were the circumstances? Have there been any other injuries? Did you ever undergo rehabilitation?*

If the individual is not employed, you will need to ask questions about their lifestyle at home. *What does a typical week entail? Who maintains the upkeep* of the home, both inside and out? What is the extent of the upkeep? Try to establish a consistent pattern of physical activity.

Decipher clues about their lifestyle to determine ability and conditioning, whether it is associated with work, or social or recreational activities. For example, if a person reports that the extent of their housecleaning is vacuuming and dusting, this suggests a particular level of ability. If another client reports that their housecleaning involves more ambitious chores, such as mopping floors, cleaning tubs and tile, and washing the windows both inside and out, you can reasonably assume a higher level of ability. A person who can maneuver their body up and down from the floor to mop or clean a tub is likely to have conditioned leg muscles and connective tissue. From a strength standpoint, they also are likely to have a stronger eccentric phase of contraction and are less likely to fall.

Direct questioning about recreational activity can be helpful because it transfers directly to the activities of the physical assessment. Try these questions: *When was the last time you went for a walk? Was it a brisk walk or a stroll? How often do you walk? How far and for how long do you walk? Do you ever experience pain while walking? If so, where and how long has it been occurring? How long does it take for the pain to subside?* People commonly over-report activity. If this is the case, it will be apparent during the physical assessment.

## Physical Assessment

The pre-screening interview is conducted through comfortable dialogue, yet in such detail as to determine what physical activity the individual has been engaged in on a *regular* basis. If you know what they have been doing, you can better determine what they're able to do. Once this has been established, you can decide the best way to proceed with the physical assessment. The information you gather

from this initial conversation will help you to be sensitive to the "weak links of the chain," thus helping to prevent new injury and/or aggravating old ones (Welch, 1996b).

## THE SPECIFIT™ WALKING TEST

Unlike most other testing protocols for cardiovascular assessment, this is simply a walk on a treadmill, or if a treadmill is not available, any flat, unobstructed walkway will suffice. While walking together, instruct the individual to walk at a normal pace. From the pre-exercise interview, you will likely know if any ambulatory problems exist. When using a treadmill, you can select a pace that is comfortable, based on your observation of their gate. The heart-rate range should already be determined using the heart-rate reserve method (HRR). Have the individual wear a portable heart-rate monitor while you hold the display portion. Now you are ready for the test.

The parameters of this walking test are common, but the approach is very unique. Begin by engaging the individual in casual conversation. This will help pass the time and give you first indication of breathlessness. Adjust the pace to first provide a warm-up and then to create various challenges. Most walking tests ignore collecting any data until the end of the test and then rely on the archaic method of palpating heart rates. Even if heart rate is not an issue due to medication (e.g., beta blockers), the remaining information—RPE, WLI, pace, and interval time—are valuable and should be gathered *throughout* the test.

Every one to three minutes, depending on interval pace, inquire as to their rate of perceived exertion (RPE). Attempt an RPE of <6 (strong to very strong), a heart-rate range of <70%, and a total test-time that does not exceed 10 minutes. The RPE values and heart rates may not always rise in a linear fashion, hence the reason for recording both. If a person states a low RPE, but the heart rate is elevated beyond

70%, then end the test. Likewise, if a person has a very low heart rate but feels their RPE is above 6, end the test.

Also ask them, on the same 0–10 scale, if there is any part of their body where they are experiencing discomfort or pain. This is the Weak Link Index (WLI). The common areas for discomfort are the shins, calves, hips, and back. Regardless of speed, if the WLI is a 3 or greater, reduce the pace and try to alleviate the discomfort. If it subsides, attempt to resume the previous speed. If the index number remains the same, then discontinue the test but record the information (i.e., time, pace, affected body part, and RPE). If the WLI remains a 1 or 2, simply ask the individual if they feel comfortable continuing the test. A test may very well be discontinued because of discomfort long before fatigue becomes an issue. Assure them that they are in control of the test at all times and do not try to convince them to push past a comfortable level of effort. Simply record the information that you have accumulated and keep it for future comparison. Programming success is vital to the adherence factor. Even though the individual might have performed at a higher level than the recommended parameters, they have accomplished an amount of measurable work that is safe, successful, and likely to be more work than they have performed recently.

## ASSESSMENT OF FUNCTIONAL STRENGTH AND ABILITY

Although walking is a common lifestyle activity, it is not always indicative of total-body functional ability. Measurement of functional ability determines what exercise is necessary to maintain and improve performance of ADL. Strength is a vital component of the older adult's functional ability, and is traditionally assessed through a one-repetition maximum (1 RM) or extrapolated 1 RM. Williams (1994) states that the use of 1 RM testing is not rec-

ommended in persons with no recent exercise history, especially in the elderly. Other test protocols include lighter resistance and maximum repetitions. Although these traditional methods provide information necessary to the eventual establishment of population-specific normative data, the information is not immediately pertinent for functional assessment. Additionally, maximum testing without a preparatory conditioning phase puts the older adult at greater risk.

When testing functional ability, it is helpful to first look at functional mobility (Welch, 1996b). The SpeciFit Assessment Method of Functional Strength and Ability bases all resistance training for the older adult around the circuit-style method. The individual is first asked to demonstrate the biomechanical patterns common to lifestyle activities, as well as to emulate patterns similar to the movements used in basic resistance-training exercises (e.g., chest press, rowing, shoulder press, leg extension, leg curl). Body weight is the only resistance used. These are simple voluntary active range-of-motion (VAROM) movements. By observing this movement in the variety of patterns suggested, you can note any difficulties in mobility that might lead to further problems if resistance is added. As part of his post-rehabilitation assessment procedures, Jones (1996b) created a scoring system for range of motion (ROM) and strength in all major joints and muscle groups:

3   Full (completes ROM against gravity)

2   Partial (completes ½ of ROM, or better, against gravity)

1   Limited (unable to complete ½ of ROM against gravity)

0   Unable (unable to perform task)

+   No pain, or pain less than 3 on a scale from 1 to 10, add ½ point

-   Pain greater than or equal to 4 on a scale from 1 to 10, subtract ½ point

To establish a resistance protocol, make an informed estimate regarding the amount of resistance to use in each separate exercise. Base your decision on three criteria:

1. Data collected during the pre-exercise interview
2. Notable difficulty in the VAROM assessment
3. An understanding of the biomechanical efficiency of the different joint angles

Free weights are preferable to machines when conducting a functional strength assessment. Observe the strength necessary to lift the weight, as well as the stabilization of the joint by the supporting musculature during the action. The range of resistance is 2 pounds to 15 pounds per dumbbell, depending on the individual and the body part being assessed.

Ask the individual to lift the weight in ranges of three to five, five to seven, and seven to 10 repetitions. These ranges promote a philosophy of programming success and allow you to observe the individual's willingness to work. If the person is asked to perform 10 repetitions, but they can only finish eight, they might feel they have failed. To avoid this feeling of defeat, select a range you are confident they will be able to achieve.

At the end of each exercise on the circuit, ask the participant for a degree of difficulty (DD) rating from 0 to 10, based solely on how hard it was to lift the weight. The ideal rating is between 4 and 6. Also ask for a WLI value to monitor any pain during or after the lifting procedure. This WLI value is particularly important if the individual has expressed any undue strain with a contorted body or grimacing face. A WLI value greater than 2 is enough to curtail the assessment of that particular muscle group. Record all values and conduct a post-exercise report in one to three days. Process the information from this report with previous test results to develop the exercise program.

# TESTS OF FUNCTION

Many valuable tests look at real-life function in different ways. Balance, coordination, speed, and agility all are important to maintain and improve the physical wellness of the older adult. You are in a position to assist other health-care professionals in the assessment of these functions. It is important to distinguish between the testing protocols as to exactly what outcome is desired.

## The Senior Fitness Test

Rikli & Jones (2001) have created The Senior Fitness Test as an answer to the need in today's marketplace for a simple, easy-to-use battery of test items that assess the functional fitness of older adults (see Appendix). It measures the key physical abilities needed to perform common everyday activities. The test, which is considered safe and enjoyable for older adults, meets scientific standards for reliability and validity, and has accompanying performance norms based on actual tests of more than 700 men and women between the ages of 60 and 94. It is the first test of its kind to provide normative data for the older adult such that an individual can see how they compare to their age-appropriate population.

## Fullerton Advanced Balance Scale

The Fullerton Advanced Balance (FAB) Scale is used to assess a variety of proprioceptive challenges (see Appendix). The following are some examples;

✓ ability to use ground cues to maintain upright balance while standing with a reduced base of support
✓ ability to lean forward to retrieve an object without a base of support
✓ ability to turn a full circle in both directions in the fewest number of steps without loss of balance

✓ ability to dynamically control center of mass with an altered base of support

✓ ability to maintain upright balance while standing on a compliant surface with eyes closed

## Multidirectional Reach Test

The purpose of the Multidirectional Reach Test (MDRT) is to measure the distance a person is able or willing to lean in a forward, backward, and lateral direction (see Appendix).

Table 4.10

**Tinetti Gait Evaluation\***

| | | |
|---|---|---|
| *Initiation of gait after told to "go"* | Any hesitancy or multiple attempts to start | =0 |
| | No hesitancy | =1 |
| *Step length and height* | *a) Right swing foot* | |
| | Does not pass left stance foot | =0 |
| | Passes left stance foot with step | =1 |
| | Right foot does not clear floor completely with step | =0 |
| | Right foot completely clears floor | =1 |
| | *b) Left swing foot* | |
| | Does not pass right stance foot | =0 |
| | Passes right stance foot with step | =1 |
| | Left foot does not clear floor completely with step | =0 |
| | Left foot completely clears floor | =1 |
| *Step symmetry* | Right and left step length not equal (estimate) | =0 |
| | Right and left step appear equal | =1 |
| *Step continuity* | Stopping or discontinuity between steps | =0 |
| | Steps appear continuous | =1 |
| *Path\*\** | Marked deviation | =0 |
| | Mild/moderate deviation or uses walking aid | =1 |
| | Straight without walking aid | =2 |
| *Trunk* | Marked sway or uses walking aid | =0 |
| | No sway but flexion of knees or back or spreads arms while walking | =1 |
| | No sway, no flexion, no use of arms, and no use of walking aid | =2 |
| *Walk stance* | Heels apart | =0 |
| | Heels almost touching while walking | =1 |

*\*Subject stands with examiner; walks down hallway or across room, first at his usual pace, then back at rapid, but safe pace (using usual walking aid such as cane, walker). Maximum Gait Score is 12.*
*\*\*Estimate path in relation to floor tiles. Observe excursion of one foot over about 10 feet of the course.*

*Modified from M. Tinetti (1986). Performance-oriented assessment of mobility problems in elderly patients. Journal of the American Geriatrics Society, 34, 119–126.*

## Berg Balance Scale

The Berg Balance Scale is an objective measure of balance abilities and is a good back-up to the FAB. It is commonly used to identify and evaluate balance impairments in older individuals. The scale consists of 14 everyday tasks that focus on reaching, bending, transferring, standing, rising, and other functional tasks (see Appendix).

## Tinetti Gait Evaluation

Tinetti (1986) devised a simple, scored screening scale to detect and quantify problems with gait (Table 4.10). It is beneficial for looking specifically at the biomechanical patterning of walking.

## SPECIAL CONSIDERATIONS

By now it should be obvious that the older adult is a complex entity when it comes to health status. Simply by virtue of their age, they hold the potential for a variety of anomalies. It has been noted that four out of 10 older adults (over 65) have a chronic disorder that may result in a functional limitation (Blocker, 1992).

You must be able to identify these and other problems through the pre-exercise screening process. Specific consent from the client's physician should be obtained if a client has any of the conditions discussed in Chapter 3, or any other medical condition that would cause exercise or physical assessment to place them at risk.

## CONCLUSION

Beginning an exercise program properly can be the first step toward a real commitment to health. Therefore, understanding the tools necessary to identify the older adult and to determine the initial exercise program for this special population is essential. This chapter has attempted to provide a variety of options for identifying what the older can actually do successfully.

There is a void, however, when designing an actual exercise program based on results from traditional strength and cardiovascular assessment. It is well established that maximal effort performed with deconditioned muscle tissue is unwise and unnecessary in the field setting. Attaining a maximal value does not detect for potential injury or even allow for movement discomfort, which is very common among the sedentary. Furthermore, when attempting to establish a total-body training program for the older adult, maximal results in a few exercises do not adequately represent the specifics of the entire body, nor will they transfer well into a precise exercise program of sets, reps, and loads.

Conducting a test is only of value if the results can be directly applied to a practical outcome. For example, if a maximal chest-press value is 40 lb, then what weight should be selected from this result for the chest press exercise? While 60 to 80% has been used as a "rule of thumb," this means the weight could vary from 16 to 24 pounds. How do you decide which weight from here? And how many repetitions should the individual perform of the exercise? Then, how many sets should be repeated? These questions must be answered just for this one exercise. How does that chest-press value carry over to the shoulder press exercise, the rowing exercise, the lat pull-down exercise, etc? There needs to be a bridge from a test result of a particular body part to the actual exercise of that body part.

A more prudent approach is to first assess the individual's voluntary active range of motion (VAROM), then add resistance. Use the individual's perception to assist in determining if the weight is proper by the "degree of difficulty" (DD) scale. Evaluate discomfort by the "weak link index" (WLI), which is based on perception as well. Record all data to illustrate the progress. Asking pertinent questions is also valuable when assessment of cardiovascular function is desired. Heart rate, RPE, and the WLI, when assessed regularly during the test, can provide information that is most beneficial to establishing an exercise protocol the individual can perform autonomously.

Using the individual's perception to help determine a prudent level of exercise has been accepted in the wellness community since Borg introduced his original RPE scale. Until now, however, it has not been utilized to its full potential. It may appear too conservative by comparison to clinical standards, but the field setting is the "real world" where individual differences tend to dictate the success of an exercise program. Relying on perception may, in fact, prevent the individual from achieving a true, baseline intensity in the beginning few weeks of the exercise program. This is acceptable because, regardless of the intensity, the exercise still represents physiological "work" and it is definitely more "work" than the individual has performed recently. Therefore, the experience is positive and adherence to the program as a change in lifestyle is more likely.

# REFERENCES AND SUGGESTED READING

American College of Sports Medicine (2000). *ACSM's Guidelines for Exercise Testing and Prescription* (6th ed.). Baltimore: Lippincott Williams & Wilkins.

American Council on Exercise (2003). *ACE Personal Trainer Manual* (3rd ed.). San Diego: American Council on Exercise.

American Geriatrics Society (1989). Assessment in geriatrics: Of caveats and names. *Journal of the American Geriatrics Society, 37,* 6, 570–572.

Anthony, J. (2003). Health screening. In *ACE Personal Trainer Manual* (3rd ed.). San Diego: American Council on Exercise.

Bemben, M.G., Kuchera, M., & Bemben, D.A. (1989). Physiological changes related to aging: Implications for health and fitness. *Journal of Osteopathic Sports Medicine, 3,* 15–19.

Blocker, W.P. (1992). Maintaining functional independence by mobilizing the aged. *Geriatrics, 47,* 42–56.

Borg, G.B. (1982). Psychological basis of perceived exertion. *Medicine and Science in Sports and Exercise, 14,* 377–381.

Bortz, W.M. (1996). How fast do we age? Exercise performance over time as a biomarker. *Journal of Gerontology: Medical Sciences, 51A,* 5, 223–225.

Brill, P. et al. (1999). The value of strength training for older adults. *Home Care Provider, 4,* 2, 62–66.

Bruce, R.A. (1984). Exercise, functional aerobic capacity and aging: Another viewpoint. *Medicine and Science in Sports and Exercise, 16,* 8.

Bryant, C.X., Franklin, B.A., & Conviser, J.M. (2002). *Exercise Testing and Program Design.* Monterey, Calif.: Healthy Learning.

Carlton, R. & Rhodes, E. (1985). A critical review of the literature on the ratings scales of perceived exertion. *Sports Medicine, 2,* 198–222.

Cartee, G.D. (1994). Aging skeletal muscle: Response to exercise. *Exercise Sport Science Review, 22,* 91.

Charette, S.L. et al. (1991). Muscle hypertrophy response to resistance training in older women. *Journal of Applied Physiology, 70,* 1912.

Cotton, R.T. (2003). Testing and evaluation. In *ACE Personal Trainer Manual* (3rd ed.). San Diego: American Council on Exercise.

Coupland, C., Wood, D., & Cooper, C. (1993). Physical inactivity is an independent risk factor for hip fracture in the elderly. *Journal of Epidemiology & Community Health, 47,* 6, 441–443.

Cumming, G.R. (1993). Children with heart disease. In J.S. Skinner (Ed.) *Exercise Testing and Exercise Prescription for Special Cases* (2nd ed.). Philadelphia: Lea & Febiger.

Diesel, W. et al. (1990). Isokinetic muscle strength predicts maximum exercise tolerance in renal patients on chronic hemodialysis. *American Journal of Kidney Disease, 16,* 109.

Dietary Guidelines Advisory Committee (2005). *Nutrition and Your Health: Dietary Guidelines for Americans.* Washington, D.C.: U.S. Departments of Health and Human Services, and Agriculture.

Dunbar, C.C. & Balanos, G.M. (1996). Ten-second pulse palpation does not accurately measure heart rate at rest or during exercise. *Medicine and Science in Sports and Exercise, 28,* S-1090, supplement.

Evans, W. & Rosenberg, I.H. (1992). *Biomarkers.* New York: Simon & Schuster.

Feinstein, A.R., Josephy, B.R., & Wells, C.K. (1986). Scientific and clinical problems in indexes of functional disability. *Annals of Internal Medicine, 105,* 413–420.

Fillenbaum, G.G. (1985). Screening the elderly: A brief instrumental activities of daily living measure. *Journal of the American Geriatric Society, 33,* 698.

Franklin, B.A. (2001). Normal cardio-respiratory responses to acute aerobic exercise. In *ACSM Resource Manual for*

*Guidelines for Exercise Testing and Prescription* (4th ed.). New York: Lippincott Williams & Wilkins.

Gilligan, C., Checovich, M.M., & Smith, E.L. (1993). Osteoporosis. In J.S. Skinner (Ed.) *Exercise Testing and Exercise Prescription for Special Cases* (2nd ed.). Philadelphia: Lea & Febiger.

Gordon, N.F. (1997). *Stroke, Your Complete Exercise Guide*. Champaign, Ill.: Human Kinetics.

Gordon, N.F. (1993a). *Arthritis, Your Complete Exercise Guide*. Champaign, Ill.: Human Kinetics.

Gordon, N.F. (1993b). *Breathing Disorders, Your Complete Exercise Guide*. Champaign, Ill.: Human Kinetics.

Hagberg, J.M. et al. (1988). Metabolic responses to exercise in young and older athletes and sedentary men. *Journal of Applied Physiology, 65,* 900.

Haskell, W.L. & Durstine, J.L. (1993). Coronary artery disease. In J.S. Skinner (Ed.) *Exercise Testing and Exercise Prescription for Special Cases* (2nd ed.). Philadelphia: Lea & Febiger.

Heath, G.W. (2001). Exercise programming for the older adult. In *ACSM Resource Manual for Guidelines for Exercise Testing and Prescription* (4th ed.). New York: Lippincott Williams & Wilkins.

Hochschild, R. (1990). Can an index of aging be constructed for evaluating treatments to retard aging rates? A 2,462-person study. *Journal of Gerontology: Biological Sciences, 45,* 6, 187–214.

Imamura, K. et al. (1983). Human major psoas muscle and scarospinalis muscle in relation to age. *Journal of Gerontology, 33,* 678.

Jones, J.C. (1986). Interactionary effects of nutrition, medication and exercise. *Southwest Journal on Aging, 3,* 2, 57–74.

Jones, M. (1996). *PERC Post Rehabilitation Protocol Assessment Manual*. San Leandro, Calif.: American Academy of Fitness Professionals.

Jones, N.L et al. (1993). Chronic obstructive respiratory disorders. In J.S. Skinner (Ed.) *Exercise Testing and Exercise Prescription for Special Cases* (2nd ed.). Philadelphia: Lea & Febiger.

Katz, S. et al. (1970). Progress in development of the index of ADL. *Gerontologist, 10,* 20.

Keller, K. & Lemberg, L. (2002). Retirement is no excuse for physical inactivity or isolation. *American Journal of Critical Care, 11,* 3, 270–272.

Leon, A.S. (1993). Diabetes. In J.S. Skinner (Ed.) *Exercise Testing and Exercise Prescription for Special Cases* (2nd ed.). Philadelphia: Lea & Febiger.

Lexel, J. (1993). Aging and human skeletal muscle: Observations from Sweden. *Canadian Journal of Applied Physiology, 18,* 2.

McArdle, W.D., Katch, F.I., & Katch, V.L. (2001). *Exercise Physiology* (5th ed.). Baltimore: Lippincott Williams & Wilkins.

Mooradian, A.D. (1990). Biomarkers of aging: Do we know what to look for? *Journal of Gerontology: Biological Sciences, 45,* 6 183–186.

Muritani, T. (1981). Training adaptations in the muscles of older men. In *Exercise and Aging: The Scientific Basis*. Hillside, Calif.: Enslow.

National Heart, Lung, and Blood Institute (1998). Clinical guidelines on the identification, evaluation, and treatment of overweight and obesity in adults: The evidence report. *Obesity Research, 6* (Suppl. 2), 51S–209S.

National Institutes of Health (2003). *The Seventh Report of the Joint Committee on Prevention, Detection, Evaluation, and Treatment of High Blood Pressure*. NIH Publication No. 03-5233.

Painter, P. (1993). End-stage renal disease. In J.S. Skinner (Ed.) *Exercise Testing and Exercise Prescription for Special Cases* (2nd ed.). Philadelphia: Lea & Febiger.

Painter, P. (1986). Exercise during hemodialysis: Participation rates. *Dialysis Transplant, 17,* 21–26.

Powell, K.E. et al. (1987). Physical activity and the incidence of coronary heart disease. *Annual Review of Public Health, 8,* 253.

Rikli, R.E. & Jones, J.C. (2001). *Senior Fitness Test Manual*. Champaign, Ill.: Human Kinetics.

Rikli, R.E. & Jones, J.C. (1997). Assessing physical performance in "independent" older adults: Issues and guidelines. *Journal of Aging and Physical Activity,* 5, 244–261.

Rimmer, J.H. (1994). *Fitness and Rehabilitation Programs for Special Populations.* Madison, Wis.: Brown & Benchmark.

Roubenoff, R. (2000). Sarcopenia and its implications for the elderly. *European Journal of Clinical Nutrition,* 54, S3, S40–47.

Sannerstedt, R. (1993). Hypertension. In J.S. Skinner (Ed.) *Exercise Testing and Exercise Prescription for Special Cases* (2nd ed.). Philadelphia: Lea & Febiger.

Skinner, J.S. (1993). *Exercise Testing and Exercise Prescription for Special Cases* (2nd ed.). Philadelphia: Lea & Febiger.

Spirduso, W.W., Francis, K.L., & MacRae, P.G. (2005). *Physical Dimensions of Aging* (2nd ed.). Champaign, Ill.: Human Kinetics.

Spirduso, W.W. (1975). Reaction and movement time as a function of age and physical activity level. *Journal of Gerontology,* 30, 435.

Spirduso, W.W. & Clifford, P. (1978). Replication of age and physical activity effects on reaction and movement time. *Journal of Gerontology,* 33, 26.

Stamford, B.A. (1988). Exercise in the elderly. In *Exercise and Sports Sciences Reviews.* New York: Macmillan.

Tinetti, M.E. (1986). Performance-oriented assessment of mobility problems in elderly patients. *Journal of the American Geriatric Society,* 34, 119–226.

Trueblood, P.R. & Rubenstein L.Z. (1991). Assessment of instability and gait in elderly persons. *Comprehensive Therapy,* 17, 8, 20–29.

Welch, G.L. (1996a). Interval training for the competitive senior. *The Senior Fitness Bulletin,* 3, 2, 15–23.

Welch, G.L. (1996b). Strengthening the weak links. *IDEA Personal Trainer,* 7, 9, 13–16.

Welch, G.L. (1995). Training goals for the older adult. *IDEA Personal Trainer,* 6, 1, 31–34.

Welch, G.L. (1995). Stabilization: An integral part of real life function. *The Senior Fitness Bulletin,* 2, 2, 8–9.

Westerterp, K. (2000). Daily physical activity and aging. Current Opinions in Clinical *Nutrition & Metabolic Care,* 3, 6, 485–488.

Wiener J.M. et al. (1990). Measuring the activities of daily living: Comparisons across national surveys. *Journal of Gerontology: Social Sciences,* 45, 6, 229–237.

Williams, M.A. (1994). *Exercise Testing and Training in the Elderly Cardiac Patient.* Champaign, Ill.: Human Kinetics.

Williams, M.A. & Sketch, M.H. (1988). Guidelines for exercise training of elderly patients following myocardial infarction and coronary bypass graft surgery. *Geriatric Cardiovascular Medicine,* 1, 107–110.

Wilmore, J.H. & Costill, D.L. (1999). *Physiology of Sport and Exercise* (2nd ed.). Champaign, Ill.: Human Kinetics.

OLDER ADULT

# Exercise Techniques

## Janie Clark

*Janie Clark, M.A., is the president of the American Senior Fitness Association (SFA), the international organization for fitness professionals who serve older adults. She is a contributing author in* Physical Activity Instruction for Older Adults *and* Exercise for Frail Elders, *the editor of* Exercise Programming for Older Adults, *and the author of* Full Life Fitness: A Complete Exercise Program for Mature Adults *and* Seniorcise: A Simple Guide to Fitness for the Elderly and Disabled. *Clark, who holds her master's degree in exercise physiology and wellness management, served on the national advisory board for the LifeSpan Project to establish functional fitness testing protocols for older adults and on the Coalition to Develop National Curriculum Standards for Senior Fitness Specialists.*

In its most basic context, the term aging simply refers to the passage of time. On another level, aging involves complicated processes that contribute to an ultimate decline in function. Complex relationships develop between the aging process itself and individual variables such as history of physical injuries or long-term behaviors involving diet, physical activity, smoking, alcohol consumption, and drug use. For these reasons, assumptions regarding "normal," "typical," or "average" individual performance abilities become less viable with increasing age. In fact, the older-adult age group is characterized by dramatic individual differences in functional capacity. For example, whereas one 75-year-old person may be unable to lift a 10-pound bag of groceries or walk around the block without assistance, another may compete successfully in marathons (Gersten, 1991; Spirduso, Francis, & MacRae, 2005). Clearly, a "one-size-fits-all" exercise program-ming approach is inappropriate for this population.

Fortunately, a variety of training options is available to older-adult fitness participants. These include group or solitary walking programs, aerobic exercise classes, chair-seated exercise, personal training, balance training, aquatics, relaxation classes, active pastimes such as gardening or square dancing, or simply integrating more physical activity into one's daily routine.

## CHOOSING AMONG FORMS OF TRAINING

There are a number of personal variables to take into account when recommending exercise modes for your older-adult clients, including:

✓ Fitness level

✓ Health status

✓ Level of mobility/physical limitations

✓ Source and degree of motivation

✓ Self-efficacy

✓ Time commitment

✓ Needs/goals

✓ Interests

A careful analysis of these variables will help guide your clients toward forms of exercise that will produce beneficial training effects while, at the same time, providing a satisfying physical activity experience that encourages prolonged compliance and adherence.

How should you determine whether to steer a new older-adult exercise client toward a low-impact aerobics class, a personal-training program, chair-seated activity, or some other form of training? Although health status and performance assessment results provide critical direction, the decision also should be based on the client's personal preference. This can be identified during an initial interview process, in which the client's goals and interests are explored. Here are some examples of potential findings and their indicated actions.

✓ Does the client have a strong interest in social opportunities for camaraderie and interaction among others in their age group? Does movement to music appeal to the client's tastes? Does the client indicate confidence in their ability to perform and enjoy group exercise? Based on the client's health history, performance assessments, and your personal observations during the interview process, is the client physically capable of successfully participating in an aerobics class? Does the class schedule fit into the client's day-to-day routine? Does the class match the client's training goals? If so, a low-impact aerobics class appears to be a good choice for this client.

✓ Is the client motivated by specific health concerns or performance goals that are best met by individualized attention? Does the client's functional capacity significantly exceed or fall below the performance level achieved in group classes? Is a personal-training regimen consistent with the individual's likes and dislikes? Does the client think that they would enjoy working with exercise machines? When the answer to any of these questions is yes, a personal-training program may be a good choice.

✓ Does the client use a wheelchair, or are they otherwise physically restricted with regard to standing, walking, or getting up and down? Has the client expressed any misgivings in connection with the ability to successfully participate in fitness training? For example, is the client concerned about the possibility of falling or not being able to get up from the floor after mat exercises? Is the client obviously frail, obese, or disabled? If so, then low-impact aerobics may not initially be a viable option for the individual. Although personal training appears to be an appropriate choice, further questions need to be answered before the client is placed in such a program. For example, does the client prefer a group environment? Will a movement-to-music format prove enjoyable and motivational for this client? If so, a chair-seated exercise class may be the best method of reintroducing the individual to a more active lifestyle.

✓ Does the client have a firm idea of what type of activity they want to try? For example, clients that have had positive experiences in aquatic exercise classes may want to re-enter a water program. Others may prefer a walking program because they view it as a non-intimidating form of exercise because it does not require learning new skills. Some may be more inclined to take a relaxation or yoga class. In every case, try to accommodate the wishes of the client, augmenting the desired form of exercise, if necessary, with additional activities to achieve a fully balanced program.

Often, a combination of modes is ideal. For example, aerobics class participants may also benefit by performing strength exercises on selected machines. Group classes might include a combination of standing aerobic work and seated muscle work. Alternatively, chair aerobics classes might include standing muscle work using the back of the chair for balance support. Accomplished group fitness instructors can supervise chair-seated and standing (or mat-exercising) participants in the same class by teaching chair-seated alternative exercises as needed. Relaxation exercises can be incorporated into the cool-down segments of other types of classes and programs. Balance training can play a part in functional-fitness programming, and elements of both can be utilized in either personal training or group settings.

Practically speaking, older-adult programming formats may incorporate elements from a number of reliable training methods, depending upon the needs and preferences of the individual involved. Examples include:
✓ Cross training (combining or periodically changing exercise modes)

✓ Interval training (alternating periods of relatively high-intensity work with periods of low-intensity work)

✓ Circuit training (interspersing aerobic exercise between strengthening activities)

Such changes in exercise mode may be made for the sake of progression. For example, although some participants must remain in chair classes because of physical limitations, others may eventually graduate to more active classes. Persons who have made muscle-conditioning progress in a class may need to increase their intensity level by moving on to a strength-machine workout. Conversely, persons with weak lower-body musculature may need to start with strength-machine workouts to condition the body before attempting a traditional aerobics class.

Variations in mode, which are virtually limitless, also may be made for variety's sake. The goal is to conduct effective programming that promotes the development of a lifelong exercise habit.

For a more in-depth discussion of principles related to matching physical needs and ability levels to appropriate training options, please refer to Chapter 7.

## TRAINING GUIDELINES

Following the principles of mode, frequency, duration, intensity, and progression helps safely produce and maintain desired training effects. The following guidelines for aerobic, strength, and flexibility training—elements essential to a balanced program—should be applied when conducting the various forms of activity addressed in this chapter. In addition, observe general safety precautions, and analyze the safety and effectiveness of specific exercises or techniques (Tables 5.1 and 5.2).

Complete programs also address balance and coordination (see Balance/Coordination Training Techniques, page 173).

Table 5.1

## General Older Adult Exercise Safety Guidelines

*The following precautions apply to all forms of exercise discussed in this chapter:*

✓ Obtain medical clearance to exercise.

✓ Never hold the breath. During strengthening exercises, exhale upon exertion and inhale during the release phase.

✓ Do not strain.

✓ Do not hyperflex (over-bend) or hyperextend (over-stretch) the joints. For example, avoid hyperflexion of the neck during curl-ups, and avoid hyperextension of the elbows during arm exercises.

✓ Do not over-grip hand weights, equipment handles, or other exercise accessories.

✓ Discourage a competitive atmosphere in group settings.

✓ Limit overhead arm work.

✓ Teach a neutral spine position.

✓ Avoid excessive vertical loading of the spine (by controlling resistance level and other training variables during strength exercise).

✓ Always provide optimal manual support for the back when bending the upper body in any direction and from any position.

✓ Separately perform moves that involve turning or bending the back, rather than combining the two activities.

✓ Use caution with regard to neck exercise. Do not move the neck quickly; avoid hyperflexion due to excessively low nodding, and hyperextension due to backward tilting of the head.

✓ Modify methods that are not well tolerated. If an exercise causes pain, modify or replace it as necessary. Reduce intensity, duration, or frequency levels that are too great.

✓ Implement slow, gradual progression.

✓ Avoid known high-risk activities and techniques (for example, straight-leg sit-ups, the hurdler's stretch, the plow, the full cobra, and any other moves identified as potentially dangerous when evaluated according to the criteria provided in Table 5.2).

✓ Remember to err on the side of safety.

## Aerobic Exercise

Cardiovascular exercise is any mode of continuous activity utilizing large muscle groups that is rhythmic and aerobic in nature (American College of Sports Medicine, 2000). For safety reasons, low-impact rather than high-impact modes of aerobic exercise are recommended for older-adult participants (Pollock et al., 1991).

The aerobic exercise training guidelines published by the American College of Sports Medicine (ACSM) (2000), the American Heart Association (Fletcher et al., 1995), and the Centers for Disease Control and Prevention in conjunction with the ACSM (Pate et al., 1995) are, for the most part, consistent (Table 5.3). In addition to improving fitness level, increased physical activity is recommended for enhancing quality of life and for reducing general health risks. The *Surgeon General's Report on Physical Activity and Health* encourages a regular, preferably daily, regimen including 30 to 45 minutes of moderate activity—brisk walking, bicycling, or even simply working around the house or yard—to lower the risks of developing coronary heart disease, hypertension, colon cancer, and

Table 5.2

**Exercise Selection: Evaluating the Advisability of Specific Exercises**

*Below are pertinent questions to answer when considering whether to conduct a specific exercise activity:*

✓ What is the purpose of the exercise? (For example, is the goal to warm up, cool down, or accomplish aerobic conditioning, flexibility improvement, or muscle strengthening? Will the exercise engage a particular muscle or muscle group?)

✓ Does the exercise effectively fulfill that purpose? (For example, does the exercise actually work the intended muscle group?)

✓ Is the exercise safe for average asymptomatic participants? (For example, does it produce excessive impact or otherwise place unnecessary stress on any joint? Does it place undue pressure on any body part, or immoderate demands on any body system?)

✓ If not, can the exercise practically be modified to an appropriate form? (For example, straight-leg sit-ups can be altered to achieve an acceptable activity by bending one knee and simply curling the trunk forward; deep squats can be replaced by shallower squats.)

✓ If an unacceptable exercise cannot be modified, with what acceptable activity can it be replaced? (For example, the plow can be replaced by leg hugs to stretch the back, gluteals, and hamstrings without distressing the neck.)

✓ Is the exercise safe for the specific individual expected to perform it? (For example, does the participant have any special condition that would preclude performing activities that are deemed safe for others in their age group?)

✓ If not, can the exercise be modified to safely accommodate the participant? (For example, should the range of motion be reduced?)

✓ If an unacceptable exercise cannot be modified to safely meet the needs of an individual with a special condition, with what acceptable activity can it be replaced? (For example, if performing floor push-ups strains a participant's wrists, then a wall push-up might be implemented; if that, too, strains the wrists, then the involved upper-body muscles can be conditioned with exercises using dumbbells or strength machines.)

*Note: When in doubt regarding the implementation of a specific exercise activity or technique, consult your participant's personal physician.*

diabetes (U.S. Department of Health and Human Services, 1996).

To establish and maintain a training intensity that is both safe and sufficient to produce beneficial physiological effects, the intensity level of aerobic exercise should be regularly monitored by rating of perceived exertion (RPE) and/or by heart-rate count (Borg, 1982; Swart, Pollock, & Brechue, 1996). The Karvonen formula can be used to determine working heart-rate goals. The formula calculates training heart-rate range based on heart-rate reserve (HRR), the difference between maximal and resting heart rates. Percentage value using the HRR method is approximately equal to percentage $\dot{V}O_2$max (i.e., a 50% intensity

prescription determined by the HRR method equals about 50% $\dot{V}O_2$max) (Pollock & Wilmore, 1990). See Tables 5.4 and 5.5.

For older participants, apply aerobic training principles in a manner that discourages potential orthopedic problems and cardiovascular complications. An intensity level of 30 to 75% $\dot{V}O_2$max [with an RPE of 11 to 13 (somewhat hard) on the Borg 6-to-20 perceived exertion scale] sustained for 30 to 60 minutes is recommended for older adults (American College of Sports Medicine, 2000; Pollock et al., 1994; Swart, Pollock, & Brechue, 1996). Total quantity of work depends upon duration and intensity, which are inversely related.

Table 5.3

**Basic Guidelines for Aerobic Exercise Training (General Population)**

*American College of Sports Medicine*

✓ Frequency: 3 to 5 days per week

✓ Intensity: 40 to 85% $\dot{V}O_2$max

✓ Duration: 15 to 60 minutes, continuous

✓ Mode: Aerobic activities

*American Heart Association*

✓ Frequency: 3 to 5 days per week

✓ Intensity: 40 to 60% $\dot{V}O_2$max

✓ Duration: 20 to 60 minutes

✓ Mode: Aerobic activities/health-promotion activities*

*American College of Sports Medicine/Centers for Disease Control and Prevention/Report of the Surgeon General on Physical Activity and Health*

✓ Frequency: Daily

✓ Intensity: Moderate

✓ Duration: Accumulate 30 minutes per day

✓ Mode: Health-promotion activities*

* Health-promotion activities may include active tasks, such as raking leaves or taking part in active leisure pastimes.

When energy costs are similar, lower-intensity, longer-duration aerobic exercise produces benefits comparable to those achieved through higher-intensity, shorter-duration exercise (Swart, Pollock, & Brechue, 1996). For previously sedentary older adults, low- to moderate-intensity exercise of longer duration is generally preferable. Initially, the exerciser's tolerance may limit duration. If so, rest periods between exercise bouts allow the exerciser to achieve the recommended duration. Accumulating the recommended exercise duration through short periods of activity, either within a single workout session or during several sessions throughout the course of a day (Pate et al., 1995), provides significant health benefits (DeBusk et al., 1990; Paffenbarger et al., 1986).

A frequency of three to five days per week (spaced throughout the week) is generally recommended (American College of Sports Medicine, 2000). Since low-fit older exercisers may be able to tolerate only very-low-intensity, short-

duration (five- to 10-minute) exercise sessions, a slight increase in frequency (four to five days per week) will help meet desirable total energy expenditure levels (approximately 1,000 kcal per week). Research suggests that the health benefits associated with physical activity are related primarily to total quantity of activity, regardless of exercise mode, duration, or intensity (American College of Sports Medicine, 2000; Pollock et al., 1994). In addition to intensity and duration, mode may have a practical impact upon frequency. For example, short- to moderate-duration, low-intensity walking can usually be safely performed seven days per week.

Progression should be implemented slowly. A two- to six-week, low-intensity starting phase permits adaptation with minimal risk for injury. The next phase (lasting approximately six months to a year for middle-aged and elderly participants, respectively) involves gradual progression by conservatively increasing both duration and intensity. Generally, duration

Table 5.4

**Karvonen Formula: Estimating Target Heart-rate Zone According to Beats Per Minute**

*Formulas should not be used to estimate target heart-rate zones for persons using medications that alter heart rate. (In that case, obtain training intensity parameters from your client's physician.)*

*In the following example, target heart-rate zone is calculated for a 65-year-old individual with a resting heart rate of 70 beats per minute. The exerciser will work at a moderate intensity level from 50 to 75% of maximum heart rate (an appropriate range for the typical asymptomatic older adult). See page 116 for a discussion of the "220-minus-age" formula.*

| | | | | |
|---|---|---|---|---|
| | 220 | | | |
| – | 65 | | | Age |
| = | 155 | | | Maximum Heart Rate |
| – | 70 | | | Resting Heart Rate |
| = | 85 | | | Heart-rate Reserve |
| X | 00.5 | X | 00.75 | Training Heart-rate Range |
| = | 43 | = | 64 | |
| + | 70 | + | 70 | Resting Heart Rate |
| = | 113 | = | 134 | Target Heart-rate Zone |

*Note: Conducting periodic 10-second pulse counts is a convenient method of monitoring heart rate during aerobic exercise. To determine the desirable 10-second count range, divide the target rate values by 6. In this example, the minimum 10-second count is 19 (113 divided by 6) and the maximum is 22 (134 divided by 6).*

can safely be increased by five-minute increments every two weeks for middle-aged participants and every three to four weeks for elderly participants. Intensity can then be adjusted as appropriate. The final phase involves maintaining the desired health/fitness level. During this stage, current or equivalent training activities are continued with an emphasis on long-term adherence (Pollock et al., 1994; Swart, Pollock, & Brechue, 1996).

## Strength Training

A number of influential research projects have been instrumental in formulating current thought on the following optimal strength-training methods (Frontera et al., 1988; Fiatarone et al., 1990; Charette et al., 1991; Fiatarone et al., 1994; Westcott, 1995).

✓ Intensity: 70 to 80% of 1 RM (one repetition maximum: the maximum amount of resistance a subject can control during one repetition of a given exercise); alternatively, an RPE of 11 to 13

✓ Repetitions: five to 15, depending on the goals of the exerciser

✓ Progression: maintenance of 70 to 80% 1 RM, reassessed every two to four weeks

✓ Sets: one to three

✓ Speed of movement: six to nine seconds per repetition

✓ Rest: one to three seconds between repetitions; 90 to 120 seconds between sets

✓ Frequency: two to three times per week (with at least 48 hours of rest between sessions)

✓ Range of motion: complete, according to individual tolerance

Keep in mind that 1 RM may be quite low for many older adults. As a result, 70 to 80% of 1 RM will not necessarily represent what is typically considered heavy resistance. Initially performing three to five repetitions at 60 to 80% 1 RM may be sufficient for the frail to activate dormant muscle fibers and enhance muscle strength and functional movement (Hyatt, 1996). Learning and mastering new exercise movements without the use of any resistance other than gravity and body

Table 5.5

**Rating of Perceived Exertion**

| RPE | | Category Ratio Scale | |
|---|---|---|---|
| 6 | | 0 | Nothing at all |
| 7 | Very, very light | 0.5 | Very, very weak |
| 8 | | 1 | Very weak |
| 9 | Very light | 2 | Weak |
| 10 | | 3 | Moderate |
| 11 | Fairly light | 4 | Somewhat strong |
| 12 | | 5 | Strong |
| 13 | Somewhat hard | 6 | |
| 14 | | 7 | Very strong |
| 15 | Hard | 8 | |
| 16 | | 9 | |
| 17 | Very hard | 10 | Very, very strong |
| 18 | | * | Maximal |
| 19 | Very, very hard | | |
| 20 | | | |

Source: Adapted, with permission, from American College of Sports Medicine (2000). *Guidelines for Exercise Testing and Prescription* (6th ed.). Philadelphia: Lippincott Williams & Wilkins.

weight may initiate progression for low-fit exercisers. In time, low-fit exercisers may graduate to the use of resistive exercise bands, dumbbells, and strength machines (Hyatt, 1996). See Chapter 6 for more information on strength training.

## Flexibility Training

Basic recommended programming parameters (American College of Sports Medicine, 2000; Ettinger, Mitchell, & Blair, 1996; Gladwin, 1996) are outlined below:

✓ Mode: static (held) stretching, rather than ballistic (bounced) stretching

✓ Frequency: two to seven days per week

✓ Duration: position held for five to 40 seconds per stretch (depending upon the muscle or muscles being stretched)

✓ Repetitions: one to five per stretch

✓ Intensity: range gently increased in each position until mild muscular tension, but not pain, is experienced

✓ Progression: develop fuller ranges naturally with time and practice

Depending upon time constraints, individualized program goals, and the specific stretches undertaken, participants may gradually progress from lower to higher ranges of frequency, duration, and repetitions provided by these parameters. The lower ranges (for example, two to three days per week frequency) may be employed for maintenance programs, whereas progression to the higher ranges (for example, five to seven days per week frequency) should be gradual to achieve significant increases in range.

## TECHNIQUES

Only the boundaries of one's creativity limit older-adult fitness programming possibilities. In this regard, there are no substitutes for practice and experience. Because no single publication includes every beneficial exercise, enjoyable dance step, or successful combination, fitness professionals must develop and rely upon their own personal skills, talents, and resourcefulness. Those faculties can, in turn, be recruited to implement and build upon the specific techniques and sample routines provided in this chapter.

## Warm-up and Cool-down Techniques

Adequate warm-up and cool-down periods are especially important to older adults because, with age, sudden vigorous work or abrupt cessation of strenuous exercise can strain the heart. Warm-up periods of approximately 10 to 15 minutes and post-aerobic cool-down/stretch periods of approximately 15 minutes are recommended for healthy participants. Beginners and persons with special conditions such as arthritis or cardiovascular problems generally need longer warm-up and cool-down sessions.

In addition to gradually increasing circulation and heart rate, the warm-up should prepare the body for movements that will be required during the workout. All of the major joints and muscles should be gently engaged. The back should be warmed up in a vertical position before lateral spinal movements are performed. As a general rule, resistive devices should not be used during the warm-up. Although mild stretches of the calves, hamstrings, back, and other body parts may be performed toward the end of the warm-up, the warm-up should primarily be devoted to continuous rhythmic movements, and intensive stretching should be saved for the cool-down. A thorough warm-up should be completed whether the training to follow is aerobic,

resistive, stretching, some combination, or a total-body workout (Table 5.6). These principles apply whether the warm-up is undertaken in a seated or standing position, or in a gym or swimming pool. Most standing land-based warm-ups can be adapted to the chair or pool. Treadmill and stationary cycle warm-ups can be augmented by a few minutes of rhythmic movements targeting the upper body.

The cool-down period following aerobic exercise should feature slowed-down movements that allow the heart rate to gradually decrease. For this purpose, the warm-up techniques described in Table 5.6 also can be used during the cool-down phase. This type of activity should be continued until pre-aerobic respiration and heart-rate states are re-established (general rule: until the heart rate descends to fewer than 100 beats per minute). If heart rate remains high despite a lengthy cool-down period, even milder movements should be undertaken until the heart rate declines, and the participant should consult his or her physician. It is also possible that the preceding aerobic work may have been too demanding; therefore, extra attention should be paid to monitoring the body's response during future aerobic activity, which should be moderated, if necessary, to help guard against overexertion. If strength-training exercises have not already been performed during the workout, they can be introduced after the active post-aerobic cool-down: Briefly stretch, then complete the strengthening routine, followed by a few minutes of gentle cool-down activity

---

Table 5.6

**Practical Warm-up Techniques**

*Provide balance support, such as the wall or the back of a sturdy chair, as necessary.*

- ✓ Easy-paced walking and/or marching (on a treadmill, in place, or moving about)

- ✓ Slow, non-strenuous pedaling on a stationary cycle

- ✓ Relaxed dancing at a conservative tempo (for example, the Charleston, small kicks, and toe touches to the front, back, or sides)

- ✓ Rhythmic, limbering exercises (for example, heel raises, knee lifts, arm reaches, and shoulder lifts and circles) working through a full, pain-free range of motion

---

and sustained stretches involving all of the body's major joints and muscles. If strength-training work was completed prior to the aerobics segment, then the post-aerobic cool-down should proceed to the complete stretch routine. The final cool-down/stretch period is a good time to include relaxation activities. Balance work should be done when partici[pants] are warmed up but not yet feeling "spent" (i.e., it may be appropriate toward the end of aerobics-only, stre[ngth]ening-only, or flexibility-only workou[ts] but should be initiated in the *middle* [of] total-body workouts).

As with aerobic exercise, the cool-down period following intensive strengt[h] work should include a few minutes of gentle cool-down activity (e.g., walking o[r] slow cycling) prior to sustained stretching activity. This is because the cardiovascular system needs a transition period after any type of strenuous activity (Westcott & Baechle, 1998).

Various workout formats require slightly different warm-up and cool-down applications (Table 5.7).

## Chair-seated Exercise Techniques

Along with low-impact aerobics, aquatic exercise, and even fitness walking programs, chair-seated exercise classes are particularly conducive to movement-to-music techniques (Table 5.8).

In muscle-conditioning programs that involve only light (or no) extrinsic resistance, it is not necessary to work the muscle groups in a particular order. For example, the chair-seated, low-impact aerobics and aquatic exercise routines provided later in this chapter generally follow top-to-bottom sequences. Engaging opposing muscles in succession is recommended. As resistance increases, it becomes more important to work larger muscle groups earlier (when participants are less fatigued).

Regarding chair-seated exercise, avoid training people in chairs without a good reason for doing so. Weightbearing activities and movements in active functional positions are generally more effective than chair-seated work. However, as discussed earlier, there are a num[ber of reasons] for havin[g] ...

... what ... [exerci]se, many chair-seated [exer]cisers use wheelchairs. Therefore, it is important to develop the ability to work effectively using arm chairs. During chair exercise, it is critical that support be provided for the participant's back, perhaps by utilizing a pillow, pad, or rolled towel if necessary. It is equally important that the participant's feet contact the floor fully, which can be accomplished by using a book, stool, or other type of platform.

Chair exercise offers wide training intensity options. An active chair exercise class might include optional standing work using the back of the chair for balance support. It might feature energetic seated aerobic activity involving all of the limbs in broad, synchronized movement patterns. The chair also provides a secure position for the use of resistive exercise accessories such as dumbbells, exercise bands, and ankle weights. On the other hand, chair classes can serve extremely disabled participants with poor prognoses who, nonetheless, will benefit from performing limited programs composed of gentle stretching, posture, and breathing exercises.

Table 5.7

## Incorporating Warm-up and Cool-down Phases into Various Workout Formats

*Aerobics-only Workout*

✓ Warm-up: at least 10 to 15 minutes

✓ Aerobic work: approximately 30 minutes or longer

✓ Active post-aerobic cool-down: at least five to 10 minutes (or longer if needed for heart-rate recovery)

✓ Stretching/relaxation: at least five to 10 minutes, longer if time permits

*Muscle Strengthening–only Workout*

✓ Warm-up: at least 10 to 15 minutes

✓ Strength training: approximately 30 to 40 minutes*

✓ Stretching/relaxation: at least five to 10 minutes, longer if time permits

*Stretch-only Workout*

✓ Warm-up: at least 10 to 15 minutes

✓ Stretching/relaxation: approximately 30 to 40 minutes, longer if desired

*Total-body Workout with Strength Work Preceding Aerobic Work*

✓ Warm-up: at least 10 to 15 minutes

✓ Strength training: approximately 15 minutes*

✓ Brief stretching: approximately two to five minutes

✓ Repeat active rhythmic warm-up activities: approximately five minutes

✓ Aerobic work: approximately 15 to 20 minutes

✓ Active post-aerobic cool-down: at least five to 10 minutes (or longer if needed for heart-rate recovery)

✓ Final stretching/relaxation: at least five to 10 minutes, longer if time permits

*Total-body Workout with Aerobic Work Preceding Strength Work*

✓ Warm-up: at least 10 to 15 minutes

✓ Aerobic work: approximately 15 to 20 minutes

✓ Active post-aerobic cool-down: at least five to 10 minutes (or longer if needed for heart-rate recovery)

✓ Brief stretching: approximately two to five minutes

✓ Strength training: approximately 15 minutes*

✓ Final stretching/relaxation: at least five to 10 minutes, longer if time permits

* Intensive strength training should be followed by a few minutes of gentle, active cool-down activity (such as walking or stationary cycling) prior to stretching.

Note: The outlines presented above represent examples of workable exercise formats, but are not intended to cover all viable training options. To keep workout length manageable, choose numbers from each range of minutes that will combine to produce a workout lasting approximately one hour (or slightly longer). Remember that balance training techniques can be incorporated into all workout formats.

Table 5.8

**Use of Music in Older Adult Movement Classes**

*Below are several important considerations for incorporating music into group fitness classes:*

✓ Music selection should always reflect the unique preferences and physiological needs of a given exercise group.

✓ Remember that the primary purpose of using music is to motivate participants. Do not detract from their exercise experience by being a perfectionist with regard to specific dance steps and precise choreography. In senior aerobics classes, more so than in other adult classes, individual participants may not always move in sync or even on the correct beat. The instructor should maintain a flexible, fun-oriented attitude.

✓ Older-adult participants tend to prefer lower volume levels than do younger adult participants.

✓ Using instrumental music may make it easier for some participants to hear the leader's instructions.

✓ Compared to land-based programs, aquatic exercise classes call for a slightly slower music tempo because water resistance tends to slow movement. Likewise, constantly trying to move in beat with the music may be less viable during water exercise than during land exercise.

✓ Certain forms of programming (including stretch and relaxation activities) are best conducted without attempting to strictly choreograph the physical movements in compliance with a specific musical beat. In such cases, pleasing music can still be played simply to create an optimal atmosphere. This exception also may apply to chair-seated exercise classes for very frail or disoriented participants.

✓ With practice and experience, accomplished instructors develop an ability to design or adapt appropriate exercise routines using nearly any type of music. However, these general recommended tempo ranges (classified by beats per minute) for land-based senior fitness classes may prove helpful: (1) warm-ups: 100s (or fewer) to 120s; (2) aerobics: 120s to 140s; (3) post-aerobic cool-downs: 100s (or fewer) to 120s; (4) muscle conditioners: 110s to 130s; and (5) stretches: 100s (or fewer).

Following are examples of the types of exercises that can be conducted in a chair-seated class:

## CHAIR WARM-UP TECHNIQUES

✓ As time permits, include gentle posture and breathing exercises. (See Chair Posture and Breathing Techniques, page 150.)

✓ Circle feet at the ankles.

✓ Alternate turn toes inward and outward (Fig. 5.1).

✓ Perform heel raises (Fig. 5.2).

✓ Perform toe raises.

✓ Alternately curl and then lift the toes.

✓ "Walk" in place.

✓ Perform knee lifts (Fig. 5.3).

✓ Perform knee extensions (optional: combine with arm extensions) (Fig. 5.4).

✓ Move knees together and apart.

✓ Lift shoulders.

✓ Circle shoulders.

✓ Move shoulders forward and backward.

✓ Reach arms forward, upward, out to the sides, and down at the sides (Fig. 5.5).

✓ Perform arm circles and sweeps.

✓ Perform elbow and wrist bends (Fig. 5.6).

✓ Open and close hands.

✓ Perform additional hand and finger work (such as moving the fingers apart and together or simulated piano playing).

✓ Perform rocking-chair motions.

✓ Perform trunk rotation (Fig. 5.7).

✓ Perform slow, gentle head turns.

FIGURE 5.1
Toes in/out

FIGURE 5.2
Heel raise

FIGURE 5.3
Knee lift

FIGURE 5.4
Knee/arm extension

FIGURE 5.5
Outward arm reach

FIGURE 5.6
Elbow bends

Wrist bends

FIGURE 5.7
Trunk rotation

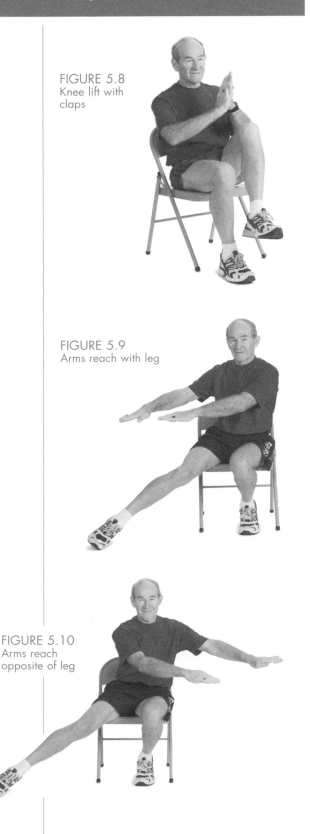

FIGURE 5.8
Knee lift with claps

FIGURE 5.9
Arms reach with leg

FIGURE 5.10
Arms reach opposite of leg

## CHAIR AEROBIC EXERCISE TECHNIQUES

Combine various leg movements with complementary arm movements. Begin the leg movements first, then add the arm motions.

✓ Alternately tap toes to the front.

✓ Alternately tap toes as far as possible out to the sides.

✓ Combine front and side toe taps to form a new leg pattern.

✓ Perform controlled kicks.

✓ Alternate knee lifts with controlled kicks.

✓ Perform crossover touches to the front.

✓ March in place, bringing knees high (be careful to touch feet to the floor lightly).

✓ Clap hands in sync with leg movements (Fig. 5.8).

✓ Snap fingers in sync with leg movements.

✓ Alternately clap hands and snap fingers in sync with leg movements.

✓ When extending either leg out to the side, reach in the same direction with both arms (Fig. 5.9).

✓ Perform the leg movement in the previous exercise, but reach in the opposite direction with both arms (Fig. 5.10).

## CHAIR POST-AEROBIC COOL-DOWN TECHNIQUES

Repeat easy-paced rhythmic movements similar to those used during the warm-up period. Then gently and briefly stretch the upper body, back, hamstrings, quadriceps, calves, and shins to prepare the joints and surrounding tissues for strength training (see Chair Stretching Techniques, page 147).

## CHAIR MUSCLE-STRENGTHENING TECHNIQUES

Resistance can be incorporated into the following exercises through the use of manual resistance (utilizing one's own hands), gentle pressure against the floor, and exercise accessories such as balls, exercise bands, and dumbbells. (Suggested means for increasing resistance are listed after each exercise.) A good alternative technique is to have participants progress to wearing ankle weights during leg work and holding them during upper-body work, especially since some participants find them easier to grasp than dumbbells.

✓ Perform upright rows (resistive tubing) if well tolerated (Fig. 5.11). This exercise is not recommended for participants who may be susceptible to shoulder impingement.

✓ Perform chest presses (resistive tubing).

✓ Perform overhead presses (resistive tubing or dumbbells).

✓ Perform overhead pull-downs (resistive tubing).

✓ Perform chin and neck retraction: Without tilting the chin upward, alternately move it back and then release (resisting with palms of hands on back of head).

✓ Perform biceps curls (resistive tubing or dumbbells) (Fig. 5.12).

✓ Perform triceps extensions (resistive tubing or dumbbells) (Fig. 5.13).

✓ Perform rotator cuff conditioning: With upper arms fixed against sides and forearms remaining parallel to the floor, alternately move hands together and then as widely apart as possible (resistive tubing or dumbbells).

✓ Perform scapular retraction: Move shoulders back bringing the shoulder blades closer together (resistance tubing).

FIGURE 5.11
Upright row

Starting position

Action

FIGURE 5.12
Biceps curl

FIGURE 5.13
Triceps extension

Starting position

Action

FIGURE 5.14
Close hands

FIGURE 5.15
Knee extension

FIGURE 5.16
Toes up as heels
press floor

✓ Perform forearm and wrist turns. For example, simulate turning a door knob (resistive tubing or dumbbells).

✓ Alternately relax and close hands (holding a soft foam ball for resistance) (Fig. 5.14).

✓ Perform hamstring curls with one side of buttocks on chair seat, thereby freeing the opposite leg for movement (resistive tubing).

✓ Perform knee extensions (resistive tubing) (Fig. 5.15).

✓ Perform thigh abduction (resistive tubing) and adduction (large ball placed between knees).

✓ Include plantarflexion and dorsiflexion by performing closed kinetic chain point/flex movements of the feet (pressing the floor for resistance) (Fig. 5.16).

## CHAIR STRETCHING TECHNIQUES

✓ Perform ear-toward-shoulder stretches: Lower ear toward shoulder, then return head to upright position (Fig. 5.17).

✓ Perform neck rotation: Turn head toward shoulder (Fig. 5.18).

✓ Perform shoulder/back release: In a slow and controlled manner, move the shoulders in a circular motion upward, back, and down, then relax (Fig. 5.19).

FIGURE 5.17
Ear toward shoulder

FIGURE 5.18
Neck rotation

FIGURE 5.19
Shoulder/back release

Starting position

Action

✓ Perform spinal extension/flexion: Begin with both hands placed on the top of the mid-thigh for spinal support, then gently extend and round the back (Fig. 5.20). (Spinal flexion is not recommended for participants with osteoporosis.)

✓ Using "ballet-styled" motions, raise both arms overhead in a high arc. Lower arms in an arc to the lap (Fig. 5.21).

✓ Stretch the trunk: Rotate torso toward one side, holding onto the same side of chair with both hands.

✓ Stretch the chest and shoulders: With arms bent at the elbows, reach behind the body trying to cross the lumbar spine (Fig. 5.22A). This can help to prepare the participant for another good exercise, the functional stretch: With hands behind the back (one elbow aimed upward and the other downward), bring the fingertips of one hand as close as possible to those of the other (Fig. 5.22B). Since many participants will not be able to touch one hand

with the other, emphasize the importance of stretching whether or not the hands actually meet.

✓ Perform hip extension: Sitting close to the front edge of the chair (positioned sideways with one side of the body facing the back of the chair, allowing free movement of the opposite hip and leg), reach foot back, angling knee down toward the floor with thigh becoming perpendicular to the floor (Fig. 5.23).

✓ Perform hamstring/gluteal stretch: With hands on thighs, extend leg forward while keeping heel on the floor. Gradually bend forward at the hips (Fig. 5.24).

✓ Stretch inner thighs: Separate knees as far apart as possible.

✓ Stretch outer thighs: Cross one leg over the opposite leg (not recommended following hip replacement surgery until specific medical clearance is granted) (Fig. 5.25).

FIGURE 5.20
Spinal extension/ flexion

Starting position

Action

FIGURE 5.21
Ballet arc

FIGURE 5.22
Chest and shoulder
stretches

A. Arms cross lumbar spine

B. Functional stretch

FIGURE 5.23
Hip extension

FIGURE 5.24
Hamstring/gluteal
stretch

FIGURE 5.25
Outer thigh stretch

✓ Stretch shins/calves with open kinetic chain point/flex: Lift foot (or both feet) and point toes (Fig. 5.26A), then slowly pull toes back toward the shin (Fig. 5.26B).

## CHAIR POSTURE AND BREATHING TECHNIQUES

The following exercises are also enjoyable relaxation activities. They may be incorporated into the warm-up and/or cool-down segments of a class. (Of course, proper breathing instructions, including cautions against breath-holding, are essential during all modes of exercise.)

✓ Achieve neutral posture by moving the pelvis forward and backward until the most comfortable position is achieved. Then move the ribs and thoracic spine forward and backward until the most comfortable position is achieved. While keeping the chin parallel to the floor (not tilted up or tucked under), move the head forward and back until the most comfortable position is achieved.

✓ Perform weight distribution exercise: With palms up, place hands under the pelvic bones (the bony tips of the ischium). Adjust so that weight feels evenly distributed on both hands.

✓ Conduct posture-awareness exercise: Alternately slouch and then sit up straight, consciously noting the difference between how the two positions feel.

✓ Stabilize the spine: Reach up toward the ceiling with one arm while reaching down toward the floor with the other. Straighten the arms as much as possible, trying to reach through the length of the fingertips. Repeat with arm positions reversed.

✓ Perform deep breathing exercise: Take a full breath, then breathe out through pursed lips, allowing the flow of air to make a soft sound as it is pushed out. Expel the last of the air by pretending to blow out a candle. After all air has been released, pause for a moment, then repeat.

✓ Inhale normally, but exhale slowly: Breathe in for a count of two, then exhale for a count of four. Breathe in for a count of two, then exhale for a count of six. Breathe in for a count of two, then exhale for a count of eight. Breathe in for a count of two, then exhale for a count of 10. Repeat.

FIGURE 5.26
Shin and calf stretches

A. Plantarflex (Point)

B. Dorsiflex (Flex)

✓ Perform intercostal breathing exercise: Place hands on the lower rib cage with fingers touching. Inhale deeply so that the rib cage expands and fingers separate. Repeat.

Note: See Aquatic Programming Techniques, page 162, and Balance/Coordination Training Techniques, page 173, for activities that may be performed while standing and using the back of a chair for balance support.

## Traditional Aerobics Class Techniques

Traditional aerobics is the cardiovascular activity of choice for many older adults. Most classes also incorporate strengthening and flexibility work. Below are specific precautions that should be observed (in addition to all basic safety guidelines) to ensure a safe and enjoyable class:

✓ When conducting a thorough warm-up, pay special attention to warming up the feet and ankles prior to conducting choreographed aerobic activities.

✓ Begin with base steps, and always return to a neutral starting position before initiating new patterns.

✓ Use gradual transitions.

✓ Cue clearly and well in advance.

✓ Teach footwork before arm work.

✓ Vary moves to avoid over-stressing weightbearing joints. Always use low-impact choreography.

✓ Balance use of the body (for example, knee lifts with leg curls).

✓ Balance directional changes (for example, front and back with right and left).

✓ Balance moving and stationary patterns.

✓ Avoid quick changes that might compromise balance.

✓ Avoid abrupt or severe turns or twisting that might compromise joints (particularly the knee joint).

✓ Avoid a competitive atmosphere.

✓ Avoid the use of resistance equipment during the aerobics portion of the workout. (Reserve it for the muscle-strengthening segment of the workout.)

## AEROBICS CLASS WARM-UP TECHNIQUES

Refer to the earlier section on warm-up and cool-down techniques. Also note that most of the warm-up activities listed in the chair-seated section can be adapted to a standing position for use in traditional aerobics classes.

## AEROBICS CLASS TECHNIQUES

Begin with the leg motions, then add the arm motions.

✓ March: Keeping fists loose, alternately swing each elbow back while marching in place or moving about (Fig. 5.27).

✓ Lift knees: Alternate raising one knee and then the other toward the front as

FIGURE 5.27
March

FIGURE 5.28
Knee lift

FIGURE 5.29
Lift-kicks

FIGURE 5.30
Touch across

FIGURE 5.31
Touch behind

FIGURE 5.32
Heel-front

FIGURE 5.33
Toe-front

FIGURE 5.34
Walking with arm swings

high as feels comfortable, while pushing both arms in various directions (Fig. 5.28).

✓ Perform lift-kicks: Without locking the knees, alternately raise one leg and then the other toward the front while sweeping both arms back and forth across the front (Fig. 5.29).

✓ Touch across: Alternately touch the toes of one foot in front of the other foot while performing alternate punches with the arms (Fig. 5.30).

✓ Touch behind: Same movement as above, but touch the toes of one foot behind the other while performing scissor motions with the arms (Fig. 5.31).

✓ Perform heel-fronts (or toe-fronts): Alternate touching one heel (or the toes of one foot) and then the other heel (or toes of the other foot) to the front while reaching forward or clapping with the hands (Figs. 5.32 & 5.33).

✓ Perform toe-outs (or heel-outs): Same as above except touch toes or heels out toward the sides while pushing with the arms or performing side arm raises.

✓ Create combinations: Mix and match the movements described above to develop new patterns and variations.

✓ Perform specific combination #1 (Fig. 5.34): Walk in place, alternately taking slow steps for a specified number of beats, then taking quick steps for a compatible number of beats. Simultaneously

FIGURE 5.35
Leg curl with elbow pull

Starting position

Action

FIGURE 5.36
Side-step

Starting position

Action

perform alternate arm swings to the front and back.

✓ Perform specific combination #2 (Fig. 5.35): Take three steps in place (foot 1, foot 2, foot 1) followed by a leg curl using leg 2; then take three steps in place (foot 2, foot 1, foot 2) followed by a leg curl using leg 1. Repeat while holding the arms bent at chest level during the steps and then pulling both elbows back during the curls. For variety, substitute knee lifts for leg curls.

✓ Perform traveling technique #1 (Fig. 5.36): Perform side-stepping by taking several side steps to the right followed by an equal number of side steps to the left (back to starting position). Add any com-

patible arm movements, such as shoulder touches.

✓ Perform traveling technique #2: Take several steps forward followed by an equal number of steps back (to starting position). Add any compatible arm movements, such as biceps curls. (Individuals with balance problems should not step backward; they should step forward in any direction, take several steps in place while turning to face a new direction, then step forward in that direction so they are always facing the direction in which they are moving.)

✓ Perform traveling technique #3: Add variety to side steps or forward-back patterns by performing a low number of knee lifts, small kicks, leg curls, shallow squats, or some other special movement while standing in place at each end of the side-stepping or forward-back pattern.

✓ Organize group maneuvers: Achieve interaction through partner or whole-group movements. For example, have couples link arms at the elbows and then switch partners square-dance style, hold hands to form a circle, and then use side steps to turn the circle like a wheel or form a conga line.

✓ Consider creative alternatives: Use the safety guidelines in Table 5.1 to modify line and folk dances, as necessary, to develop senior-appropriate aerobic dance patterns.

## AEROBICS CLASS POST-AEROBICS COOL-DOWN TECHNIQUES

Perform easy-paced rhythmic movements similar to those performed during the warm-up period. Then gently and briefly stretch the upper body, back, hamstrings, quadriceps, calves, and shins to prepare the joints and surrounding tissues for strength training (see Aerobics Class Standing and Floor Exercises for Stretching, page 159).

## AEROBICS CLASS STANDING AND FLOOR EXERCISES FOR MUSCLE STRENGTHENING

Note: See Aquatic Programming Techniques, page 162, and Balance/Coordination Training Techniques, page 173, for standing exercises that can be performed during aerobics classes by using a ballet barre, the wall, or another stable means of balance support. Also, see the chair-seated section for exercise band activities and additional muscle-strengthening exercises that can be adapted to a floor-seated and/or standing position.

Many older adults can safely benefit by progressing to the use of dumbbells during the following shoulder, back, arm, and chest exercises:

✓ Perform shoulder lifts and circles (Fig. 5.37).

✓ Perform side lateral raises (only to a height below shoulder level and if well tolerated) (Fig. 5.38).

FIGURE 5.37
Shoulder lift

FIGURE 5.38
Lateral raise

FIGURE 5.39
Upright row

Starting position

Action

FIGURE 5.40
Military press

Starting position

Action

✓ Include upright rowing if well tolerated (not recommended for participants who may be susceptible to shoulder impingement) (Fig. 5.39).

✓ Perform military presses (being cautious not to permit excessive vertical loading of the spine, particularly for participants with back problems) (Fig. 5.40).

✓ Perform biceps curls (Fig. 5.41).

✓ Perform triceps extensions (to the back for lighter intensity; higher intensities can be achieved through upward extension) (Fig. 5.42).

✓ Perform supine chest presses (Fig. 5.43).

✓ Incorporate chest/back exercise variations: Additional chest and back exercises that do not require the use of weights, bands, or other forms of resistive equipment include bent-knee push-ups on the floor, wall push-ups, and cat curls on the floor or in a back-supported standing position. It is not uncommon for older adults to experience discomfort in an all-fours position due to compression of the knee joints.

FIGURE 5.41
Biceps curl

FIGURE 5.42
Beginner's triceps
extension

Starting position

Action

FIGURE 5.43
Chest press

Starting position

Action

FIGURE 5.44
Diagonal curl-up

FIGURE 5.45
Buttocks lift

FIGURE 5.46
Buttocks squeeze

FIGURE
5.47
Prone leg lift

✓ Perform modified vertical and diagonal curl-ups (smoothly rolling the upper body forward to raise it just high enough to clear the shoulder blades off the floor). Take care not to hyperflex the neck (Fig. 5.44).

✓ Include lower abdominal exercise: Lie on back with arms at sides, palms on the floor, and legs held above the body. Being careful not to swing or rock the legs, lift buttocks slightly off the floor, then return to the starting position (Fig. 5.45). If an easier alternative is needed, perform pelvic tilts: With knees bent and feet on the floor, lift the buttocks slightly while pressing the lower back to the floor and contracting the abdominals.

✓ Perform buttocks squeezes: Alternately squeeze and relax the buttocks muscles (Fig. 5.46).

Many older adults can safely benefit by progressing to the use of leg weights during the following five exercises:

✓ Condition back of the thigh: In a prone position, perform small leg lifts. The knee also may be flexed and extended in this position. If needed, a towel or thin pillow may be placed beneath the abdominal/hip area to help maintain a neutral spine position (Fig. 5.47).

✓ Condition front of the thigh: Alternately flex and extend the leg forward (Fig. 5.48).

FIGURE 5.48
Flex/extend forward

✓ Condition the inner thigh: From a side-lying position, perform lifts with the lower leg (not recommended following hip replacement surgery until specific medical clearance is granted) (Fig. 5.49).

✓ Condition the outer thigh: From a side-lying position, perform lifts with the upper leg (Fig. 5.50).

✓ Condition shins and calves: Alternately raise heels and then toes (utilizing balance support as necessary) (Fig. 5.51).

## AEROBICS CLASS STANDING AND FLOOR EXERCISES FOR STRETCHING

Note: Many of the stretches described in the Chair Stretching Techniques section (page 147) can be adapted to a standing and/or floor-exercise position.

✓ Perform range-of-motion work for the neck: Perform head turns, tilts to the sides (but not back, which may over-compress the cervical vertebrae), and nods (Fig. 5.52). Nods should be performed conservatively without pressing the chin all the way toward the chest (which may put excessive pressure on the neck area or over-stretch muscles of the cervical spine area). The safest approach for persons with cervical spinal osteoporosis or arthritis is to avoid nodding exercises.

✓ Perform shoulder stretch: While resting one arm in the bend of the opposite elbow, allow it to stretch gently across the chest (Fig. 5.53).

✓ Perform chest stretch: With fingertips touching shoulders, move elbows back (Fig. 5.54).

FIGURE 5.49
Lower-leg lift

FIGURE 5.50
Upper-leg lift

FIGURE 5.51
Heel raise

FIGURE 5.52
Nod

FIGURE 5.53
Shoulder stretch

FIGURE 5.54
Chest stretch

✓ Perform biceps stretch: Extend both arms upward or downward (Fig. 5.55).

✓ Perform triceps stretch: Place one hand at the back of the neck. Grasp the elbow with the opposite hand, then pull it gently and slowly toward the back of the head (only so far as feels comfortable) (Fig. 5.56).

✓ Perform midsection and back stretch: With knees bent, reach both arms overhead. Older adults who are able to keep their lower back from arching upward from the floor can maximize this stretch by simultaneously stretching the legs and pointing the toes in the opposite direction on the floor (Fig. 5.57).

✓ Perform hamstrings/buttocks stretch: Gently pull the legs toward the chest (being careful to place hands behind, rather than around, the knees) (Fig. 5.58).

✓ Perform quadriceps stretch: Lying on the stomach, bend one leg upward until a pleasant stretch is felt at the front of the thigh. It is easier to relax into an effective stretch if one holds the foot of the bent leg with the hand on the same side of the body; however, trying to do so may exceed arm reach and thereby hyperflex the knee joint. A practical alternative is to loop a towel around the leg to extend the participant's range of motion and allow the control necessary to ease into

FIGURE 5.55
Biceps stretch

FIGURE 5.56
Triceps stretch

FIGURE 5.57
Supine stretch

Figure 5.58
Leg hug

an optimally stretched position. The quadriceps may also be stretched in a side-lying position (Fig. 5.59).

✓ Perform standing calf stretch: With both hands on the back of a chair, lean forward while keeping both heels on or near the floor (Fig. 5.60). (Avoid sinking into a swayback posture and hyperextending the knees or elbows.) The shins and calves can be stretched in a floor-exercise position by slowly performing and holding open kinetic chain point/flex movements with the feet (Fig. 5.61). Likewise, ankle range of motion can be promoted in various positions, including on the floor, by performing slow open kinetic chain circular movements of the feet.

✓ Perform inner-thigh stretch: With relaxed knees, separate legs as far apart as feels natural. If this position is uncomfortable, extend one leg at a time slightly toward the side while bending (but not hyperflexing) the opposite knee toward the front. Stretch several parts of the body by placing both hands on the floor in front of you for support while relaxing the upper body slightly forward (Fig. 5.62).

✓ Perform outer-thigh stretch: With one leg bent and crossed over the other, press the knee gently toward the floor with the opposite hand. Press conservatively so that only a pleasant stretch, not a pulling sensation, is felt along the outer thigh. Variation #1: If the hip is allowed to cross over, the lower back will be stretched (Fig. 5.63). Variation #2: Increase the stretch for the hip area by gently pulling the bent, crossed leg toward the chest (a supine piriformis stretch). This exercise is not recommended following hip replacement surgery until specific medical clearance is granted.

Note: If desired, incorporate activities from Chair Posture and Breathing Techniques, page 150, Relaxation Class Techniques, page 171, and Balance/Coordination Training Techniques, page 173, into the final cool-down stretch period.

FIGURE 5.59
Side-lying quadriceps stretch. A towel or resistance band can be used to slightly increase range of motion.

FIGURE 5.60
Standing calf stretch

FIGURE 5.61
Toes-pointed stretch

FIGURE 5.62
Wide-leg stretch

FIGURE 5.63
Cross-over stretch

# Aquatic Programming Techniques

While the same principles and safety guidelines that govern other forms of exercise pertain to aquatic exercise as well, several special considerations also apply:

✓ Complete lifeguard certification or have a qualified lifeguard present during classes.

✓ Remove unnecessary obstacles from the pool deck and sweep it free of slippery water spots. Regularly inspect the condition of the pool and its railings, ladders, and shower areas.

✓ Never touch electronic sound equipment while wet or when standing on a damp surface.

✓ A flat pool floor surface is preferable to one that slopes. Wearing non-skid aqua shoes can help prevent slipping and may offer extra cushioning for the joints.

✓ In outdoor pools, the skin should be protected by sunscreen. Sunglasses can safeguard the eyes, and tinted goggles are available for those whose eyes are sensitive to pool chemicals.

✓ A water temperature of 87 to 88° F (30 to 31° C) works well for most older adult group class designs.

✓ Instructors who teach on the pool deck (instead of in the water) can see, and be seen better by, participants. A good view of the instructor is important because pool areas often have poor acoustics and are made noisy by splashing water. Also, some participants who normally use hearing aids will not wear them during water classes.

✓ It is generally considered more viable to monitor intensity level during water aerobics by RPE rather than by heart-rate counting (Sanders, 2002).

✓ Accessories made for in-pool use such as water bells, paddles, webbed gloves, and ankle cuffs can be incorporated to increase intensity and/or to help participants float during selected activities.

✓ Exercises that require holding onto the wall to keep both feet above the pool floor can strain the upper body. Seek alternative positions in which the participant floats or keeps at least one foot in contact with the pool floor.

✓ As in all older adult training, avoid needlessly hyperextending the joints. During standing leg lifts, for example, remind participants not to support their body weight on a hyperextended knee.

✓ As always, emphasize neutral spine techniques; one swimming pool exercise that can aggravate a bad back is flutter kicks with unsafe hyperextension of the back.

✓ Because water's buoyancy takes most of the impact out of exercise, many older adults who cannot safely jog, jump, or kick on land can successfully do so in the pool. Still, all senior adults should monitor the response of joint tissue to movements that involve hopping or bouncing—even in water. If joint stress or pain is experienced, substitute lower-impact activities.

## AQUATIC WARM-UP TECHNIQUES

Refer to the foregoing section on warm-up and cool-down techniques. Also note that most of the warm-up activities listed in the chair-seated section can be adapted to a standing position for use in aquatic exercise classes. The water-walking activities described below can be used during the warm-up or the aerobic segment, depending upon participant performance level. The warm-up period is an excellent time to practice personal safety skills such as sculling for balance and recovering in-balance posture (with both feet securely positioned beneath the body).

## AQUATIC AEROBIC-TRAINING TECHNIQUES

The aerobics segment of the workout can consist of water walking, choreographed aerobic movements, or some

combination of both. To control intensity, a general rule is to alternate periods of more strenuous work (such as energetic knee lifts) that last up to approximately one minute with periods of less strenuous work (such as jogging in place) lasting approximately 30 seconds. If at all possible, it may be desirable to conduct more than one class to accommodate the training needs of participants at different fitness levels.
Note: Some movement combinations from Traditional Aerobics Class Techniques, page 151, can be adapted for use in the water. Coordinate arm and leg movement for optimal balance and stabilization.

Water walking activities and variations:
✓ Walk in the center of the pool or while touching the pool wall for balance support.

✓ Walk in place, forward, back, sideways, diagonally, in a circular pattern, or from one side of the pool to the other and back.

✓ Walk on the entire foot, on the toes, on the heels, with toes aimed straight ahead, turned out, or turned in.

✓ Walk with legs in a naturally extended position, or with knees slightly bent.

✓ Walk in a natural forward-moving fashion, as though walking a line, with high knee lifts, knee lifts out toward the sides, extra long strides, or with controlled kicking motions.

✓ Rather than walking, jog, run, or leap through the water.

✓ Along with lower-body movements, perform various arm motions such as the crawl stroke, the back stroke, the breast stroke, the dog paddle, punches, pushes, and sweeps.

✓ Choose a depth at which the participant can control their body's buoyancy in the water while maintaining an effective speed of movement.

Other aquatic aerobic moves:
✓ Hop on both feet (touching down as lightly as possible without hyperextending the knees upon landing) (Fig. 5.64).

✓ Alternately hop on one foot, then the other (without exceeding four consecutive hops per foot for joint safety).

FIGURE 5.64
Hop

Starting position                    Action

✓ Perform chorus-line-style kicks (Fig. 5.65).

✓ Perform jumping jacks with different types of arm movements and jumping jack variations, such as alternately extending one leg and then the other upon landing (Fig. 5.66).

✓ Perform alternate high knee lifts to the front and/or sides.

✓ Perform frog jumps: With knees to the sides, pull both feet up as high as possible under the body, then return to standing posture (Fig. 5.67).

✓ Perform bobbing movements: Extend left leg back while right knee remains bent to the front, then quickly reverse leg positions. Continue alternating, being careful to keep the front knee behind the front toes and the back knee relaxed upon landing (Fig. 5.68).

✓ Practice skilled movements: If participants can swim and tread water, consider including lap swimming or treading in shallow water so that it is possible to stand occasionally as necessary.

FIGURE 5.65
Kick

FIGURE 5.66
Jumping jack variation

Starting position

Action

## AQUATIC POST-AEROBICS COOL-DOWN TECHNIQUES

Perform easy-paced rhythmic movements similar to those performed during the warm-up period. In general, broad sweeping movements are better than short, reduced-range movements. Gently and briefly stretch the upper body, back, hamstrings, quadriceps, calves, and shins to prepare the joints and surrounding tissues for strength training. (See Aquatic Stretching Techniques, page 168.) Keep active enough for participants to stay warm; for example, alternate stretching exercises with lower-body movements such as walking or easy-paced jogging.

## AQUATIC MUSCLE-STRENGTH-ENING TECHNIQUES

For upper-body work, participants should assume a stance in which they feel stable and balanced. Many older adults feel most secure with feet a comfortable distance apart and one foot in front of the other.

FIGURE 5.67
Frog jump

FIGURE 5.68
Bob

✓ Perform biceps/triceps strengthener: Alternately flex and extend the elbow against water resistance. Start with arms at sides, palms up; with upper arms remaining against the body and elbows remaining pointed downward, bend the elbows and raise the hands toward the shoulders; while hands are at shoulder level, turn the palms forward and straighten the elbows, pressing hands down to starting position. Then turn palms up and repeat (Fig. 5.69).

✓ Incorporate shoulder strengtheners: Perform arm lifts in various directions (e.g., toward the front or back).

✓ Include chest/upper-back strengthener #1: In a scissor-like manner, cross arms in front of the body, open out to the sides, then cross behind the back. Continue alternating. To add resistance, turn palms as necessary to ensure maximum water displacement throughout the movements (Fig. 5.70).

✓ Include chest/upper-back strengthener #2: Start with arms out to the sides, palms forward; move arms together in front of the body; return to starting position, consciously squeezing shoulder blades together as arms move back (Fig. 5.71).

FIGURE 5.69
Biceps/triceps strengthener

FIGURE 5.70
Arm scissors

✓ Include upper-body multi-muscle strengthener: Perform pool wall push-ups.

✓ Perform trunk stabilizer: Start with both arms extended together in front of the chest with palms touching; pull arms toward one side and then the other, allowing the torso to turn gently from side to side with the arms (Fig. 5.72).

✓ Perform abdominal/back strengthener: Simply undertake walking activities in relatively shallow water (e.g., waist deep) while focusing intently on maintaining optimal posture.

The following exercises, which use the pool wall as a ballet barre are suitable for beginners. Progression may involve performing increasingly more challenging variations of the work: (1) without touching the wall, (2) while holding foam dumbbells, (3) while wearing webbed gloves, (4) while traveling, and (5) while keeping hands out of the water.

✓ Perform front-of-thigh strengthener: Using the pool wall as a ballet barre (touch the wall for balance, but do not lean on it), perform bent-knee leg lifts to the front as well as knee flexion/extension to the front (Fig. 5.73).

FIGURE 5.71
Arms out/in

FIGURE 5.72
Turn

FIGURE 5.73
Bent-knee lift

FIGURE 5.74
Leg bend toward back

FIGURE 5.75
Side lift

Figure 5.76
Cross lift

✓ Perform back-of-thigh strengthener: Using the pool wall as a ballet barre, perform backward leg lifts by bending at the knee to raise the foot up toward the buttocks (Fig. 5.74).

✓ Perform outer-thigh strengthener: Using the pool wall as a ballet barre, perform leg lifts to the side (Fig. 5.75).

✓ Perform inner-thigh strengthener: Using the pool wall as a ballet barre, perform leg lifts in front of the opposite leg (not recommended following hip replacement surgery until specific medical clearance is granted) (Fig. 5.76).

✓ Perform shin/calf strengthener: Using the pool wall as a ballet barre, alternately raise the toes, then the heels (Fig. 5.77).

Note: Some of the strengthening and stretching exercises from Chair-seated Exercise Techniques, page 139, and Traditional Aerobics Class Techniques, page 151, also can be adapted for use in the water.

## AQUATIC STRETCHING TECHNIQUES

During flexibility work, keep active enough to stay warm; for example, alternate stretching exercises with lower-body movements such as walking or easy-paced jogging.

✓ Stretch the neck: Perform head turns, tilts, and/or nods.

✓ Stretch biceps: Fully extend both arms, either overhead or down in the water.

✓ Stretch triceps: Place one hand on the nape of the neck and the other on the opposite elbow. Slowly slide the hand down the neck until the elbow points up (Fig. 5.78). To vary this exercise, slide the hand down the forearm to meet the other hand at the nape of the neck. Reach both hands down the back.

✓ Stretch upper-back/shoulders: Interlace fingers, palms facing forward, and stretch both arms to the front. Then relax arms down by the sides and perform slow shoulder circles, first backward, then forward (Fig. 5.79).

FIGURE 5.77
Toe/heel raises

FIGURE 5.78
Elbows-up stretch

FIGURE 5.79
Upper-body stretch

✓ Perform back/posture stretch: Press the back to the pool wall while standing as tall as possible. Keeping the rib cage elevated, press the shoulders back and down while reaching toward the floor with the fingers.

✓ Stretch chest: With hands on hips, gently press shoulders back.

✓ Stretch trunk: Stand with side to the pool wall and feet together at arm's length from the edge. Touch wall with the arm closest to the wall (extended but relaxed). First pull hips away from the wall while reaching in overhead with the outside arm. Then, with the rib cage elevated, reach up toward midline. Finally, pull hips toward wall while reaching down and out with the same arm. Repeat facing opposite direction (Fig. 5.80).

✓ Stretch quadriceps: With the knee aimed downward, raise the foot to the back. To better relax into the stretch, grasp the ankle with the hand that is on the same side of the body. If grasping the ankle is difficult, try grasping the heel. Do not hyperextend the back or

FIGURE 5.80
Trunk stretch

Starting position

Action

FIGURE 5.81
Standing leg hug

FIGURE 5.82
Stretch-over

touch the heel to the buttock (which hyperflexes the knee).

✓ Perform hamstring/gluteal stretch: With hands placed behind (not around) the knee, first perform a gentle leg hug, then extend the leg at the knee until a pleasant stretch is felt along the back of the thigh (Fig. 5.81). (If balance support is needed, stand with back to the pool wall.)

✓ Stretch outer thigh: Cross one leg in front of the other until a pleasant stretch is felt along the outer thigh (not recommended following hip replacement surgery until specific medical clearance is granted) (Fig. 5.82).

✓ Stretch inner thigh: Facing the wall with feet apart, shift hips to the side, causing one leg to bend as the other stretches. Repeat in opposite direction (Fig. 5.83).

✓ Stretch shin: Using the pool wall as a ballet barre, point toes (Fig. 5.84).

✓ Stretch calf: Using the pool wall as a ballet barre, flex foot (Fig. 5.85).

## Relaxation Class Techniques

Relaxation activities can be incorporated into any type of fitness programming format, whether it be a seated exercise class, a low-impact aerobics class, aquatic exercise, fitness walking, or personal training. They are best included at the end of the exercise session. On the other hand, you can conduct classes fully devoted to relaxation. However, it should be made clear to participants that relaxation programming alone does not constitute a complete, well-balanced fitness regimen and that they will need to augment the class with other forms of exercise.

It is important to create an atmosphere conducive to relaxation programming. If practical, dim the lighting somewhat and block out sounds from outside the immediate area. Use smooth, calming music such as symphonic selections. Or try audiotapes or CDs featuring captured

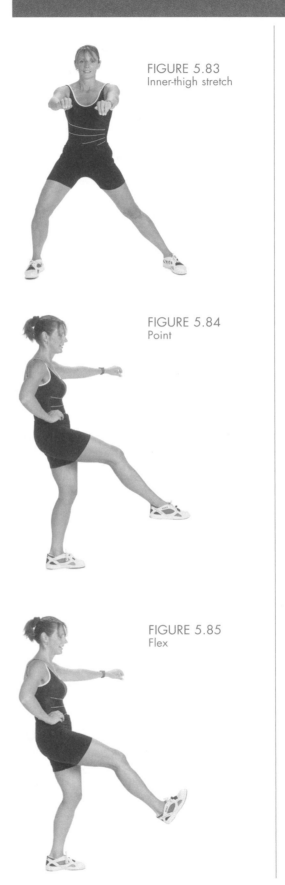

FIGURE 5.83
Inner-thigh stretch

FIGURE 5.84
Point

FIGURE 5.85
Flex

nature sounds such as wind, rain, muted thunder, and rolling waves. Probably the most essential key to success will be the instructor's voice and demeanor. Speak slowly, quietly, and soothingly. Avoid sudden or unnecessary movements, and any tendency to rush. Do not allow any hurried sense to arise during relaxation activity.

Elements of the following relaxation techniques can be used singly during the final cool-down/stretch segment of an exercise session or in combination within the context of a more comprehensive relaxation program.

✓ In aquatic settings, the water itself can be a relaxation programming device. Water has a pleasurable stroking effect as it surrounds, massages, and laps against the body. Setting aside several minutes for complete personal relaxation at the end of aquatics class is a good way to capitalize on the water's natural properties. Allow participants a peaceful, unstructured period to simply float or lounge in the water, or perform breathing exercises or their choice of quiet activity.

✓ Stretching and gentle range-of-motion activities can be especially relaxing. Refer to all of the stretches described in this chapter as a resource. Also, yoga-styled classes are renowned for their ability to relax and de-stress participants.

✓ Soft, tactile, or aromatic accessories can be utilized to promote reposeful, enjoyable sensations. For example, sensory-based activities might include luxuriously applying hand lotion or handling a plush, feathery, or fur-like fabric or object.

✓ Relaxation methods can involve techniques as simple as including poignant lines of poetry, brief inspirational quotations, thoughts for the day, simple stress-management tips, or positive self-talk activities during the final moments of a class.

✓ Relaxing self-massage can be performed in a number of ways. For example, have participants lightly sweep their fingers through their hair, gently rub their skeletal muscles, and softly caress their skin. Do not massage the neck (except quite lightly at the very back) since this can interrupt blood flow.

Note: Gentle posture and breathing exercises can be a valuable addition to relaxation programming. For seven good activity examples, refer to Chair Posture and Breathing Techniques, page 150.

Below are some additional specific techniques:

✓ Perform gentle posture activity #1: In a chair-seated position, sit back on the hips. With both hands placed on top of the thighs to provide support for the spine, lean forward and back several times (bending from the hips, not from the waist), then lean from side to side several times. Continue adjusting the position until the upper-body weight feels evenly distributed.

✓ Perform gentle posture activity #2: In a chair or floor-seated position, interlace fingers with palms facing forward. Raise arms overhead. Hold for one or two long breaths, then relax and lower arms. Repeat.

✓ Perform gentle posture activity #3: In a chair or floor-seated position, place hands behind head. Move elbows back while pulling the chin in. Keeping chin parallel to the floor (not tipped upward or tucked down), gently move the head back into the hands. Slowly turn head to the right, then to the left. Repeat.

✓ Perform breathing exercise #1: In a chair or floor-seated position, inhale deeply, attempting to fill the lungs. Note the pressure of the breath on the chest and abdomen as the air moves toward the lungs. Slowly exhale. Repeat.

✓ Perform breathing exercise #2: In a chair or floor-seated position, with both hands placed on the top of the thighs to support the spine, lean forward from the hips while exhaling as fully as possible. While returning to an upright position, attempt to refill the lungs with air by sniffing "like a dog" five or six times. Repeat.

✓ Perform breathing exercise #3: In a chair or floor-seated position, pull both elbows backward while inhaling deeply. With back slightly arched, hold breath for a count of five. Push air out by gently contracting the abdominal muscles. Repeat several times.

✓ Conduct simple, progressive muscle relaxation activities. For example, while lying flat on the back with eyes closed, begin with the head and move down to the toes. Mentally focus on one muscle group at a time, first noting any tightness present, then inhaling fully. While slowly exhaling, envision the tension flowing out of the muscles and completely out of the body along with the breath. When the procedure is completed, rest quietly for a few minutes before getting up.

✓ Another method of progressive relaxation: While seated or lying down, focus on each muscle group, working down from head to toe. First, tense the muscle for approximately two seconds, noticing how this feels; second, release the tension, again noticing how this feels; third, pause and reflect upon the difference between the two sensations before moving on to the next muscle group.

✓ Incorporate pleasurable mental imagery to help participants relax. Developing effective graphic description skills may take practice. Have participants recline and close their eyes. Remember to speak in a slow, soothing manner. Note that in the following example references to the senses of touch, sight, hearing, and smell are all woven into the imaginary scenario: *Feel yourself gliding easily on your back down a broad, lazy stream in the forest. The stream is so clear and pure that if you turn your head only slightly, you can discern through its shear, emerald waters thousands of tiny polished stones scattered like precious jewels on the stream bed. Without a care in the world, you can feel the sunlight warming your skin and the cool water caressing your arms, your legs, your back, and your sides as you float peacefully along the shimmering stream. Feel the gentle tickle of a light breeze playfully teasing at your face. Hear the echo of a bird's song as it drifts down from the thick, green foliage of the surrounding forest. Breathe deeply the fresh, sweet fragrance of the velvety moss and ferns that grace the water's edge; breathe deeply the heavy perfume of exotic flora blooming recklessly along the stream's verdant banks. Just float and dream ... float and dream ... as the forest's natural treasures lull you into a peaceful reverie.*

## Balance/Coordination Training Techniques

As in other forms of senior fitness programming, balance training's possibilities are limited only by the fitness professional's skills and creativity. Certain types of sports, such as tennis, promote balance skills in people who can safely enjoy them. Even equine therapy is used by qualified professionals to increase the balance and coordination of disabled participants. Various types of ball play, such as tossing, catching, batting, and aiming, can be implemented for coordination and balance purposes. (In chair-seated classes, a partially inflated beach ball works particularly well.) Tai chi is another excellent means of balance/coordination training.

Performing balance work in a swimming pool can lessen participants' fear of falling. Land-based balance activities can be undertaken while facing a wall, ballet barre, or the back of a sturdy chair for support. In some land-based exercise groups, participants are capable of providing one another with mutual support during balance training by working as partners or standing in a circle while holding hands.

Many factors can contribute to imbalance. Therefore, various interventions ranging from disease management, medication adjustments, glasses/eyesight correction, and many forms of physical activity training may be appropriate in addressing such problems. Participating in a complete, well-balanced fitness program is probably the most critical factor for maintaining and preserving adequate balance. However, there are certain techniques that can be employed that are specifically designed to recruit and sharpen balance mechanisms. Several of these are listed below.

Balance work should be conducted *after* participants are thoroughly warmed up but *before* they are noticeably fatigued (e.g., at about the midpoint of total-body workouts). The following exercises should be done in a standing position with balance support available. Safety should be the primary consideration during balance training and in all other forms of older adult physical training.

✓ Stand with feet approximately shoulder-width apart and extend arms out, slightly forward and lower than the shoulders. Lift both heels off the floor and try to hold the position for 10 seconds.

✓ Standing with feet together, hold arms in the same position as described in the previous exercise. Place one foot on the inside of the opposing ankle and try to hold the position for 10 seconds (Fig. 5.86). Repeat with hands behind the back.

✓ Perform a one-legged stand with one foot raised to the back (the non-weight-bearing knee flexed 90°). Try to maintain the position for a minimum of three seconds. The long-term goal is to decrease the need for balance support and to hold the position for 10 seconds. However, as necessary, allow the hands to contact the provided support apparatus.

✓ Perform the same exercise as above, but raise one foot to the front (the non-weight-bearing knee flexed and lifted approximately as high as the hip) (Fig. 5.87).

✓ Transfer body weight onto one foot and lift the other slightly off the floor. Reverse, then continue alternating weight-shift/foot-lift movements from one side to the other.

✓ With the knee straight but not hyperextended, execute single (relatively small) leg raises to the front, then the back. Continue alternating front to back (Fig. 5.88).

✓ Assume the same position as in the previous exercise, but alternate small leg rais-

FIGURE 5.86
Foot on opposite ankle

FIGURE 5.87
Knee flexed to front

FIGURE 5.88
Front/back lifts

es to the side with raises toward the inside (slightly past the central axis of the body if no hip range restrictions exist).

✓ Design a balance-training program based on scientific research findings, such as those derived from a sensory-training project conducted by noted motor control specialist Marjorie Woollacott (1995). In that study, older adults were instructed to stand under eight different conditions, 10 seconds in each stance, five times each, 10 different times per day, for 10 days. The eight conditions involved standing:

1. on a firm surface, eyes open, head neutral

2. on a firm surface, eyes closed, head neutral

3. on a firm surface, eyes open, head tilted back

4. on a firm surface, eyes closed, head tilted back

5. on a foam surface, eyes open, head neutral

6. on a foam surface, eyes closed, head neutral

7. on a foam surface, eyes open, head tilted back

8. on a foam surface, eyes closed, head tilted back

Balance mechanisms were called upon as progressively more difficult conditions provided lesser degrees of accurate sensory feedback from the environment. At the end of the trial, sway had decreased under all conditions, significantly so in the most difficult positions. Improvement occurred in the ability to stand on one leg, a skill that transfers into routine tasks of daily living.

The investigators' experience suggests that this training should be ongoing. When the study ended, the subjects' performance levels declined after four weeks without training. Incorporating the activity into year-round older adult fitness programs may enhance clients' balance and lower their risk for falls.

For obvious reasons, great care must be taken to ensure client safety during such activity. Whereas tilting the head backward and standing with one's eyes closed both are highly questionable activities in other older adult exercise situations, both are integral to this balance training design. Therefore, this type of training is not for everyone. It requires cautious screening as well as a carefully controlled, well-supervised environment that reflects the provision that all potential safety issues have been anticipated, analyzed, and addressed in advance to ensure the individual client's continuing physical safety. Examples of risk-reducing precautions include: (1) omitting the backward head tilt for participants with neck problems; and (2) reminding all participants to open their eyes and/or utilize balance support as frequently as they deem personally necessary.

## Fitness Walking Techniques

The general guidelines for aerobic training as outlined earlier in this chapter should be applied to older adult fitness walking programs. In addition to those basic criteria, several special considerations also should be kept in mind when planning walking activities for older participants:

✓ Environmental considerations: Do not conduct outdoor walking activities when the temperature exceeds 85° F (29° C) or the humidity exceeds approximately 60%. Do not walk in extreme cold (which can cause lung discomfort or hypothermia), when wind chill is immoderate, when air pollution levels pose a risk, or when lightning threatens. Have an indoor alternative ready for bad weather days. Avoid walking on dangerous surfaces such as those with holes, obstructions, icy patches, or broken sidewalks.

✓ Apparel and accessories: Make certain that participants are wearing comfortable, supportive walking shoes and clothing appropriate to existing weather conditions. Layered clothing can be removed as the body warms or added if the weather grows cooler. Protect the eyes and skin with sunglasses, visors, and sunscreen. Have drinking water available and consume it liberally, especially in hot weather. If possible, walk during daylight hours. If it is necessary to walk after sundown, wear reflective attire. (Individuals should carry identification; those who are not members of a group should walk with a friend whenever possible.)

✓ Warming up and cooling down: Avoid the common mistake of conducting walking-only warm-up and cool-down periods before and after fitness walking sessions. While it is effective to begin with slow walking and progressively increase the pace to limber up and gradually increase circulation, additional warm-up activities should be included to provide a complete warm-up period as described earlier in this chapter. A structured, total-body warm-up may help participants lift their feet slightly higher or swing the arms and legs with greater ease, which can help prevent tripping and add pleasure to the walking experience. Likewise, gradually reducing one's pace toward the end of a walking session is an excellent cool-down component. Walking also should be followed by stretching to foster joint range of motion and to discourage unnecessary soreness or cramping.

✓ Ensuring an effective aerobic workout: A watch and inexpensive pedometer are useful for tracking time and distance. To maintain an adequate aerobic-intensity level, however, it also is important to rate perceived exertion and/or periodically monitor heart rate. Energy expenditure can be increased by increasing duration or frequency. Speed also may be increased within safe and sensible limits. (Approximately 3 mph is a good goal for most participants.) Persons who do not have problems related to balance, the lower back, or the knees can increase intensity by walking on a variable terrain surface including gradual inclines. The use of weights during fitness walking for older adults is generally not recommended. Ankle weights should not be used because they can overstress the back, hips, and knees. Wrist weights that are no heavier than 1 pound each may be used safely by some individuals; however, they may overstress the back, neck, shoulders, and elbows in others. In general, the most prudent approach is to reserve the use of weights for conventional strength-training sessions.

✓ Walking technique: With each step, the heel should touch the ground just before the ball of the foot followed by the toes, effecting a heel-to-toe rolling action. Maintain good posture with relatively loose shoulders and low arms. When the arms are carried too high, unnecessary neck and shoulder tension can result. Allow the arms to swing naturally at sides. Work toward preserving or increasing stride length, as needed.

✓ Special program-planning consideration #1: It is good to vary outdoor walking routes when possible, using local features such as beaches, mountains, parks, wooden walkways, long fishing piers, well-maintained outdoor stairways with railings, bridges, scenic parks and neighborhoods, and interesting historical districts. Only crime-safe walking routes that are free of dangerous traffic conditions should be taken. Regarding any route chosen, advance provisions (such as carrying a cellular telephone) that enable the instructor to summon emergency assistance promptly, if needed, must be in place.

✓ Special program-planning consideration #2: Team teaching works well for outdoor groups with members at different fitness levels. While one instructor sets a pace for the fast walkers (and can lead them on a longer route that eventually circles back to rejoin the other participants), another instructor stays with the slower walkers.

✓ Special program-planning consideration #3: Although indoor walking programs may lack the variety, stimulation, and fresh-air qualities of outdoor programs, they do have certain advantages. These include temperature and climate control, no exposure to ultraviolet rays, smooth, unobstructed walking surfaces, and ready access to rest benches, water fountains, rest rooms, and telephones. Music can be conveniently incorporated, if desired. Various walking patterns (such as large figure eights and criss-cross

routes) may be combined with lap walking for variety.

## Personal-training Techniques

Personal trainers are in a special position that allows them to utilize any techniques from previous sections that they deem beneficial. In addition, they can supervise extremely effective forms of training that are best conducted on a one-to-one basis, such as individualized functional-fitness training and strength-machine work.

Note: In personal training settings, the treadmill and stationary cycle are convenient means for gradually increasing circulation during the warm-up phase and for conducting aerobic training.

## Functional-fitness Training

Functional fitness, which defines the parameters of one's ability to perform basic activities of daily living, should influence the practical objectives of older-adult exercise programming. Ideally, fitness specialists seek to train elderly clients for optimal functional performance.

Functional fitness relates to an individual's physical independence in terms of:

✓ Mobility (e.g., standing and walking)

✓ Self-care (e.g., bathing, grooming, and toileting)

✓ Exerting adequate control over one's living environment (e.g., driving and shopping, preparing meals, and performing household maintenance tasks)

✓ Preserving specific physical abilities needed for pursuits that enhance quality of life (e.g., entertaining grandchildren, volunteering, gardening, playing golf, and traveling)

Through effective functional-fitness training, older adults may be able to avoid, postpone, reduce, or reverse declines in physical-performance level. When the training succeeds in decreasing an individual's risk for falling, its value is incalculable.

Personal trainers are in an excellent position to help clients maintain and improve their functional-fitness level. As a general guideline, functional-fitness training should simulate selected real-life tasks. In choosing exercises, consider the day-to-day activities each individual client needs to perform successfully. Specific functional exercises should be undertaken within the broader context of a complete, well-balanced training program. Below are several especially effective functional-fitness training techniques:

✓ Perform gentle neck rotation.

✓ Perform upper-body exercises involving the arms, hands, and trunk in lifting, reaching, turning, pulling, and pushing.

✓ Simulate everyday stair-climbing tasks by stepping up and stepping down on a low platform (with balance support available).

✓ Perform sit-to-stand activities (moving from a chair-seated position to a standing posture and vice versa).

✓ Perform squats (observing the safety cautions provided in Chapter 6).

✓ Perform additional lower-extremity strengtheners (such as heel raises).

✓ Perform balance-training activity.

✓ Perform walking activity.

## Strength Training

Personal training provides the most efficient means for ensuring that an adequate strength-training intensity is achieved. Remember, the personal trainer is free to use any of the techniques shown in this chapter, adapting them as appropriate to a participant's personal-training program.

For more information on strength training and program design, see Chapter 6.

# CONCLUSION

There is no single best method of training older adults. The best approach is the one that meets the participant's goals and needs and that they will perform consistently. Developing an effective, balanced, well-tolerated program that enhances quality of life is a realistic goal. All of the methods described in this chapter are viable, depending upon the individual to be trained. The professional's challenge, as well as the key to success for all involved, is determining and implementing the most appropriate training method or methods for each participant.

# REFERENCES AND RECOMMENDED READING

American College of Sports Medicine (2000). *Guidelines for Exercise Testing and Prescription* (6th ed.). Baltimore: Lippincott Williams & Wilkins.

American Senior Fitness Association (2003). *Long Term Care Fitness Leader Training Manual* (3rd ed.). New Smyrna Beach, Fla.: SFA.*

American Senior Fitness Association (2003). *Senior Fitness Instructor Training Manual* (3rd ed.). New Smyrna Beach, Fla.: SFA.*

American Senior Fitness Association (2003). *Senior Personal Trainer Training Manual* (3rd ed.). New Smyrna Beach, Fla.: SFA.*

Best-Martini, E. & Botenhagen-DiGenova, K.A. (2003). *Exercise for Frail Elders.* Champaign, Ill.: Human Kinetics.

Borg, G.A.V. (1982). Psychophysical bases of perceived exertion. *Medicine and Science in Sports and Exercise,* 14, 377–381.

Charette, S.L. et al. (1991). *Muscle Hypertrophy Response to Resistance Training in Older Women.* Palo Alto, Calif.: American Physiological Society.

Clark, J. (2002). *Seniorcise: A Simple Guide to Fitness for the Elderly and Disabled* (2nd ed.). New Smyrna Beach, Fla.: SFA.*

Clark, J. (Ed.). (1996). *Exercise Programming for Older Adults.* New York: Haworth Press.

Clark, J. (1993). *Full Life Fitness: A Complete Exercise Program for Mature Adults.* Champaign, Ill.: Human Kinetics.

Coven, E. (1992). *Seniorobics: The Fitness Guide for People 55+.* Jericho, N.Y.: FitWise Programs, Inc.**

DeBusk, R.F. et al. (1990). Training effects of long versus short bouts of exercise in healthy subjects. *American Journal of Cardiology,* 65, 1010–1013.

Ettinger, W., Jr., Mitchell, B., & Blair, S. (1996). *Fitness after Fifty: Never Too Late to Start.* St. Louis: Beverly Cracom.

Fiatarone, M.A. et al. (1994). Exercise training and nutritional supplementation for physical frailty in very elderly people. *New England Journal of Medicine,* 330, 1769–1775.

Fiatarone, M.A. et al. (1990). High-intensity strength training in nonagenarians. *Journal of the American Medical Association,* 263, 3029–3034.

Fletcher, G.F. et al. (1995). Exercise standards: A statement for healthcare professionals from the American Heart Association. *Circulation,* 91, 580–615.

Frontera, W.R. et al. (1988). *Strength Conditioning in Older Men: Skeletal Muscle Hypertrophy and Improved Function.* Palo Alto, Calif.: American Physiological Society.

Gersten, J.W. (1991). Effect of exercise on muscle function decline with aging. *Western Journal of Medicine,* 154, 579–582.

Gladwin, L.A. (1996). Stretching: A valuable component of functional mobility training in the elderly. *Activities, Adaptation & Aging,* 20, 3, 37–47.

Hyatt, G. (1996). Strength training for the aging adult. *Activities, Adaptation & Aging,* 20, 3, 27–36.

Jones, C.J. & Rose, D. (Eds.) (2004). *Physical Activity Instruction for Older Adults.* Champaign, Ill.: Human Kinetics.

Paffenbarger, R.S. et al. (1986). Physical activity, all-cause mortality, and longevity of college alumni. *New England Journal of Medicine,* 314, 605–613.

Pate, R.R. et al. (1995). Physical activity and public health: A recommendation from the Centers for Disease Control and Prevention and the American College of Sports Medicine. *Journal of the American Medical Association,* 273, 402–407.

Pollock, M.L., & Wilmore, J.H. (1990). *Exercise in Health and Disease* (2nd ed.). Philadelphia: Saunders.

Pollock, M.L. et al. (1994). Exercise training and prescription for the elderly. *Southern Medical Journal,* 87, 5, S88–S95.

Pollock, M.L. et al. (1991). Injuries and adherence to walk/jog and resistance training programs in the elderly. *Medicine and Science in Sports and Exercise,* 23, 1194–1200.

Sanders, M.E. (2002). Aquatic exercise. In L.A. Gladwin (Ed.) *Fitness Theory & Practice* (4th ed.). Sherman Oaks, Calif.:

Aerobics and Fitness Association of America.

Sanders, M. & Rippee, N. (1993) (videos). *Speedo Aquatic Fitness System: Instructor Training Course Video.* ***

Spirduso, W.W., Francis, K.L., & MacRae, P.G. (2005). *Physical Dimensions of Aging.* (2nd ed.). Champaign, Ill.: Human Kinetics.

Swart, D.L., Pollock, M.L., & Brechue, W.F. (1996). Aerobic exercise for older participants. *Activities, Adaptation & Aging,* 20, 3, 9–25.

U.S. Department of Health and Human Services (1996). *Physical Activity and Health: A Report of the Surgeon General.* Washington, D.C.: U.S. Government Printing Office.

Van Norman, K.A. (1995). *Exercise Programming for Older Adults.* Champaign, Ill.: Human Kinetics.

Westcott, W.L. (2003). *Building Strength and Stamina: New Nautilus Training for Total Fitness* (2nd ed.). Champaign, Ill.: Human Kinetics/Nautilus International.

Westcott, W.L. (1995). *Strength Fitness: Physiological Principles and Training Techniques* (4th ed.). Dubuque, Iowa: William C. Brown.

Westcott, W.L. & Baechle, T.R. (1998). *Strength Training Past 50.* Champaign, Ill.: Human Kinetics.

Wilson, M.A. (1996). *Caregiver's Guide to Exercise.* Spokane, Wash.: Sit and Be Fit.****

Woollacott, M. (October 6, 1995). Changes in balance control in the older adult: Effects of balance training programs. (Lecture given at International Conference on Aging and Physical Activity; available on audiotape from Human Kinetics, P.O. Box 5076, Champaign, IL 61825).


*Available from the American Senior Fitness Association, P.O. Box 2575, New Smyrna Beach, FL 32170 (telephone 800-243-1478, fax 904-427-0613).

**Available from FitWise Programs, P.O. Box 759, Jericho, NY 11753 (telephone 516-822-6306).

*** Available from Speedo International, Ltd., 5591 E. Rainbow Ridge Ct., Reno, NV 89523 (telephone 800-999-4332).

**** Available from Sit and Be Fit, P.O. Box 8033, Spokane, WA 99203-0033 (telephone 509-448-9438).

## Acknowledgments

The author wishes to extend special thanks to Wayne Westcott, Ph.D., Laura Gladwin, M.S., Mary Sanders, M.S., Mary Ann Wilson, R.N., Ellen Coven, M.A., Kay Van Norman, M.S., and Gwen Hyatt, M.S., whose publications provided many of the specific exercise techniques described in this chapter.

BASIC STRENGTH-TRAINING

# Guidelines for Older Adults

## James A. Peterson

James A. Peterson, *Ph.D., FACSM, is a sports medicine consultant who resides in Monterey, Calif. Dr. Peterson is a prolific writer, having authored 63 books and more than 200 articles on a variety of sports medicine, fitness, and management topics. Among the books he has co-authored are* Finding the Winning Edge *with Bill Walsh and Brian Billick and* Competitive Leadership *with Brian Billick. In addition, he was the co-editor for the second edition of ACSM's Standards and Guidelines for Health/Fitness Facilities. An active member and fellow of the American College of Sports Medicine, Dr. Peterson currently serves as the associate editor-in-chief for ACSM's Health and Fitness Journal. He lectures nationally at a variety of sports medicine and coaching venues and has appeared on a number of national television shows, including* CBS Evening News, *ABC's* Good Morning America, *and ABC's* Nightline.

## Barry A. Franklin

Barry Franklin, *Ph.D., FACSM, is director of cardiac rehabilitation and exercise laboratories at William Beaumont Hospital. He holds adjunct faculty appointments as clinical professor of exercise science at Oakland University, professor of physiology at Wayne State University School of Medicine, and clinical professor, department of family medicine, at the University of Michigan Medical School. Dr. Franklin served as president of the AACVPR in 1988 and president of ACSM in 1999, and has held multiple leadership positions with the American Heart Association. He currently serves as the editor for the* American Journal of Medicine and Sports *and holds editorial positions with 17 other scientific and clinical journals, including the* American Journal of Cardiology *and* Medicine and Science in Sports and Exercise. *Dr. Franklin's latest book, co-authored with Joseph C. Piscatella, is entitled* Take a Load Off Your Heart.

Aging involves at least two basic truths. The first truth is that everybody ages. The second truth is that everybody ages somewhat differently. In other words, a "typical" older adult does not exist. According to the National Institute on Aging's Gerontology Research Center in Baltimore, Maryland: "Aging is a highly unique, individualized process. There is no such thing as a typical elderly person. People age at markedly different rates. Some individuals even show improvements over time for certain physiological functions. Declines in older men and women occur most frequently during incidents or periods of stress."

What does exist, however, is ample evidence that exercise can help slow the deleterious biological changes that occur over an adult's lifetime (Franklin & Munnings, 1995). While much of the investigative efforts involving the impact of exercise on the "aging process" has focused on aerobic exercise, more recent studies have examined the effects of resistance training on older individuals and has shown that proper strength training can complement endurance exercise (Wood et al., 2001) and help forestall the rate of deterioration of the musculoskeletal system in older adults.

In fact, strength training has been found to have a positive impact on almost all of the numerous changes that the musculoskeletal system undergoes as individuals age. For example, a progressive, steady decline in muscle mass and strength (especially of the lower extremities) occurs with age, leading to deficiencies in gait and balance, loss of functional mobility, increased risk of falling, and ultimately a loss of independence. Muscle mitochondrial and enzymatic changes, which reduce muscle respiratory capacity (the muscle's ability to extract oxygen from the blood), also occur as a result of aging. Aging is also associated with a decrease in bone mineral content and mass (this occurs in both sexes), thereby increasing the older person's risk for osteoporosis and bone fractures. Furthermore, as we age, increased stiffness of connective tissue results in a loss of joint flexibility and mobility.

As the next section emphasizes, strength training on a regular basis provides numerous benefits to older adults, attenuating many of the age-associated physiological declines that are commonly attributed to aging.

## RATIONALE FOR STRENGTH TRAINING

Strength training offers numerous benefits to older adults and considerable research shows that a properly designed strength-training program can meet a wide array of needs and interests of older individuals. More simply stated, the rationale for engaging in strength training is compelling. Following are some of the primary benefits of strength training:

*Increases muscular strength and walking endurance.* Numerous studies demonstrate that inactive individuals typically incur a 20 to 30% loss in strength levels by age 65. Research also shows that adults who engage in a resistance-training program are able to increase their muscular strength and walking endurance (Ades et al., 1996), even with little or no improvement in aerobic capacity (Hickson, Rosenkoetter, & Brown, 1980).

*Helps maintain or increase joint flexibility.* Strength training enhances joint flexibility in older adults when they exercise through a full range of motion (American College of Sports Medicine, 1998).

*Helps preserve muscle mass.* Research shows that proper strength training helps individuals preserve their muscle tissue during aging, as opposed to the roughly 20 to 40% loss in muscle mass that inactive individuals may experience. Although aerobic exercise has been shown to improve cardiorespiratory fitness, it does not prevent the age-related loss of muscle tissue. Only regular participation in strength training has been shown to effectively maintain lean body mass levels throughout an individual's mid-life and senior years.

*Helps maintain resting metabolic rate.* Research indicates that the average adult experiences an approximately 2 to 5% decrease in metabolic rate every decade of life (Evans & Rosenberg, 1992; Keyes, Taylor, & Grande et al., 1973). This reduction in resting metabolism is closely linked to the decrease in muscle mass associated with aging. Because regular strength training prevents muscle loss, it helps individuals maintain resting metabolic rates at or near normal levels as they age.

*Helps manage or reduce arthritic pain.* Proper strength training is believed to ease the pain associated with osteoarthritis. It is generally accepted that the strength training–induced improvements in the strength and function of muscles, bones, and connective tissue decrease the amount of stress on the joints, resulting in a reduction in arthritic pain.

*Has favorable effects on selected health and fitness variables (Table 6.1).* Although the full extent of these effects tends to vary from person to person, regular progressive exercise has been shown to have a positive effect on bone mineral density, body composition, glucose metabolism, resting blood pressure, lipid

Table 6.1

**Effects of Resistance Exercise on Selected Health and Fitness Variables**

| Variable | Training Adaptation |
|---|---|
| Bone mineral density | ↑↑ |
| Body composition | |
| % fat | ↓ |
| Lean body mass | ↑↑ |
| Strength | ↑↑↑ |
| Glucose metabolism | |
| Insulin response to glucose challenge | ↓↓ |
| Basal insulin levels | ↓ |
| Insulin sensitivity | ↑↑ |
| Serum Lipids | |
| HDL | ↑↔ |
| LDL | ↓↔ |
| Blood pressure at rest | |
| Systolic | ↓↔ |
| Diastolic | ↓↔ |
| VO$_2$max | ↑ |
| Endurance | ↑↑ |
| Physical function | ↑↑↑ |
| Basal metabolism | ↑↑ |

**Legend:** ↑ = increase; ↓ = decrease; ↔ = unchanged; ↑ or ↓ = small effect; ↑↑ or ↓↓ = moderate effect; ↑↑↑ or ↓↓↓ = large effect

HDL = high-density lipoprotein cholesterol; LDL = low-density lipoprotein cholesterol.

Adapted from Pollock, M.L. & Vincent, K.R. (1996). Resistance training for health. *The President's Council on Physical Fitness and Sports Research Digest, 2,* 8.

and lipoprotein levels, and cardiovascular and physical function (Pollock & Vincent, 1996). Furthermore, the heart-rate and blood-pressure responses of individuals who strength train regularly have been found to be lower when they lift any given load (e.g., carrying groceries, lifting moderate-to-heavy objects) (McCartney et al., 1993). Thus, strength training can decrease the demands on the heart during daily activities.

*Improves the ability to perform the activities of daily living—at home, work, or play.* As a result, individuals are better able to maintain a physically active and relatively challenging lifestyle. One of the cornerstones of independent living is having enough muscular fitness to perform daily tasks (e.g., climbing stairs at home, carrying groceries, getting out of a soft chair without using the armrests, rearranging furniture). Studies, however, suggest that variable-resistance training may be better than high-resistance training for decreasing the muscle activation needed to carry objects (Hunter et al., 2001).

*Enriches overall health.* A higher level of muscular fitness can greatly reduce an individual's chances of suffering either muscle-related or skeletal injuries. It is estimated that approximately half of the various injuries that occur during physical activity could be prevented through higher levels of muscular fitness. Strength training can also help individuals who suffer from a particular medical condition or physical problem. For example, strength training improves the upper-body muscular fitness of cardiac patients whose muscles have lost tone and function due to physical inactivity, coronary artery bypass surgery, or cardiac transplantation (Graves & Franklin, 2001). Performed over an extended period of time, strength training can also help maintain or increase the density of an individual's bones—an adaptation that helps to lower their risk of suffering osteoporosis-related falls and fractures. In addition, it helps provide pain relief to people with osteoarthritic conditions by reducing the stress on their joints. Finally, strength training appears to play an important role in treating and preventing lower-back pain.

*Boosts mental health.* Having a higher level of muscular fitness can improve how individuals feel about themselves (i.e., their self-efficacy). Research conducted at Harvard University demonstrated that strength training is very effective at reducing depression in older adults (Singh, Clements, & Fiatarone, 1997). In fact, more than 85% of the participants who completed the 10-week strength-training program no longer met the clinical criteria for depression. This finding suggests that improved levels of muscular fitness may be associated with greater levels of self-confidence and a more positive overall outlook on life.

*Enhances appearance.* Strength training can provide individuals of all ages (especially older persons) with readily apparent feedback on their exercise efforts. Substantial changes in muscle strength and tone can occur over a relatively brief period of time. A fit, healthy appearance is generally a matter of body composition, which can be favorably affected by proper strength training.

# OVERCOMING BARRIERS TO PARTICIPATION

Despite its documented benefits, strength training is often a difficult "sell" to older adults because many of these individuals simply cannot see themselves "pumping iron." As such, one of your initial tasks must be to fully understand, and be responsive to, the reasons (real and perceived) that might keep older adults from engaging in a strength-training program. In that regard, fitness professionals have a responsibility to address the various barriers that might impede the motivation for someone to strength train.

Most (if not all) of the more commonly proposed reasons concerning why many older adults may be reluctant to participate in a strength-training program stem from a lack of sufficient understanding about resistance exercise. Their reluctance may be grounded in a plethora of myths, misconceptions, and unfounded claims that are commonly associated with strength training. In other instances, their aversion can be related to personal anxiety over whether strength training is both safe and appropriate (health-wise) for them. In yet other circumstances, their hesitancy appears to arise from apprehension that strength training may be beyond their personal capabilities. Whatever the situation, be proactive in your efforts to help individuals deal with their misgivings about strength training.

## General Safety and Health-related Concerns

Some older adults are hesitant to engage in a strength-training program because of safety concerns, while other individuals are apprehensive about the impact that resistance training might have on a particular existing medical condition. A better understanding of the nuances of proper strength training can help alleviate their concerns.

## SAFETY CONCERNS

Among the various factors involved in strength training (by individuals of any age), none is more important than safety. Fortunately, strength training is a relatively safe activity if the exerciser adheres to certain guidelines and uses common sense. Indeed, research has shown that weight-lifting exercises can be conducted by healthy older adults who do not have clinical, electrical, and biological signs of cardiac muscle injury, if appropriate selection criteria and proper breathing techniques are applied (Bermon, Rama, & Dolisi, 2000). Consider the following guidelines:

*Engage in a strength-training program that is designed to achieve muscle balance.* Train the muscles that oppose each other—the quadriceps muscles (front thigh), for example, are opposed by the hamstring muscles (rear thigh). If one is too strong for the other, the weaker muscle is more likely to be injured at some point in time. Pairs of opposing muscles should have about a 1:1 strength relationship. The exception is the quadriceps and hamstrings, which should be 3:2 (i.e., the quadriceps should be 150% stronger than the hamstrings). As such, achieving an appropriate level of muscle balance is crucial. One of the easiest ways to work on muscle balance is to have the exerciser alternate pushing exercises with pulling exercises (e.g., do a leg press, then a leg curl).

*Perform every exercise through a full, pain-free range of motion (the degree to which there is normal movement around a joint).* If a person does not exercise through a full range of motion, less work is being performed. Furthermore, eventually the level of flexibility in the joints

involved in the exercise will be decreased (a factor that may lead to an increased risk of injury).

*Perform every exercise at a controlled rate of speed.* If an individual raises and lowers a weight slowly (about two seconds on the lifting phase and four seconds on the lowering phase), that individual's muscles will do effective work throughout the exercise. On the other hand, if the exerciser throws or jerks the weight, the muscles involved in the exercise will be working only at the beginning and at the end of the lift. In addition, the rapid deceleration in throwing a weight increases the exerciser's chances of being injured.

*Warm up properly.* Common sense suggests that the individual should spend a few minutes before strength training to prepare for the demands of rigorous activity. Warming up serves several purposes. The primary purpose is to slowly elevate the exerciser's pulse to an aerobic level, thereby increasing the exerciser's cardiac output. As a result, both body and muscle temperature are raised. This factor increases the activity of the enzymes in the working skeletal muscles, which increases the metabolism of those muscles. The viscosity in the muscle is reduced, and muscle blood flow is increased. Therefore, more oxygen and fuel reach the muscles involved in the activity.

A proper warm-up also improves the mechanical efficiency and power of the working muscles. Furthermore, the time necessary to transmit nervous impulses is decreased, augmenting the exerciser's reaction time and coordination. In addition, warming up decreases the likelihood of injuries to the muscles and the supporting connective tissues involved in the activity. The increase in temperature and blood flow to these muscles and supporting tissues is particularly beneficial for older adults, who often have muscles and connective tissues that are less elastic.

A warm-up session should last at least five minutes, raise the core temperature of the body (signaled by the fact that the exerciser perspires), and involve the major joints. A typical warm-up session might include performing an aerobic activity at a very low level and then doing a set of strength exercises using very light resistance.

*Respond to muscle soreness in an appropriate manner.* Several different theories exist about the cause of muscle soreness that persists for two or three days after a strength-training workout, especially for individuals new to strength training. The most widely accepted theory is that muscle soreness results from microtears to the muscle and its tendinous attachments. Usually, this damage occurs during the beginning of a program when the relatively under-stressed muscle fibers have not adapted to the new demands imposed on them. Soreness can also occur when exercisers dramatically increase the intensity of their training or incorporate new exercises into their workout. One of the most commonly employed ways to minimize muscle soreness is to have the exerciser strength train on two to three consecutive days when initiating a resistance-training program. A more common-sense step is to strictly limit the degree to which the exerciser increases the level of intensity from one workout to another. Older adults, in particular, should engage in a strength-training program that is progressive in nature. However, muscle soreness that lasts longer than three to four days may indicate that either the exerciser is trying to do too much too soon or that he or she may need to be referred to a physician. It should also be noted that some cholesterol-lowering drugs (statins), which are taken by many middle-aged and older adults, have been linked to unusual muscle weakness or fatigue, called **rhabdomyolysis**. This is a potentially serious condition that requires immediate medical attention.

*Older adults should always have a spotter.* A spotter's job is to assist exercisers while they are performing resistance training and ensure that they are not injured by having a weight fall on them. If the exerciser cannot complete a repetition, take the weight from them (if asked). Another purpose of spotters is to give constant verbal feedback to the exerciser—either to motivate them or to ensure that they use the proper techniques. Spotters can also help an exerciser bring a heavy weight into the starting position for an exercise (particularly for negative-only training).

*Encourage older adults to avoid breath-holding during strength training.* Older adults should never hold their breath while strength training. Holding the breath while exerting force can cause dangerous increases in intra-thoracic pressure. The process, called the "Valsalva maneuver," can cause marked fluctuations in heart rate and blood pressure (American College of Sports Medicine, 2000). In normal subjects the blood pressure rises and the heart rate slows automatically with the onset of straining (phase 1); the blood pressure falls and the heart rate sympathetically rises during the period of sustained straining (phase 2); with sudden release of straining (phase 3) the blood pressure drops and the heart rate increases; in phase 4 there is an overshoot of blood pressure that induces a marked reflex slowing of the heart rate.

Two theories are generally advocated concerning the proper approach to breathing while strength training. The simplest and most sensible guideline suggests that exercisers should breathe normally and regularly as they train. A second and more involved theory contends that exercisers should control their breathing pattern while they exercise. Proponents of this theory recommend that the exerciser should inhale during the negative (lowering) phase of the exercise and exhale during the positive (lifting) phase of the exercise, because the lifting phase requires greater exertion and results in the highest levels of intra-abdominal and intra-thoracic pressure.

## HEALTH-RELATED CONCERNS

Older adults who suffer from varied medical conditions are frequently concerned about whether strength training is an appropriate exercise modality for them. Understandably, these adults may be somewhat apprehensive about participating in an activity that might aggravate their condition. These individuals (particularly those who are classified as high-risk patients) should consult with their physician before embarking on a strength-training regimen. Fortunately, the somewhat limited amount of research that has been conducted in this area has shown that a properly conducted strength-training program can have a positive impact on the quality of the lives of those with selected medical conditions, including coronary heart disease, osteoarthritis, and osteoporosis. Modest improvements in functional performance and disability have also been reported in older women after high- and low-velocity resistance training (Sayers et al., 2003).

### Coronary Heart Disease

Individuals with coronary heart disease (CHD)—similar to those without CHD—require a minimum level of muscular fitness for daily living and functional independence. Many individuals who have CHD, however, lack the physical strength required to perform common tasks (e.g., rising from a chair, carrying groceries, opening windows). Strength training is a safe, effective method for improving the muscular strength and endurance levels in clinically stable patients with coronary heart disease (Franklin et al., 1991). Proper strength training has also been found to favorably modify selected coronary risk factors in cardiac patients. Because the hemodynamic response to resistance

exercise is largely proportionate to the percent of maximal voluntary contraction (MVC) (Lind & McNicol, 1967), as well as the muscle mass involved (Mitchell et al., 1980), increased muscle strength results in an attenuated heart rate and blood pressure response to any given load, because the load now represents a lower percentage of the MVC. Stated simply, strength training can decrease the cardiac demands on an individual during daily activities requiring upper-extremity efforts.

### Osteoarthritis

Strength training may help individuals with osteoarthritis effectively manage their condition. Because stronger muscles absorb more (relatively speaking) of the attendant stress on a joint, the stress on affected joint surfaces is reduced. Furthermore, the functional ability of an osteoarthritic individual can be improved if surrounding muscles and unaffected joints share stress with affected joints.

### Osteoporosis

Available research indicates that strength training can have a positive affect on individuals with osteoporosis—a condition that is characterized by decreased bone mineral content (i.e., decreased density). Strength training has been shown to slow bone loss and increase bone density. In addition, training-induced improvements in muscular strength and balance may help prevent falls that cause fractures among individuals with osteoporosis, particularly elderly women. Fractures of the hip and wrist are the most common; fractures of the hip, however, are the most devastating. Persons who have hip fractures have a 5 to 20% greater risk of dying within a year than do others their age, and 15 to 25% or more of those who have lived independently before a hip fracture need long-term care after the fracture (Franklin & Munnings, 1995). Thus, strength training may, at least indirectly, serve to increase survival and functional independence.

## SELF-CONFIDENCE CONCERNS

Some older adults may hold negative attitudes about engaging in strength training simply because they feel that they will be unable to do whatever will be required of them. Their uneasiness is often grounded in either a fear of the unknown or anxiety over the possibility of embarrassing themselves because of some inadequacy on their part (real or imagined). In such situations, you need to convince these individuals that their "muscles do matter" and that it is never too late to pursue the potential benefits of strength training. Furthermore, you need to inform them that you will design a strength-training regimen that not only meets their needs and interests, but also one that is well within their capabilities.

## ORGANIZING THE STRENGTH-TRAINING PROGRAM

The key to ensuring that older adults achieve maximum benefits from their resistance-training efforts is to design a strength-training program that not only meets their needs, but also addresses the physiological characteristics of this unique population.

Designing a strength-training program for older adults involves seven basic variables:
✓ Selecting the exercises
✓ Ordering the exercises
✓ Determining repetitions
✓ Determining sets
✓ Determining resistance level
✓ Limiting the time between exercises
✓ Allowing time between workouts

## Selecting the Exercises

As a general rule of thumb, a strength-training workout for older adults should be limited to eight to 10 exercises. Doing more than 10 exercises can be counter-productive physiologically and psychologically (American College of Sports Medicine, 2000). Individuals reach a point where additional work is simply not worth the effort. The workout should include exercises to develop major muscle groups in the body, plus specific exercises to meet a person's particular needs or interests. For example, if a client is prone to back pain, consider including resistance exercises that are designed to develop the lower back (erector spinae) and abdominal muscles. See pages 198–215 for sample workouts.

## Ordering the Exercises

A strength-training program should begin with exercises that involve the largest muscles in the body and progress to those using the smallest muscles. The recommended order in which muscles should be addressed is: lower back and buttocks, legs, upper torso, arms, and abdominals. Neck exercises, if included at all, should be performed last. Accordingly, most strength-training exercises are designed to develop the largest muscle involved in the movement. If individuals stop performing an exercise because a smaller muscle has become fatigued before a larger one, then they have compromised the possible gains that could be achieved by the larger muscle. For example, if individuals start their workout with modified sit-ups, they will exhaust their abdominal muscles—muscles that should be exercised last. Fatigue may prematurely occur when they perform an exercise (such as a squat) in which their abdominals act as stabilizers. They will have to either lift less weight during the exercise (thereby decreasing their need for stabilization), or subject themselves to a heightened risk of injury (by exercising at a level of intensity that their abdominals cannot safely support). Either way, they have compromised their efforts.

## Determining Repetitions, Sets, and Resistance Level

These three variables—repetitions, sets, and resistance level—constitute the numbers crunch of strength training. A repetition is doing a specific exercise one time. A set is doing a particular number of repetitions in a row, before stopping. The weight used is the level of resistance (demand) that individuals put on their muscles while exercising. You have several choices about how to structure the way in which you incorporate repetitions, sets, and resistance into a client's strength-training program. Two of the most commonly employed methods are the multiple- and single-set approaches.

The traditional approach to strength training suggests that individuals:

✓ complete three sets of five to eight repetitions to develop muscle strength
✓ complete three sets of nine to 15 repetitions to develop muscle endurance

When taking a multiple-set approach, choose a level of resistance that will enable the client to perform all sets somewhere between the minimum and maximum number of repetitions before reaching muscle failure (i.e., unable to complete another repetition). As an alternative, select a weight based on the "one-rep-max system" by determining the maximum amount that the client can lift in one repetition of an exercise, and then lift a certain percentage (usually between 50 and 75%) of that amount during each set of the exercise. Considerable research, however, suggests that multiple sets may have limited additional value, unless high-level performance (e.g., master athletes) is the objective (Kraemer et al., 2002).

## Limiting the Time Between Exercises

As a general rule, the time between exercises should be limited to less than one minute to make the most of a per-son's available time in the weight room. No science involved here, just sound time management. Utilize active rest between exercises. Minimizing rest periods helps individuals focus on exerting maximum effort while training.

## Allowing Time Between Workouts

Unless individuals are doing a split-routine workout (i.e., upper-body exercises one day, lower-body exercises the next day), they should allow at least one full day between their workouts. An alternate-day schedule (Monday-Wednesday-Friday or Tuesday-Thursday-Saturday) is the most commonly followed system. Keep in mind that as individuals get older, more rest is usually needed between workouts. Accordingly, older adults may sometimes want to give themselves two or three full days of rest between workouts instead of one.

## STRENGTH-TRAINING PRINCIPLES

You should become familiar with the essential training principles to make sure that your clients get the most out of their strength-training workouts. Among the more critical factors are progression and recovery time. In addition, the American College of Sports Medicine (ACSM) has developed recommendations for an appropriate strength-training protocol for older adults that specifies how to treat the three primary training variables—intensity, frequency, and duration (American College of Sports Medicine, 1998; 2000).

## Intensity

A muscle becomes stronger when a greater demand than normal is regularly placed on it. Considerable debate, however, exists about what level of intensity is needed to achieve maximum results. One theory suggests that anything less than an all-out effort will produce less than maximum gains. Another theory suggests that an appropriate demand is achieved by training at a predetermined percentage of an individual's maximum level of strength with each exercise.

ACSM recommends that, at a minimum, an individual perform one set of eight to 10 exercises that train the major muscle groups. Each set should involve eight to 12 repetitions that elicit a perceived exertion rating of 3 to 5 (on the 0 to 10 scale)—moderate to strong (Table 6.2). Depending on the fitness and experience levels of the exerciser, however, it may be more appropriate for persons 50 to 60 years and older to perform 10 to 15 repetitions of an exercise, using lighter weights (Figure 6.1). The reason for the increased repetition range at a lower relative effort for the older, more frail individual is injury prevention (Pollock et al., 1994). Select exercises that ensure that all of the major muscle groups are included in each training session.

Table 6.2
**Ratings of Perceived Exertion**

| RPE | | Category Ratio Scale |
|---|---|---|
| 6 | 0 | Nothing at all |
| 7 Very, very light | 0.5 | Very, very weak |
| 8 | 1 | Very weak |
| 9 Very light | 2 | Weak |
| 10 | 3 | Moderate |
| 11 Fairly light | 4 | Somewhat strong |
| 12 | 5 | Strong |
| 13 Somewhat hard | 6 | |
| 14 | 7 | Very strong |
| 15 Hard | 8 | |
| 16 | 9 | |
| 17 Very hard | 10 | Very, very strong |
| 18 | * | Maximal |
| 19 Very, very hard | | |
| 20 | | |

Source: Adapted, with permission, from American College of Sports Medicine (2000). *Guidelines for Exercise Testing and Prescription* (6th ed.). Philadelphia: Lippincott Williams & Wilkins.

Figure 6.1

Using weightloads that permit eight to 15 repetitions will generally facilitate improvements in muscular strength and endurance, regardless of age or health status.

## Progression

A strength-training program should be progressive in nature. Too much, too soon will lead to an injury, muscle failure, or both. Individuals should gradually increase the stress they place on their muscles as they are able to meet the imposed demand. As muscles adapt to a point where they can handle the stresses imposed on them (by getting stronger), encourage your client to gradually increase the resistance level to stimulate new growth and development.

## Recovery Time

When a muscle is stressed beyond what it can normally handle, some rest is needed for the muscle tissues, tendons, and ligaments to recover. If the time between exercise sessions is too brief, the muscle may be unable to make the adaptations needed before being stressed again. In this instance, the muscle either will not develop to the extent possible or may suffer a decrease in strength. Conversely, if too much time is taken between workouts, the muscles will gradually return to their untrained state.

## Frequency

ACSM recommends that resistance training be performed at least twice a week, with at least 48 hours of rest between workouts (American College of Sports Medicine, 2000). Research indicates that as an individual becomes older, the need for sufficient time to recover increases.

## Duration

ACSM suggests that resistance training sessions lasting longer than 60 minutes may have detrimental effects on an individual's exercise adherence. ACSM guidelines allow individuals to complete total-body strength-training sessions within 20 to 25 minutes (American College of Sports Medicine, 2000).

## SPECIAL PROGRAM CONSIDERATIONS AND TRAINING GUIDELINES

Keep the following guidelines in mind when developing and implementing a training regimen for older adults:

✓ Have potential participants complete a health status questionnaire prior to starting a program (Table 6.3).

✓ Assess relative muscular fitness by having clients complete a functional capacity questionnaire (Table 6.4).

✓ Set a goal to develop sufficient muscular strength and endurance to enable an individual to live a physically independent lifestyle.

✓ Closely supervise and monitor the first several training sessions, being particularly sensitive to the special needs and capabilities of an older individual.

✓ Start out (the first eight weeks) with minimal levels of resistance to allow for adaptations of the connective tissue elements.

✓ Teach every participant the proper training techniques for all of the exercises in the program, including avoidance of the Valsalva maneuver.

✓ As a training effect occurs, achieve an overload initially by increasing the number of repetitions, and then by increasing the amount of resistance lifted.

✓ Never use a resistance so heavy that the exerciser cannot perform at least eight repetitions per set. Heavy weights can be dangerous and can damage the skeletal and joint structures of an older individual.

✓ Have clients perform all exercises in a slow, controlled manner. To prevent orthopedic trauma to joint structures, do not allow ballistic (fast and jerky) movements.

Table 6.3

**Health Screening Survey for Older Adults**

*Questions to ask adults over the age of 65 who are beginning a training program:*

1. Do you get chest pains while at rest and/or during exertion?

2. If the answer to Question 1 is "yes": Is it true that you have not had a physician diagnose those pains yet?

3. Have you ever had a heart attack?

4. If the answer to Question 3 is "yes": Was your heart attack within the last year?

5. Do you have high blood pressure?

6. If you do not know the answer to Question 5: Was your last blood pressure reading more than 150/100?

7. Do you have diabetes?

8. If the answer to Question 7 is "yes": Are you presently being treated for diabetes?

9. Are you short of breath after extremely mild exertion, at rest, or at night in bed?

10. Do you have any ulcerated wounds or cuts on your feet that do not seem to heal?

11. Have you experienced an unexplained loss of 10 pounds or more in the past six months?

12. Do you get pain in your buttocks, thighs (front or back), or calves when you walk?

13. While at rest, do you frequently experience fast, irregular heartbeats? Or, at the other extreme, very slow beats? (While a low heart rate can be a sign of an efficient and well-conditioned heart, a very low rate can also indicate a cardiac problem.)

14. Are you currently being treated for any heart or circulatory condition, such as vascular disease, stroke, angina, hypertension, congestive heart failure, poor circulation to the legs, valvular disease, blood clots, or pulmonary disease?

15. Have you previously undergone either coronary angioplasty or heart bypass surgery, or both?

16. As an adult, have you ever had a fracture of the hip, spine, or wrist?

17. Have you fallen more than twice in the past year (no matter what the reason)?

*If you answered "yes" to any of the above questions, you should discuss exercise goals with your physician before starting a resistance-training program.*

Adapted from Evans, W., Ph.D., FACSM, a 1994 presentation titled "Exercise & Aging."

Table 6.4

**Functional Capacity Questionnaire**

✓ Do you have difficulty picking up a small child?

✓ Do you have difficulty carrying a 10-lb bag of groceries?

✓ Do you have difficulty performing household chores (e.g., vacuuming, mopping, washing windows)?

✓ Do you have difficulty climbing a flight of stairs?

✓ Do you have difficulty getting in and out of a car or the bathtub?

✓ Do you have difficulty rising from a sofa or a low chair without using your arms for assistance?

✓ Do you have difficulty opening a jar of food?

*If you answered "yes" to any of these questions, it may be an indication that you have already experienced significant losses of muscular strength. The decline in your level of muscle strength can be partially countered or offset by participation in a well-designed strength-training program.*

Adapted from Evans, W., Ph.D., FACSM, a 1994 presentation titled "Exercise & Aging."

✓ Instruct clients to perform every exercise through a range of motion that is within a "pain-free arc" (i.e., the maximum range of motion that does not elicit pain or discomfort). As favorable adaptations and improvements occur, gradually increase the exercise range of motion to enhance flexibility.

✓ Have clients perform multijoint exercises (as opposed to single-joint exercises), because they tend to develop overall muscular fitness.

✓ Given a choice, use machines rather than free weights. Machines require less skill, provide some spotter functions (to reduce the potential for injury), protect the back by stabilizing body position, allow the user to start with lower resistance and increase it by smaller increments (not true for all strength-training machines), and permit easier control of the exercise range of motion.

✓ Teach clients to perform a minimum of two strength-training sessions per week. This is the frequency required to produce beneficial physiological adaptations. More frequent sessions may be neither desirable nor productive.

✓ Never permit arthritic individuals to participate in strength training during active periods of pain or inflammation, since exercise could exacerbate the condition.

✓ Have clients engage in a year-round resistance-training program, since the cessation of resistance training can result in a rapid, significant loss of strength. When returning from a break in training, individuals should start with weights that are equal to or less than 50% of the intensity at which they had been training, and gradually increase the resistance over time.

✓ Keep accurate records of your client's workouts [e.g., what exercises were performed, how many reps and sets of each exercise were done, how much resistance was used, and any other relevant information (i.e., factors that may have affected the workout, such as an injury)]. This information can be used to help identify flaws in the training regimen, measure improvements, motivate the exerciser, etc.

## EQUIPMENT OPTIONS

One of the many positive benefits of strength training is that a program can be tailored to meet an individual's needs. As such, individuals typically have real choices about what equipment and what training environments are best for them.

At the beginning of a program, utilize the type of equipment the client is most comfortable with, as this will increase adherence and motivation levels. As the individual progresses, incorporate additional forms of resistance as needed to enhance the workout regimen and help the client reach his or her goals. In many cases, equipment selection will be dictated by availability.

See pages 198–215 for sample workouts using machines, free weights, elastic resistance, and common household items. Remember, it is essential that older adults feel comfortable and safe throughout their workouts. Incorporating stability balls, for example, could de-motivate certain clients if the workout becomes too difficult, and, in some cases, could prove dangerous. Instead, focus on targeting all major muscles groups, progressing slowly, and working through a full range of motion.

## Workout Environment

Deciding where to strength train involves a number of factors, including accessibility to desired equipment, availability of professional assistance and advice, safety, cost, and personal preference. Older adults will likely weigh the relative importance of each factor before making their decision, so it is up to you to make them comfortable in your facility and satisfied with your services. Refer to the Participant Recruitment section that begins on page 235 for more complete coverage of this topic.

## SUMMARY

One of the best lifestyle and health-related choices an older adult will ever make is to engage in a strength-training program on a regular basis. The rationale for, and potential benefits of, strength training for older adults are well-documented (Franklin, 1998), so you can be confident that your efforts to ensure that they achieve those benefits are worthwhile.

# WEIGHTSTACK MACHINE

## LOWER BODY

Every workout, regardless of the type of resistance used, should include exercises for the torso. See page 215 for a description of a curl-up exercise.

### Seated Leg Press
### (gluteals, quadriceps, hamstrings)

*Performance recommendations*

Sit on a leg press machine with feet hip-width apart. Hold the handles and contract the abdominals. Flex the knees to approximately 90 degrees, keeping them aligned with the ankles, and keep the entire foot in contact with the foot-plate. Extend the legs until they are straight but not locked. Pause and then slowly return to the starting position.

*Training points to emphasize*

✓ Avoid hyperextension of the knee at the end of the movement.
✓ Push through the heels, not the toes.
✓ Do not allow the knees to travel past the toes during the lowering phase.
✓ Position the feet to create a 90-degree angle at the ankles.

### Seated Leg Extension
### (quadriceps)

*Performance recommendations*

Sit on the leg extension machine and hook the tops of the feet behind the roller pad. Flex your feet, and lightly grip the handles. Extend the legs, lifting the pad upward until the knees are straight but not locked. Pause and then slowly return to the starting position.

*Training points to emphasize*

✓ Do not allow the gluteals to lift off the seat as the legs move up and down.
✓ Use slow, controlled movement (do not "drop or bounce" the weightstack between reps).
✓ Maintain alignment between the neck and spine throughout the exercise movement.
✓ If the machine allows, begin with the knees flexed 90 degrees.

## Standing Single-leg Hamstring Curl (hamstrings)

*Performance recommendations*

Stand with the upper pad above the knee and the lower pad just below the calf. Maintain a neutral spine and hold onto the machine with one hand as needed for balance. Slowly curl the weight through a full, pain-free range of motion. Pause and then slowly return to the starting position.

*Training points to emphasize*
- ✓ Lift and lower the weight in a slow, controlled fashion.
- ✓ Do not lean forward or backward during the exercise.
- ✓ Do not arch the back during the movement.

## UPPER BODY

## Chest Press (pectorals, anterior deltoids, triceps)

*Performance recommendations*

Adjust seat so hand grips are at chest level. Sit on seat with shoulders back and chest lifted. Exhale while pushing the hand grips out. Extend the arms until the elbows are relatively straight but not locked out. Pause and then slowly return to the starting position.

*Training points to emphasize*
- ✓ Keep chest lifted and maintain a neutral spine.
- ✓ Maintain alignment of the hands, wrists, and forearms.
- ✓ Lift and lower the weight in a slow, controlled fashion.

## Lat Pull-down
(latissimus dorsi, biceps)

*Performance recommendations*

Sit facing the weight stack with knees under the thigh pad, feet flat on the floor, and arms extended. Grasp the handles slightly wider than shoulder-width apart with a pronated grip. Maintain a neutral spine, keep abdominals contracted, and lean back slightly so that the handles are aligned with the clavicle. Retract the scapula and pull the handles toward the chest. Pause and then slowly return to the starting position.

*Training points to emphasize*

- ✓ Avoid hyperextension of the lumbar spine.
- ✓ Maintain a neutral wrist position throughout the exercise.
- ✓ Avoid performing behind-the-neck lat pull-downs, which increase the chances of injury to the shoulder joint.

## Seated Row
(latissimus dorsi, biceps, rhomboids, posterior deltoids)

*Performance recommendations*

Sit facing the weightstack with knees bent and feet flat on the floor. Grasp the handles with a neutral grip. Keep the chest lifted, shoulders back, and head and neck aligned with the spine. Retract the scapula and pull the handles toward the rib cage. Pause and then slowly return to the starting position.

*Training points to emphasize*

- ✓ Keep chest lifted, shoulders back, and do not round the upper back when the arms extend.
- ✓ Do not initiate the pulling with the arms and shoulders—"lead with the elbows."
- ✓ Avoid hyperextension of the lumbar spine (i.e., do not arch the back).

## Standing Cable Side Lateral Raise
### (medial deltoids)

*Performance recommendations*

Stand in a "ready" position with a neutral spinal posture. The body is upright and the hips and knees are slightly flexed. Grasp the handle with an overhand grip. With a slightly flexed elbow, raise the arm out and up until it is approximately parallel to the floor. Pause and then slowly lower the arm back down to the starting position.

*Training points to emphasize*

- ✓ Keep the hand slightly in front of the shoulder with the elbow directly in line with the shoulder.
- ✓ Keep the wrist neutral with the palm oriented to the floor at the end of the range of motion.
- ✓ Avoid internally or externally rotating the shoulder, or supinating or pronating the elbow.
- ✓ Lower the arm back down to the starting position with control.

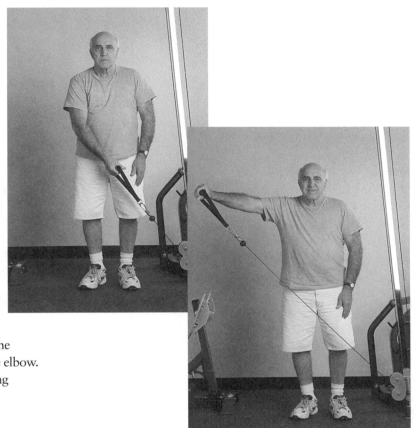

## Standing Cable Biceps Curl
### (biceps)

*Performance recommendations*

Stand in a "ready" position with a neutral spine. The body is upright and the hips and knees are slightly flexed. Grasp the handle with an underhand grip. Bring the hands toward the shoulders and flex the elbows through a full, pain-free range of motion. Pause and then slowly lower the arms back down to the starting position.

*Training points to emphasize*

- ✓ Initiate the movement at the elbow (do not "swing" the handle up to lift the weight).
- ✓ Keep the wrists neutral throughout the exercise.
- ✓ Retract the shoulder blades and maintain the same shoulder position throughout the exercise.
- ✓ Do not lean forward or backward during the exercise.

## Standing Cable Triceps Press
## (triceps)

*Performance recommendations*

Stand in a "ready" position with feet shoulder-width apart or in a staggered stance. The body is upright and the hips and knees are slightly flexed. Grasp the handle with an overhand grip and place the elbows alongside the body. Hold the handle so that an approximately 90-degree angle is formed at the elbow. Extend the elbows and press the handle toward the floor. Pause and then slowly return to the starting position.

*Training points to emphasize*

✓ Initiate the movement at the elbow (do not "hunch over" or pull with the shoulders).
✓ Keep the wrists neutral throughout the exercise.
✓ Retract the shoulder blades and maintain the same shoulder position throughout the exercise.
✓ Do not allow the elbows to flare away from the body.

# WEIGHT MACHINES

## LOWER BODY

### Seated Leg Press
(gluteals, quadriceps, hamstrings)

*Performance recommendations*

Sit on a leg press machine with feet hip-width apart. Hold the handles and contract the abdominals. Flex the knees to approximately 90 degrees, keeping them aligned with the ankles, and keep the entire foot in contact with the foot-plate. Extend the legs until they are straight but not locked. Pause and then slowly return to the starting position.

*Training points to emphasize*
- ✓ Avoid hyperextension of the knee at the end of the movement.
- ✓ Push through the heels, not the toes.
- ✓ Do not allow the knees to travel past the toes during the lowering phase.

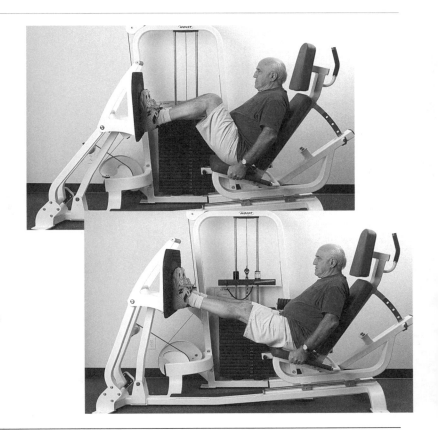

## UPPER BODY

### Incline Chest Press
(pectorals, anterior deltoids, triceps)

*Performance recommendations*

Adjust seat so the hand grips are at chest level. Sit on seat with shoulders back and chest lifted. Exhale while pushing the hand grips out. Extend the arms until the elbows are relatively straight but not locked out. Pause and then slowly return to the starting position.

*Training points to emphasize*
- ✓ Keep the chest lifted and maintain a neutral spine.
- ✓ Maintain alignment of the hands, wrists, and forearms.
- ✓ Lift and lower the weight in a slow, controlled fashion.

## Lat Pull-down
### (latissimus dorsi, biceps)

*Performance recommendations*

Sit facing the weightstack with knees bent under the thigh pad, feet flat on the floor, and arms extended. Grasp the bar slightly wider than shoulder-width apart with a pronated grip. Maintain a neutral spine, keep abdominals contracted, and lean back slightly so that the bar is aligned with the clavicle. Retract the scapula and pull the bar toward the chest. Pause and then slowly return to the starting position.

*Training points to emphasize*

✓ Avoid hyperextension of the lumbar spine.

✓ Maintain a neutral wrist position throughout the exercise.

✓ Avoid performing behind-the-neck lat pull-downs, which increase the chances of injury to the shoulder joint.

## Seated Lat Row
### (latissimus dorsi, biceps, rhomboids, posterior deltoids)

*Performance recommendations*

Sit facing the weightstack with knees bent 90 degrees and feet flat on the floor. Grasp the handles with a neutral grip. Keep the chest lifted, shoulders back, and head and neck aligned with the spine. Retract the scapula and pull the handles toward the rib cage. Pause and then slowly return to the starting position.

*Training points to emphasize*

✓ Keep chest lifted, shoulders back, and do not round the upper back when the arms extend.

✓ Do not initiate the pulling with the arms and shoulders—"lead with the elbows."

✓ Avoid hyperextension of the lumbar spine (i.e., do not arch the back).

## Shoulder Press
(anterior deltoids, triceps, trapezius)

*Performance recommendations*
Sit with knees bent 90 degrees and feet flat on the floor, and grasp the handles with palms facing in. Press the weight overhead. Pause and then slowly return to the starting position.

*Training points to emphasize*
- ✓ Begin with the handles at, or slightly above, shoulder level.
- ✓ Do not arch the back.
- ✓ Keep the shoulder blades retracted with the torso and head erect.
- ✓ Do not "lock out" the elbows at the top of the movement.

## Machine-assisted Pull-up
(latissimus dorsi, teres major, posterior deltoids, biceps)

*Performance recommendations*
Kneel on the machine platform with an upright, neutral spinal posture. Place the hands on the parallel grips overhead, with the hands directly in line with slightly flexed elbows, and using a neutral grip. Maintain a body position that is almost perpendicular to the floor. Initiate the movement by contracting the latissimus dorsi, and pull the body up until the chin is even with, or slightly above, the grips. Pause and then slowly return to the starting position.

*Training points to emphasize*
- ✓ Do not allow the body to swing forward or backward.
- ✓ Maintain neutral lumbar and cervical posture.
- ✓ Retract and depress the scapulae throughout the exercise movement.

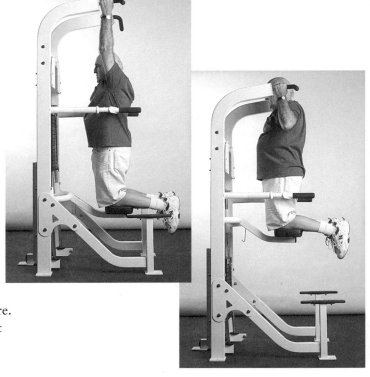

## Machine-assisted Dip Movement
(pectorals, anterior deltoids, triceps)

*Performance recommendations*

Kneel on the machine platform with an upright posture and neutral spine. Place the hands on the support handles with a neutral grip and slightly retract the scapula. Maintain a body position that is almost perpendicular to the floor during the descent phase. Pause and then slowly return to the starting position.

*Training points to emphasize*

✓ During the descent phase, the elbows should not flex more than 90 degrees.

✓ Keep the head and shoulders aligned over the hips.

✓ Upon returning to the straight-arm start position, depress the scapula without hyperextending the elbows.

# FREE WEIGHTS

## LOWER BODY

### Standing Dumbbell Squat (gluteals, quadriceps, hamstrings)

*Performance recommendations*

Hold a dumbbell with both hands and stand with a neutral spine and feet shoulder-width apart. Slowly start the descent with hips back, keeping the bodyweight centered over the heels or mid-foot. Lower to approximately 90 degrees of knee flexion. Pause and slowly return to the starting position.

*Training points to emphasize:*
- ✓ Do not allow the knees to travel past the toes during the lowering phase.
- ✓ Do not "drop" the gluteals lower than the knees.
- ✓ Avoid use of a block or board under the heels.
- ✓ Maintain a neutral spinal posture throughout the exercise movement.

### Standing Dumbbell Heel Raise (gastrocnemius, soleus)

*Performance recommendations*

Holding a dumbbell in each hand, stand upright with neutral spinal alignment. Slowly lift the body vertically by contracting the gastrocnemius and soleus muscles. Raise the heels up until full, pain-free range of motion is achieved. Pause and then slowly lower the heels back down until they are almost touching the floor.

*Training points to emphasize*
- ✓ Keep weight on the balls of the feet.
- ✓ Keep the toes pointed straight ahead.
- ✓ To increase the exercise range of motion, stand on a block or platform and let the heels drop below the edge.
- ✓ Retract the scapulae throughout the movement.

# UPPER BODY

### Dumbbell Bench Press
### (pectorals, anterior deltoids)

*Performance recommendations*

Lie supine on a bench to allow free movement of the shoulders and place the feet flat on the floor or up on the bench, whichever is more comfortable. Hold a dumbbell in each hand with the arms extended. Lower the dumbbells until they are at shoulder level. Pause and then raise the dumbbells back up to the starting position.

*Training points to emphasize*

- ✓ Maintain alignment of the hands, wrists, and forearms.
- ✓ Lift and lower the weights in a slow, controlled fashion.
- ✓ Do not arch the back.
- ✓ Keep the head, neck, and spine aligned.

### Kneeling Single-arm Dumbbell Lat Row
### (latissimus dorsi, teres major, posterior deltoids, biceps)

*Performance recommendations*

Place one knee on the bench with the same-side hip aligned directly over it. The knee of the other leg should be at approximately the same height and slightly flexed. Place the non-working hand on the bench and position the upper body so that it is parallel to the floor. Slowly flex the elbow and pull the arm up until the upper arm is parallel to the floor or slightly higher and the elbow forms an approximately 90-degree angle. Pause and then slowly lower the arm back down to the starting position.

*Training points to emphasize*

- ✓ Keep the elbow close to the side of the body.
- ✓ Maintain neutral lumbar and cervical posture.
- ✓ Keep the chest "square" to the floor throughout the exercise movement.

## Dumbbell Shoulder Press
(anterior deltoids, triceps, trapezius)

*Performance recommendations*

Sit on a bench with the back erect and a dumbbell in each hand. The upper arms are shoulder height and elbows are bent to 90 degrees. The palms face forward with neutral, stable wrist position. Press the dumbbells up overhead. Pause and then slowly return to the starting position.

*Training points to emphasize*
- ✓ Do not arch the back.
- ✓ Keep the shoulder blades retracted with the torso and head erect.
- ✓ Do not "lock out" the elbows at the top of the movement.
- ✓ Perform the exercise standing up to reduce compression stress on the spine.

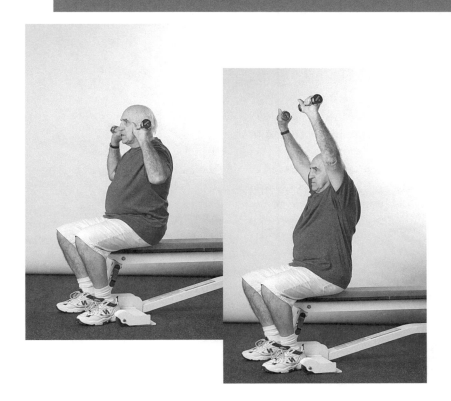

## Dumbbell Biceps Curl
(biceps)

*Performance recommendations*

Stand in a "ready" position with a neutral spine. The body is upright and the hips and knees are slightly flexed. Grasp a dumbbell in each hand with an underhand grip. Bring the hands toward the shoulders and flex the elbows through a full, pain-free range of motion. Pause and then slowly lower the arms back down to the starting position.

*Training points to emphasize*
- ✓ Initiate the movement at the elbows (do not "swing" to lift the weight).
- ✓ Keep the wrists neutral throughout the exercise.
- ✓ Retract the shoulder blades and maintain the same shoulder position throughout the exercise.
- ✓ Do not lean forward or backward during the exercise.

## Kneeling Single-arm Dumbbell Triceps Extension (triceps)

*Performance recommendations*

Place one knee on the bench with the same-side hip aligned directly over it. The knee of the other leg should be at approximately the same height and slightly flexed. Place the non-working hand on the bench. Position the upper body so that it is parallel to the floor. Flex the elbow and extend the shoulder until the upper arm is parallel with the floor. Slowly extend the elbow until the forearm is parallel to the floor. Pause and then slowly lower the arm back down to the starting position.

*Training points to emphasize*

✓ Do not allow the elbow to flare away from the body.

✓ Keep the wrist stabilized, not allowing the top of the dumbbell to tip toward the floor.

✓ Retract the shoulder blades and maintain the same shoulder position throughout the exercise.

✓ Do not arch the back.

# HOUSEHOLD ITEMS

The following exercises are offered as a low-cost alternative for home-based workouts. The items used as resistance include water jugs, juice cartons, plastic juice bottles, and soup or vegetable cans. The exerciser should choose an unbreakable item that provides appropriate resistance for the movement being performed (e.g., gallon water jugs for standing squats, but half-liter water bottles for standing side lateral raises). For the sake of simplicity, the resistance in each exercise is described as a "weight."

## LOWER BODY

### Standing Squat
(gluteals, quadriceps, hamstrings)

*Performance recommendations*

Hold a "weight" with both hands and stand with a neutral spine and your feet shoulder-width apart. Slowly start the descent with hips back, keeping the bodyweight centered over the heels or mid-foot. Lower to approximately 90 degrees of knee flexion. Pause and slowly return to the starting position.

*Training points to emphasize:*
- ✓ Do not allow the knees to travel past the toes during the lowering phase.
- ✓ Do not "drop" the gluteals lower than the knees.
- ✓ Avoid use of a block or board under the heels.
- ✓ Maintain a neutral spinal posture throughout the exercise movement.

### Standing Heel Raise
(gastrocnemius, soleus)

*Performance recommendations*

Holding a "weight" in each hand, stand upright with neutral spinal alignment. Slowly lift the body vertically by contracting the gastrocnemius and soleus muscles. Raise the heels up until full, pain-free range of motion is achieved. Pause and then slowly lower the heels back down until they are almost touching the floor.

*Training points to emphasize*
- ✓ Keep weight on the balls of the feet.
- ✓ Keep the toes pointed straight ahead.
- ✓ To increase the exercise range of motion, stand on a block or platform and let the heels drop below the edge.
- ✓ Retract the scapulae throughout the movement.

## Seated Elastic Chest Press
(pectorals, anterior deltoids, triceps)

*Performance recommendations*

Sit in a chair with a resistance band wrapped around the back at chest level. Holding the handles with neutral wrists, sit with the shoulders back and chest lifted. Exhale while pushing the handles out. Extend the arms until the elbows are relatively straight but not locked out. Pause and then slowly return to the starting position.

*Training points to emphasize*

✓ Keep chest lifted and maintain a neutral spine.

✓ Maintain alignment of the hands, wrists, and forearms.

✓ Perform this movement in a slow, controlled fashion.

## Kneeling Single-arm Lat Row
(latissimus dorsi, teres major, posterior deltoids, biceps)

*Performance recommendations*

Place one knee on a bench or chair with the same-side hip aligned directly over it. The knee of the other leg should be at approximately the same height and slightly flexed. Place the non-working hand at the front of the chair and position the upper body so that it is parallel to the floor. Slowly flex the elbow and pull the arm up until the upper arm is parallel to the floor or slightly higher and the elbow forms an approximately 90-degree angle. Pause and then slowly lower the arm back down to the starting position.

*Training points to emphasize*

✓ Keep the elbow close to the side of the body.

✓ Maintain neutral lumbar and cervical posture.

✓ Keep the chest "square" to the floor throughout the exercise movement.

## Standing Side Lateral Raise
(medial deltoids)

*Performance recommendations*

Stand in a "ready" position with a neutral spinal posture. The body is upright and the hips and knees are slightly flexed. Grasp the "weight" with an overhand grip. With the elbows slightly flexed, raise the arms out and up until they are approximately parallel to the floor. Pause and then slowly lower the arms back down to the starting position.

*Training points to emphasize*

- ✓ Keep the hands slightly in front of the shoulders with the elbows directly in line with the shoulders.
- ✓ Keep the wrists neutral with the palms oriented to the floor at the end of the range of motion.
- ✓ Avoid internally or externally rotating the shoulders, or supinating or pronating the elbows.
- ✓ Lower the arms back down to the starting position with control.

## Standing Biceps Curl
(biceps)

*Performance recommendations*

Stand in a "ready" position with a neutral spine. The body is upright and the hips and knees are slightly flexed. Grasp the "weight" with an underhand grip. Bring the hands toward the shoulders and flex the elbows through a full, pain-free range of motion. Pause and then slowly lower the arms back down to the starting position.

*Training points to emphasize*

- ✓ Initiate the movement at the elbows (do not "swing" to lift the weight).
- ✓ Keep the wrists neutral throughout the exercise.
- ✓ Retract the shoulder blades and maintain the same shoulder position throughout the exercise.
- ✓ Do not lean forward or backward during the exercise.

## Kneeling Single-arm Triceps Extension (triceps)

*Performance recommendations*

Place one knee on a chair or bench with the same-side hip aligned directly over it. The knee of the other leg should be at approximately the same height and slightly flexed. Place the non-working hand on the chair. Position the upper body so that it is parallel to the floor. Flex the elbow and extend the shoulder until the upper arm is parallel with the floor. Slowly extend the elbow until the forearm is parallel to the floor. Pause and then slowly lower the arm back down to the starting position.

*Training points to emphasize*

- ✓ Do not allow the elbow to flare away from the body.
- ✓ Keep the wrist stabilized, not allowing the top of the dumbbell to tip toward the floor.
- ✓ Retract the shoulder blades and maintain the same shoulder position throughout the exercise.
- ✓ Do not arch the back.

## TORSO

### Curl-up
(rectus abdominis)

*Performance recommendations*

In a supine position, place the hands across the chest (the behind-the-head position is not appropriate for many older adults due to a limited range of motion in the shoulder girdle) and flex one knee as shown. Raise the head and shoulders off the floor while maintaining a neutral spine. Pause and then slowly return to the starting position. Alternate the bent leg midway through each set of repetitions.

*Training points to emphasize*

- ✓ Do not flex the cervical spine by curling the neck.
- ✓ Do not elevate the head and shoulders a large distance off the floor.
- ✓ Move the head, neck, and shoulders as one unit.

# REFERENCES

Ades, P.A. et al. (1996). Weight training improves walking endurance in healthy elderly persons. *Annals of Internal Medicine,* 124, 568–572.

American College of Sports Medicine (2000). *ACSM's Guidelines for Exercise Testing and Prescription,* 6th ed. Baltimore, Md: Lippincott Williams & Wilkins.

American College of Sports Medicine (1998). Position stand: The recommended quantity and quality of exercise for developing and maintaining cardiorespiratory and muscular fitness and flexibility in healthy adults. *Medicine and Science in Sports and Exercise,* 30, 975–991.

Bermon, S., Rama, D., & Dolisi, C. (2000). Cardiovascular tolerance of healthy elderly subjects to weight-lifting exercises. *Medicine and Science in Sports and Exercise,* 32, 1845–1848.

Evans, W. & Rosenberg, I. (1992). *Biomarkers.* New York: Simon & Schuster.

Fiatarone, M.A. et al. (1990). High-intensity strength training in nonagenarians. *Journal of the American Medical Association,* 263, 3029–3034.

Franklin, B.A. et al. (1991). Resistance training in cardiac rehabilitation. *Journal of Cardiopulmonary Rehabilitation,* 11, 99–107.

Franklin, B.A. & Munnings, F. (1995). Rejuvenation through exercise. *Encyclopedia Britannica: Medical and Health Annual,* 263–268.

Franklin, B.A. (1998). Pumping iron: Rationale, benefits, safety, and prescription. *ACSM's Health and Fitness Journal,* 2, 5, 12–15.

Graves, J.E. & Franklin, B.A., Eds. (2001). *Resistance Training for Health and Rehabilitation.* Champaign, Ill.: Human Kinetics.

Hickson, R.C., Rosenkoetter, M.A., & Brown, M.M. (1980). Strength training effects on aerobic power and short-term endurance. *Medicine and Science in Sports and Exercise,* 12, 336–339.

Hunter, G.R. et al. (2001). High-resistance versus variable-resistance training in older adults. *Medicine and Science in Sports and Exercise,* 33, 1759–1764.

Hunter, G.R. et al. (2002). Resistance training and intra-abdominal adipose tissue in older men and women. *Medicine and Science in Sports and Exercise,* 34, 1023–1028.

Keyes, A., Taylor, H., & Grande, F. (1973). Basal metabolism and age of adult men. *Metabolism,* 22, 579–587.

Kraemer, W.J. et al. (2002). Progression models in resistance training for healthy adults. *Medicine and Science in Sports and Exercise,* 34, 364–380.

Lind, A.R. & McNicol, G.W. (1967). Muscular factors which determine the cardiovascular responses to sustained and rhythmic exercise. *Canadian Medical Association Journal,* 96, 706–715.

McCartney, N. et al. (1993). Weight-training-induced attenuation of the circulatory response of older males to weight lifting. *Journal of Applied Physiology,* 74, 1056–1060.

Mitchell, J.H. et al. (1980). The role of muscle mass in the cardiovascular response to static contractions. *Journal of Physiology,* 309, 45–54.

Pollock, M.L. et al. (1994). Exercise training and prescription for the elderly. *Southern Medical Journal,* 87, S88–S95.

Pollock, M.L. & Vincent, K.R. (1996) Resistance training for health. *The President's Council on Physical Fitness and Sports Research Digest,* 2, 8.

Pollock, M.L. et al. (2000). Resistance exercise in individuals with and without cardiovascular disease: benefits, rationale, safety, and prescription. *Circulation,* 101, 828–833.

Sayers, S.P. et al. (2003). Changes in function and disability after resistance training: Does velocity matter? *American Journal of Physical Medicine and Rehabilitation,* 82, 605–613.

Singh, N., Clements, K. & Fiatarone, M. (1997). A randomized controlled trial of progressive resistance training in depressed elders. *Journal of Gerontology,* 52A, 1, M27–M35.

Wood, R.H. et al. (2001). Concurrent cardiovascular and resistance training in healthy older adults. *Medicine and Science in Sports and Exercise,* 33, 1751–1758.

EXERCISE

# Programming and Leadership

## Kay Van Norman

*Kay Van Norman, M.S., is the founder and president of SENioRS Unlimited, a consulting firm specializing in older adult wellness programming. She currently serves as a delegate for the Health Promotion Institute of the National Council on Aging, and on the boards of the International Council on Active Aging and the American Senior Fitness Association.*

*Ms. Van Norman has served as director of the Keiser Institute on Aging, an international effort to bridge the gap between research and practice in the field of older adult wellness. She has taught for the Department of Health & Human Development at Montana State University and directed MSU's "Young At Heart" exercise program for older adults. Van Norman is a former national chair of the Council on Aging and Adult Development within the American Alliance for Health, Physical Education, Recreation and Dance, and received the 1998 Rosabel Koss Honor Award for her service to the profession of older adult health. In 2003 she received a Best Practices award from the National Council on Aging for her innovative products meeting the needs of older adults. Van Norman is the author of Exercise Programming for Older Adults, numerous chapters, and more than 20 national and international journal articles on the subject.*

Safe and effective programming for older adults requires integrating knowledge of their special needs with appropriate assessment procedures and exercise techniques, giving special attention to program implementation, as well as marketability. This chapter facilitates this integration of concepts by first providing specific strategies for determining current levels of function, identifying and prioritizing specific needs at each functional level, and then designing programming that effectively meets these needs without exposing participants to unnecessary risks. This integration requires one to carefully form a bridge between the current research on physical activity and aging and exercise programming. This bridge can be built with function-based programming that reflects the practical application of proven concepts (Figure 7.1).

In addition, this chapter provides strategies for applying exercise principles in a way that meets the special needs of seniors, and outlines methods for developing programs to attract seniors from various levels of functional ability. Finally, strategies for the recruitment and motivation of seniors are addressed, along with low-cost equipment options for increasing exercise effectiveness and enjoyment.

# DETERMINING THE LEVELS OF FUNCTION

The range of functional ability within the older adult population can be categorized into five different levels. Spirduso, Francis, and MacRae (2005), in their book *Physical Dimensions of Aging,* second edition, identify these levels as: Physically Dependent, Physically Frail, Physically Independent, Physically Fit, and Physically Elite. Her definitions provide a useful framework for identifying the functional abilities and needs of individuals at each level.

## Physically Dependent

The physically dependent older adult cannot execute some or all of the Basic Activities of Daily Living (BADL), including self-dressing, bathing, transferring, using the toilet, feeding, and walking. These individuals are dependent on others for food and for basic functions of living.

## Physically Frail

Physically frail seniors can perform BADL, but cannot perform some or all of the activities necessary to live independently. This is generally due to a debilitating disease or condition that physically challenges them on a daily basis.

## Physically Independent

The physically independent older adult lives independently, usually without debilitating symptoms of major chronic diseases, but has low health and fitness reserves. For many such individuals, a brief illness or injury can mean a rapid loss of physical function and, thus, a loss of independence. Even after recovery from the initial illness or injury, their loss of function results in physical frailty.

## Physically Fit

The physically fit senior exercises at least twice per week for their health, enjoyment, and well-being, or works regularly at a physically demanding job or hobby. Their health and fitness reserves put them at low risk for falling into the physically frail category.

## Physically Elite

The physically elite older adult trains on an almost daily basis to compete in sport tournaments, work in a physically demanding job, or participate in recreational activities.

# IDENTIFYING AND ADDRESSING NEEDS

Pre-screening and physical assessments help you determine each individual's level of physical function. Pre-screening

FIGURE 7.1

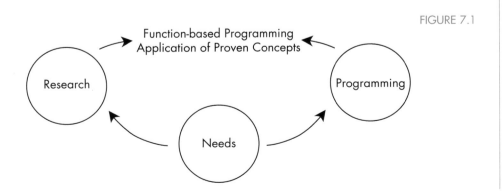

includes inquiring about medical background, medications, and pre-existing health conditions.

Refer to Chapter 4 for specific pre-screening and physical assessment strategies. Also, you may refer to Table 7.1 for a list of commonly used tests of physical function. Using the appropriate physical assessments will help you identify the client's current level of functional ability and any physical deficits that must be addressed.

Chapter 4 also provides strategies for assessing psychological responses to exercise, including expectations and goals. The psychological aspect of assessment is a critical, but often overlooked, component of developing programming that addresses needs, as well as personal objectives related to exercise participation.

Using both physical and psychological assessments will help you identify the most immediate needs for each individual or group, and allow you to prioritize program goals. For example, whereas aerobic conditioning is very beneficial for older adults, it is of little or no use to someone within the first two levels of functional ability who are struggling to perform BADL. This is where the concept of "movement that matters" becomes useful (i.e., prioritizing and addressing the most immediate physical and psychological needs). Chapter 4 makes reference to this same concept by stating that "assessments should be specific to each client's needs, abilities, and objectives."

## Physically Dependent

Movement that helps maintain or improve physical function for basic self-care is important to this group. Physically dependent older adults need the strength, range of motion, balance, and coordination necessary for self-feeding, bathing, dressing, going to the bathroom, transferring, and walking. Concentrate on activities to improve finger and hand strength and agility, arm strength, shoulder and hip range of motion, leg strength (especially in the quadriceps and ankle flexors), ankle strength and range of motion, and foot and toe mobility.

## IDENTIFYING NEEDS

To provide programming that addresses BADL, it is important to understand the specific physical function necessary for each of the activities. The following outline will help you determine these necessary functions:

### Self-toileting

Self-toileting requires enough strength and range of motion in the legs and hips to go from a standing to seated position and from a seated to standing position. In the case of a wheelchair-bound individual, it requires upper-body strength for transferring from the chair to the toilet and back. Self-toileting also requires enough strength and range of motion in the hands and arms to remove and replace clothing.
✓ R.O.M.—in the hips, knees, ankles, shoulders, and wrists

✓ STRENGTH—in the legs, hips, arms, and hands

### Self-bathing

Self-bathing requires strength and range of motion in the hips and legs to get in and out of the tub. It also requires enough strength and range of motion in the hands and arms to remove and replace clothing and wash all areas of the body.
✓ R.O.M.—in the hips, knees, ankles, shoulders, and wrists

✓ STRENGTH—in the legs, hips, arms, and hands

### Self-transferring

Successful self-transferring requires strength and range of motion in the legs, and balance to sit on, and stand up from, a chair, or transfer to or from a bed. In the case of wheelchair-bound individuals, it requires enough strength in the upper body to transfer from the chair to a bed and from a bed to the chair.

Table 7.1
**Tests of Physical Function**

| Category of Physical Function | Sample Tests | Sources |
|---|---|---|
| Physically elite | $\dot{V}O_2$max; modified Balke treadmill | ACSM, 1991 |
| Physically fit | Bruce treadmill protocol | Bruce et al., 1973 |
| Physically independent (some) | Resistance strength tests (dynamometry) | McArdle et al., 2001 |
| | Routine flexibility and agility tests | |
| | Senior fitness test | Rikli & Jones, 1998 |
| | AAHPERD functional fitness test | Osness, 1987 |
| | Fitness tests: | |
| |     Jumping, hand strength, flexion | Kimura et al., 1990 |
| |     Balance, agility, power, flexibility | Kuo, 1990 |
| |     Jumping, side-step, flexion, reaction time | Tahara et al., 1990 |
| Physically independent | AAHPERD field test | Osness, 1987 |
| | AADL | Reuben et al., 1990 |
| | Continuous-scale physical functional performance test | Cress et al., 1996 |
| Physically frail | Physical performance test | Reuben & Siu, 1990 |
| | Tinetti's mobility assessment | Tinetti, 1986 |
| | IADL | Lawton & Brody, 1969 |
| | Hierarchical ADL-IADL | Kempen & Suurmeijer, 1990 |
| | Classification schema for upper-extremity function and mobility | Williams & Greene, 1990 |
| | Geri-AIMS | Hughes et al., 1991 |
| | Physical impairment scale | Jette, Branch, & Berlin, 1990 |
| | Functional independence measure | Granger et al., 1986 |
| Physically dependent | ADL | Katz et al., 1963 |
| | Mobility test | Schnelle et al., 1995 |
| | Physical disability index | Gerety et al., 1993 |
| | Physical performance and mobility exam | Lemsky et al., 1991 |
| | Physical function scale of MOS SF-36 | Ware & Sherbourne, 1992 |

*Note:* ACSM = American College of Sports Medicine; AAHPERD = American Alliance for Health, Physical Education, Recreation and Dance; AADL = advanced activities of daily living; IADL = instrumental activities of daily living; ADL = activities of daily living; MOS SF-36 = Medical Outcomes Short Study Form

*From W.W. Spirduso, Physical Dimensions of Aging, 2nd ed., Table 11.1 (in press). © 2005 by Waneen W. Spirduso. Reprinted with permission from Human Kinetics (Champaign, Ill.).*

✓ R.O.M.—in the ankles, knees, and hips

✓ STRENGTH—in the legs, hips, and arms (to aid in rising)

✓ BALANCE—enough to accomplish transfers without falling

## Walking

Walking requires strength and range of motion in the lower body and enough balance to get from one place to another without falling. Walking with an assistive device also requires strength in the upper body to effectively use the device.

✓ R.O.M. —in the ankles, hips, and knees

✓ STRENGTH—in the ankles, hips, and legs. There is a secondary concern for strength in the upper back to help maintain posture, proper alignment, and balance. If an assistive device is being used, additional upper-body strength is necessary.

✓ BALANCE—to transfer weight from one foot to the other, sustain a one-footed stance, and maintain an appropriate stride length and normal gait

✓ CONFIDENCE—in their ability to walk without falling

When choosing exercises to improve performance of BADL, ask yourself three questions:
1) Does this exercise address an immediate need?
2) Will it help improve function?
3) Is there a safer alternative?

When determining programming for individuals in the dependent category who have multiple physical impairments, it is always important to weigh the benefits of an exercise against its possible risks. Sometimes a measured amount of risk is acceptable if the benefits are significant. For example, it is extremely important for an individual to maintain the ability to self-toilet. Quadriceps strength plays a large role in this aspect of self-care and personal independence. Knee extensions against resistance can significantly improve quadriceps strength but, for some individuals, may also cause discomfort in the knee joint. If modifications do not alleviate the discomfort, but the discomfort is temporary and manageable, the benefits of maintaining enough quadriceps strength for self-toileting are likely to outweigh the risks. Refer to Table 7.2 for programming appropriate for physically dependent older adults.

## Physically Frail

Physically frail seniors need exercise that helps them maintain or improve

Table 7.2

### Programming for the Physically Dependent

✓ Chair-based exercises that specifically address each of the BADL

✓ One-on-one water-based exercise (water walking, and range-of-motion and strength work)

✓ Resistance exercise for the upper and lower body

✓ Individualized "home-based" exercises

✓ Breathing and relaxation

✓ Hand function exercises

their ability to perform BADL and Instrumental Activities of Daily Living (IADL). IADL are more complex physical abilities such as preparing meals, housecleaning, shopping, and mobility in and out of the home. Exercise programming will focus on muscular strength, endurance, flexibility, joint range of motion, balance, and coordination.

## IDENTIFYING NEEDS

Leg strength significantly contributes to improved balance and the ability to recover from near falls. It also helps clients regain or maintain a normal gait pattern, which includes ankle flexion with heel strike, a full stride length, and appropriate gait speed. Programming that focuses on strengthening the upper back and stabilizing the shoulder blades in a neutral position (instead of rounded forward), will help improve posture. For example, encouraging clients to routinely perform scapular retraction (i.e., pulling the shoulder blades together in back) throughout the day can help improve posture. Improved posture in turn promotes better balance and gait.

Additional areas to address include foot mobility and agility, which also impact balance and gait. This can be accomplished by utilizing low-cost manipulatives. While this may seem to be a small component of functional ability, it should not be overlooked. Research indicates that loss of agility in the feet and toes contributes significantly to diminished balance (Perkins-Carpenter, 1991; Spirduso, Francis, & MacRae, 2005).

Special attention also should be paid to helping frail seniors overcome the fear of injury. Many frail seniors perceive exercise as potentially harmful, and may in fact have been injured in the past trying to perform inappropriate exercise. Pre-assessments and attention to their personal needs and objectives will help you define program content and objectives that are easily attainable. Success in movement is essential to help

Table 7.3

**Programming for the Physically Frail**

✓ Chair-based exercises that specifically address the basic and instrumental activities of daily living

✓ One-on-one water-based exercise (water walking, and range-of-motion and strength work)

✓ Resistance exercise to improve upper- and lower-body strength

✓ Breathing and relaxation

✓ Chair exercise and chair-assisted exercise that practice balance and coordination

✓ Group water-based programming that addresses strength, range of motion, balance, and coordination

✓ Individualized "home-based" exercise

frail seniors gain confidence in their ability to be physically active without injury. Refer to Table 7.3 for programming appropriate for frail seniors.

## Physically Independent

This category of older adults ranges from individuals who are barely functionally independent and maintaining lifestyles that ask very little of them physically, to seniors who are fairly active, but are not engaged in exercise, work, or recreation that keeps them physically "fit." Physically independent seniors need exercise that helps them maintain and improve their physical function, remain independent, and prevent illness, disability, or injury that could lead to physical frailty. Exercise programming for independent seniors should focus on muscular strength and endurance, flexibility, joint range of motion, balance, coordination, and cardiovascular endurance.

### IDENTIFYING NEEDS

For an exercise to be considered aerobic it must have the capacity to improve cardiovascular conditioning. Therefore, a chair aerobics class for independent seniors must include an aerobic component. For many clients this can be accomplished through vigorous movement of the arms and the legs. Exercises such as rhythmic knee lifts and kicks to the front and sides, as well as frequently standing up from, and sitting down on, a chair can be a part of that aerobic component. Chair "dancing" using continuous rhythmic movement of the arms and legs in set patterns also can be a fun way to achieve aerobic conditioning.

Another primary goal is to educate the physically independent senior on the importance of prevention of functional loss, thus motivating them to significantly increase their health and fitness reserves (Barry & Eathorne, 1994; Carter et al., 1991; Resnick, 1991; Schilke, 1991; Shephard, 1993).

One way to do this is to make your program's wellness and fitness messages personally relevant to your clients. For example, if your program's messages are all exercise-based, those individuals who have always thought of themselves as non-exercisers will likely find the messages irrelevant. A large number of older adults (especially older women) do not consider themselves the exercise/fitness type. Therefore, focus your exercise and wellness messages on topics such as maintaining bone strength to combat the effects of osteoporosis, and maintaining leg strength to prevent falls and retain the ability to walk, climb stairs, golf, and enjoy travel. In short, messages related to maintaining an independent lifestyle are most appropriate. These messages are relevant to the older adult whether they consider themselves to be an exerciser or non-exerciser. Refer to Table 7.4 for activities appropriate for physically independent seniors.

## Physically Fit

Physically fit older adults require exercise programming that maintains their level of fitness, which in turn allows

## Table 7.4

### Programming for the Physically Independent

✓ Chair aerobics

✓ Low-impact aerobics

✓ Modified line dancing and folk dancing

✓ Water aerobics

✓ Lap swimming

✓ Walking programs

✓ Circuit training

✓ Resistance training

✓ Recreational activities

✓ Tai chi

✓ Stretching

✓ Relaxation

them to live an active, independent lifestyle, work in their chosen professions, and/or participate in a wide range of recreational activities. Programming should focus on muscular strength and endurance, flexibility, joint range of motion, balance, coordination, agility, and cardiovascular endurance. The primary goal in working with physically fit seniors is to provide them with current health information and various opportunities to maintain their level of fitness.

## IDENTIFYING NEEDS

This group of seniors is generally very self-motivated. They have already determined that physical activity is important to their quality of life. Therefore, your focus will be on providing convenient and safe "maintenance" programming that addresses each component of fitness. Emphasize safety because many physically fit seniors are motivated to keep doing more and more without regard for safety. Education on the benefits of appropriate exercise intensity, as well as the risks of inappropriate intensity, is important. Again, it is necessary to emphasize the importance of strength in maintaining functional independence and overall physical fitness. Even those who are involved

in water aerobics and low-impact aerobics will notice significant gains in strength through resistance training.

Finally, this group of seniors should be provided with information about the Senior Olympics and other opportunities to challenge their physical abilities. Refer to Table 7.5 for activities appropriate for physically fit seniors.

## Physically Elite

Physically elite seniors require exercise programming that helps them maintain their fitness levels, and provides conditioning for improved performance in competition or in strenuous vocational or recreational activities. Programming should include general conditioning for muscular strength and endurance, flexibility, agility, and cardiovascular endurance. It also may include sport- or activity-specific training.

## IDENTIFYING NEEDS

Exercise programming for the physically elite often is focused on improving performance in a desired area or areas. Many times this includes intensive

## Table 7.5

### Programming for the Physically Fit

✓ Low-impact aerobics

✓ Line dancing and folk dancing

✓ Water aerobics

✓ Lap swimming

✓ Walking programs

✓ Circuit training

✓ Resistance training

✓ Recreational activities

✓ Tai chi

✓ Yoga

✓ Stretching

✓ Relaxation

✓ Sports and games (golf, tennis, etc.)

Table 7.6

**Programming for the Physically Elite**

✓ Low-impact aerobics

✓ Line dancing and folk dancing

✓ Water aerobics

✓ Lap swimming

✓ Walking programs (possibly race walking)

✓ Circuit training

✓ Interval training

✓ Resistance training

✓ Recreational activities

✓ Tai chi

✓ Yoga

✓ Stretching

✓ Relaxation

✓ Sports and games

✓ Sport- or activity-specific training for competition

strength training. Your role is to provide the physically elite senior access to appropriate resources and equipment and to offer reinforcement of proper exercise intensity and techniques. Supplying the elite senior with information concerning the adverse effects of overtraining and the need for appropriate recovery periods between workouts will give them the tools to prevent injury while training and competing. In addition, it is important to provide strategies for addressing injuries if they do occur. Refer to Table 7.6 for a list of activities appropriate for physically elite seniors.

# LEVELED PROGRAMMING

Leveled programming refers to offering a range of classes to meet the needs of various levels of functional ability. If you are teaching in a fitness facility, you may only be providing programming for older adults from the upper level of the physically independent category through the

physically elite. However, an exercise program at a senior residence facility would require that you provide entry-level activity classes that allow someone in the dependent or frail category to be successful in your program, as well as classes that challenge independent to physically fit older adults. The needs of the physically elite older adult for general conditioning can be met in the upper-level aerobics, circuit, and resistance classes. However, the sport- or activity-specific training would be done on an individual basis.

The following pages identify suggestions for appropriate classes using the leveling concept. For detailed descriptions and photographs of specific land- and water-based exercises, please refer to Chapters 5 and 6 of this text, and to *Exercise Programming for Older Adults* in the suggested reading list.

## Land-based Programming

Land-based programming includes movement opportunities such as chair exercise, walking, dancing, low-impact aerobics, circuit training, strength training, tai chi, yoga, functionally specific stations, recreational activities, and a variety of sports and games.

### ENTRY LEVEL

Options for entry-level land-based programming include functional-fitness-based chair exercise, resistance training, and the use of home-based exercise brochures or videos. Function-based chair exercise programs consist of exercises that meet the needs of dependent and frail seniors. These exercises help them maintain and improve their ability to perform BADL. Many times, activities programs in senior residence facilities offer a series of games and activities for fun and socialization with little regard for functional needs. Functional-fitness-based programming is equally as important as social activities. Take steps to ensure that your program addresses functional needs and look for

## Developing an Individualized Exercise Program

Eleanor is a 76-year-old woman with poor vision. She used to enjoy walking several times a week, but hasn't been able to walk alone for almost a year due to fear of falling and, as a result, has become sedentary.

Pre-assessments indicate that she has a history of lower-back pain, has lost most of her sight to glaucoma, and is on blood-pressure medication. Physical assessments indicate that her functional status is in the physically frail category. In particular, she is having difficulty getting up from a seated position and her gait demonstrates a very short stride, flat-footed placement with almost no heel strike, and unsteady balance. The assessments show that this is partly due to weakness in the ankles and legs, and low range of motion in the hips. However, Eleanor's gait abnormality is exaggerated by her extreme fear of falling. She is anxious to regain function, but is fearful of being injured. Eleanor's goals are to rise from a seated position more easily, improve balance, and regain the ability to take a walk.

### PROGRAM DESIGN

Eleanor's most immediate needs are for increased lower-body strength to facilitate a more normal gait pattern and ease in rising from a seated position. This can be accomplished through resistance training on machines and/or with ankle weights. Focus on ankle dorsiflexion (to facilitate an appropriate heel-strike pattern) and quadriceps strength (for rising from a chair). Because of her poor vision, Eleanor will need close supervision in the weight room to facilitate success in movement, alleviate fear, and prevent injury.

In addition to strength work, she needs to improve flexibility of the gastrocnemius muscle and the hip extensors to improve her gait pattern.

A secondary need is to address her fear of injury by ensuring that she feels safe in all aspects of the walking movement. Water walking can facilitate balance, coordination, and range-of-motion work, and remove the fear of falling. Land-based balance work also is important for Eleanor to regain the ability to walk for enjoyment, but should be addressed gradually after she has gained confidence and strength. Aerobic conditioning is a secondary concern that should be addressed after she has gained strength and confidence in her ability to exercise without injury. Any aerobic conditioning should be done in water or in a chair, as her poor vision places her at high risk for falling.

ways to add functional tasks to social games and activities whenever possible.

Strength training is such an important part of improving and maintaining function that even very frail older adults can gain significant benefits (Fiatarone et al., 1994; Fielding et al., 2002). Resistance training can involve light weights and resistance bands or strength-training machines. After frail seniors become accustomed to the idea of resistance training with light, hand-held weights

and resistance bands, allow them to utilize senior-appropriate strength-training machines if possible. Sometimes, when these individuals get a better sense of movement and how it can benefit them, they will be more motivated to utilize strength machines. It is critical for strength-training machines used in senior programming to be "senior appropriate." This means they must be fully adjustable to body size, and allow for beginning at minimal weight and for small increments of increased resistance. Keiser air-resistance machines are especially suited to seniors because they meet all these criteria, and are non-intimidating and easy to operate.

In skilled nursing facilities, assisted-living facilities, and senior housing centers, the home-based exercise concept can be useful. This refers to exercises that focus on maintenance of BADL and can be performed by the individual on a regular basis without supervision. Utilize a variety of simple exercise brochures, each designed to meet the needs of different levels of function. The Permission to M.O.V.E. (Motivation, Opportunity, Verification, & Education) campaign, for example, outlines specific strategies for motivating seniors to take an active role in maintaining their functional independence by performing simple, safe exercises daily (See page 247 for more information). This type of programming allows everyone to become involved regardless of whether or not they are motivated to come to a regularly scheduled class. Once you give even very unmotivated older adults the opportunity to move on a regular basis and offer reinforcement for their efforts, they typically become more inclined to further increase their level of physical activity. Some even progress to choosing to participate in structured classes.

## LEVEL II

Options for Level II programming include walking, functional-fitness-based station work, more vigorous chair exercise (involving some aerobic conditioning), circuit training, flexibility training, and strength training. Walking programs can include walking trails (indoor or outdoor), as well as station formats. In addition to getting residents walking, emphasize the importance of maintaining or normalizing posture and gait patterns while walking. The stations format allows residents to walk from one functional-fitness station to the next and is advantageous because it is available on a

continuous basis. When using the stations format at senior residence facilities, choose exercises carefully to incorporate a level of basic functional ability, posing minimal risks to potentially unsupervised participants.

Chair exercise can incorporate functional fitness activities with a higher level of coordination, flexibility, balance, and strength work. In addition, an aerobic phase is gradually added to improve cardiovascular health.

A supervised circuit- or strength-training program also is appropriate at this level. Circuit training involves alternating between a strength machine and an aerobic machine throughout a pre-set circuit. The strength-training program utilizes strength equipment alone with specific goals for improving strength in both the lower and upper body.

Tai chi also is a good choice for Level II programming. Its slow, controlled movement with concentration on breathing and internalizing balance and coordination is appropriate for older adults. The challenge with tai chi may be the preconceived idea of what the practice of tai chi means. Many older adults relate it to some type of religion and, therefore, are reluctant to become involved with this type of activity. Try incorporating some of the tai chi movement techniques into a class they are already comfortable with, such as low-impact aerobics. The movements become balance and coordination work rather than formalized tai chi training.

## LEVEL III

The third level of land-based programming should include activities such as low-impact aerobics, walking or jogging, circuit training, strength training, line and folk dancing, and a variety of recreational activities.

Low-impact aerobic programs should consist of gentle movement to music as a warm-up; continuous, simple movement to music for an aerobics phase; a resistance phase; and a cool-down and stretch phase. One sound approach to a balanced program, for example, includes approximately 10 to 20 minutes of warm-up, coordination, and balance work; 20 to 25 minutes of aerobics; and 15 to 20 minutes of cool-down, strengthening, and stretching. Focus on safety by weighing the benefits against the risks for each choice. Movement choices and class format also must be structured in a way that allows all clients to feel successful. Your program structure should exhibit simple patterns—without complicated combinations, surprise direction changes, or fast cross-over steps that can put clients at risk for a fall. Embrace a teaching style that relays information about what is coming next (e.g., hand signals and voice cueing before a change). In addition, return often to simple steps (such as marching in place) to ensure that all participants are successful in movement at least some of the time, and most are successful the majority of the time. For specific exercise descriptions, please refer to Chapter 5 of this text and *Exercise Programming for Older Adults* in the suggested reading list.

Note that classes such as tai chi, circuit training, strength training, and functionally specific fitness stations can be used at several levels of programming. With proper supervision, these classes can be structured to simultaneously meet the needs of seniors from a variety of functional ability levels.

## Water-based Programming

Water-based programming refers to any activities that are conducted in the water, such as water walking, one-on-one water exercise, water aerobics, water circuit training, games such as water polo, and swimming. Water-based programming at each level can simultaneously meet the needs of seniors at a variety of levels of functional ability. An individual can work as hard or as gently as they choose to in the water. This allows a water aerobics class, for example, to be a gentle workout for some, or a vigorous workout for the person who chooses to resist the water with the arms and lift the knees more quickly and/or higher than average. For detailed descriptions and examples, refer to Chapter 5 of this text, and *Exercise Programming for Older Adults* and ACE's *Aquatic Exercise* in the suggested reading list.

### ENTRY LEVEL

Entry-level classes in water-based programming include one-on-one water exercise and group or individual water walking. In one-on-one water exercise, an instructor helps a student move through a set of goal-specific exercises in the pool. Water walking engages participants in walking forward, backward, and sideways across the pool. Variations are numerous and include using long strides, short strides, cross-over steps, a heel-strike pattern, walking on tip toes, and walking with bent or straight knees. Emphasis can be placed on using these variations to improve coordination and balance. This class also should include a strength segment, a flexibility segment, and a cool-down and relaxation segment. Water walking classes usually are designed to improve strength, range of motion, coordination, and balance for older adults who are not ready for an aerobic program, or who simply prefer a workout with less impact.

### LEVEL II

The second level of water-based programming includes a Water Aerobics Level I class. This class commonly includes a 20- to 25-minute warm-up; a range-of-motion, coordination, and strength phase; a 15- to 20-minute cardiovascular conditioning (aerobic) phase; and a 20- to 25-minute cool-down and stretch phase. Another option within this level of programming is to provide an opportunity for those who enjoy lap swimming.

## LEVEL III

The third level includes Water Aerobics Level II, which generally uses the same format as Level I, except the aerobic segment is increased to 20 to 25 minutes. It also could include more repetitions or more difficult exercises in the strength segment, and more complicated coordination work. It is still important, however, to provide a balanced class with 15 to 20 minutes of warm-up; range-of-motion, strength, and coordination work; and 15 to 20 minutes of cool-down and stretching. Lap swimming also is appropriate for this level of programming.

## Warm-up

Regardless of the mode of exercise chosen (i.e., land, water, chair), never begin a senior exercise class with aggressive stretching. Seniors tend to have diminished flexibility of the tendons, ligaments, and muscles, resulting in a higher potential for muscle and tendon strain and tears (Spirduso, Francis, & MacRae, 2005). Begin your classes with a combination of gentle continuous movement and easy range-of-motion activities to increase circulation. Gentle static stretching and preparatory stretching also can be part of a senior warm-up. When incorporating static stretching into a warm-up, have seniors stretch to a comfortable range of motion and hold that stretch. Stretching to the point of mild discomfort for the purpose of increasing flexibility should only be performed at the end of a class when muscles are thoroughly warmed.

The warm-up phase is a good time to teach any new movement sequence you plan to use later in the aerobic phase of class. This gives students a chance to try the movement slowly and gain confidence before attempting to execute the movement in time with the music during aerobics. Have your students go through the ranges of motion they will be using during the aerobics phase. For example, if you plan to push the arms overhead during the aerobic phase then it is a good idea to perform the same action more slowly during the warm-up.

## Safe Movements

When choosing movement possibilities, weigh the risks against the benefits of each type of exercise. Choose smooth rather than jerky arm movements, and completed movements rather than choppy or abrupt starts and stops. Smooth, complete movements reduce the risk of joint stress and injury to participants. In land-based exercise classes, low-impact movements are the only appropriate choice for an older adult class, as high-impact movements pose an unacceptably high level of risk. Simple movements and movement combinations are safer and promote self-confidence by allowing participants to be successful. Many seniors may have lost a significant amount of coordination if they have not been participating regularly in a coordination-promoting activity. Therefore, rapid changes of direction and complicated movement patterns increase both anxiety and the danger of falling. They also decrease self-esteem and the overall enjoyment of those who are unsuccessful in the movement. While keeping movements simple, you must also make an effort to use a variety of movement combinations, music, and teaching formations to keep classes fun and interesting. In strength-training classes, be very conscientious about ensuring proper body alignment and exercise techniques. Teach clients to perform resistance work through their pain-free range of motion. In addition, be aware of machines that allow hyperextension or hyperflexion of the joints, and make sure seniors know how to adjust these machines to prevent joint stress and injury.

## Managing Aerobic Training Risks

Due to the high incidence of cardiovascular dysfunction in the older adult population, it is important to use a variety of methods to help ensure that your participants are exercising at an appropriate aerobic level. This can be achieved by determining individual target heart-rate zones, using the rating of perceived exertion scale, and frequent heart-rate checks. A combination of methods will help your students learn how intense their exercise should be.

### DETERMINING INTENSITY

As a fitness professional, it is your job to make sure each individual participating in cardiovascular conditioning activities knows their individually determined target heart-rate range. Research shows that even moderate- to low-intensity aerobic exercise provides a training benefit for many seniors (Barry & Eathorne, 1994). Use the Karvonen formula for your students without heart disease and vary the intensity of your aerobics from the low end (50%) to the high end (75%) of the aerobic range throughout the workout. To facilitate this varied intensity, arrange your aerobic music at alternating tempos within 120 to 140 beats per minute. For example, after the warm-up phase, arrange music to play slow (120 bpm), medium (130 bpm), fast (140 bpm), medium (130 bpm), slow (120 bpm), medium (130 bpm), fast (140 bpm), and then medium (130 bpm). This method provides aerobic-training benefits while reducing the risks associated with bringing seniors to the higher end of their aerobic range and having them stay there the entire aerobic phase.

Make certain that each senior knows their target heart-rate range and what their 10-second count should be. To effectively use the target heart-rate range, use a simple and consistent method to check heart rates. This helps ensure that all class members can successfully find and count their pulse. It is a good practice to use the same cues each time you take an exercise pulse rate. Make the cues clear and direct: *Stop and find your pulse.* Then pause for two to three seconds, and say, *Ready, start,* having them count for 10 seconds, and then say, *Stop.* As soon as the 10-second count is completed, participants can march in place while each person tells you their heart rate. If you practice taking exercise and recovery pulse rates with your students, it will only take moments for each heart-rate check. When they all feel comfortable and confident with the procedure, they will provide you with more accurate feedback on their heart rates.

Your senior students with known heart disease should exercise at a heart rate recommended by their physician that corresponds to a comfortable exertion. It is critical to note that medications that regulate the heart rate invalidate target heart-rate calculations. Therefore, you must know which of your students take medication. Clients on this type of medication should rely on perceived exertion ratings. Exercisers should learn to work at a level they can identify as somewhere between moderate to moderately hard during the aerobic phase of the class. While exercising, an individual should be able to carry on a conversation without gasping for air. Even clients who are not on medications that alter heart rates should learn to use the rating of perceived exertion method because it provides one more safeguard to maintaining an appropriate exercise intensity, as well as important information about how an individual is responding to exercise that day. The body's response to exercise is affected by many things, including heat, cold, medications, stress, or illness. Due to many outside factors, an individual may be exercising below their target zone, but feel as though they are working moderately hard to hard. Giving as much importance to the rate of perceived exertion as to the calculated target heart-rate zone helps to ensure that participants are exercising at a safe level that is in line with their body's response to exercise that day.

## MONITORING INTENSITY

Again, it is a good practice to check heart rates after the warm-up since this will tell clients how their bodies are responding to exercise that day. Monitor exercise intensity frequently by checking heart rates twice during the aerobic phase and asking each person to tell you their 10-second count or their perceived exertion rating. This only takes a matter of seconds during a class, and gives you immediate feedback to determine if someone is exercising at a potentially unsafe rate. It also continually reinforces the concept that appropriate exercise intensity is essential to safe, effective exercise.

In low-impact aerobics, the circle formation used for variety and interest also provides a valuable opportunity for you to examine each individual's response to the exercise intensity. Look for signs of overexertion such as a flushed face and unusually rapid breathing. You also can ask everyone how they are doing, how the temperature in the room feels, and casually give someone the talk test by asking them a direct question requiring more than a one-word answer.

At the end of the aerobic phase, check their final exercise heart rates. Have clients reduce exercise intensity (walking slowly or a similar activity) for one minute, then take their recovery pulse for 10 seconds. Ask each student how many beats they decreased in the one-minute recovery period. If you have a student whose pulse does not decrease after one minute, take their pulse again one minute later to determine if it has decreased. Failure of the heart to noticeably recover after aerobic exercise can be an indication of a variety of problems. This individual should be monitored throughout the rest of the class to determine if their heart rate is responding. Clients whose heart rate does not return to their pre-exercise level five to 10 minutes after completing the exercise should be referred to a physician.

During the cool-down phase, ask each student, regardless of whether or not they are on heart-rate medication, to indicate their perceived exertion rating. This will help your students begin to understand how they feel when they are exercising within their target heart-rate zone.

## RECORDING EXERCISE INTENSITY

Write each student's predetermined 10-second count, or an indication of reliance on the perceived exertion rating, next to their names on the roll sheet or a chart for easy referral. An effective strategy is to keep a record of each student's exercise heart rate, recovery heart rate,

FIGURE 7.2
Sample record-keeping chart

| Date | | | | | | | | | | | | | | | |
|---|---|---|---|---|---|---|---|---|---|---|---|---|---|---|---|
| Name | EHR/R | RPE | EHR/R | RPE | EHR/R | RPE | EHR/R | RPE | EHR/R | RPE | EHR/R | RPE | EHR/R | RPE |
| | | | | | | | | | | | | | | |
| | | | | | | | | | | | | | | |
| | | | | | | | | | | | | | | |
| | | | | | | | | | | | | | | |
| | | | | | | | | | | | | | | |

EHR=exercise heart rate; R=recovery heart rate; RPE=rating of perceived exertion
From K. Van Norman, Exercise Programming for Older Adults, page 35, Figure 3.4. © 1995 by Kay Van Norman. Reprinted with permission from Human Kinetics (Champaign, Ill.).

and perceived exertion rating for every exercise period during the first several weeks of class. Refer to Figure 7.2 for a sample chart that can be used in this manner. Recording these figures will help you to become familiar with each individual's response to exercise and alert you to potential problems such as excessively high exercise heart rates or failure of the heart to recover after one minute. It also will help reinforce to your students the importance of monitoring exercise intensity with both the target heart rate and rating of perceived exertion. After you become familiar with your class members and their responses to exercise, continue to ask each participant for these numbers even if you no longer take the time to record them.

## ATTENTION TO DETAIL

When developing programs for older adults, a little attention to detail goes a long way toward effectively meeting their needs. Refer to Chapter 5 for movement strategies to meet the needs and objectives of your particular class population. However, regardless of the strategies or the level of programming used, you must understand the importance of fostering a social atmosphere in your classes. This begins with your ability to project a friendly, interested attitude to each class member. Learning participants' names, greeting them as they enter class, introducing new participants to others in the group, and checking on regulars who miss class are all effective ways to show concern for individuals in the group. Enjoying the social interaction is consistently listed as one of the top reasons seniors continue to attend group exercise classes, so look for ways to encourage and support social interaction among participants. Rather than always having participants face the front, have them face each other or arrange the class in a circle to provide opportunities for participants to exchange comments and smiles while they exercise. During a low-impact aero-bics class, for example, the circle formation often results in someone sharing a joke or anecdote.

Give special attention to the tempo and type of music to make your class "senior friendly." A range of 120 to 140 beats per minute is appropriate for the aerobic portion of the class. Music should have a steady, easily distinguishable beat, with simple instrumentals and mid-range vocals. Slower music (that also has a steady beat) works well for the warm-up. Music for the cool-down and stretch phase of the class can be similar to the warm-up music or it can be of the easy-listening or relaxation variety. The type of music used is just as important as the tempo. Music that was popular during the time your class participants were young adults may bring back good memories and increase their enjoyment. Ask your seniors what music they like. Many will be happy to suggest favorite records and tapes to you. Inappropriate music can result in a very unenthusiastic group or no group at all! There are currently a number of music companies that produce senior exercise recordings.

Keep in mind that one of a fitness professional's major legal responsibilities is compliance with copyright law. All forms of commercially produced creative expression are protected by copyright law, but music is the area most pertinent to exercise instructors. Simply stated, almost all musical compositions that one can hear on the radio or television or buy in a music store or via the Internet are owned by artists and studios and are protected by federal copyright law. Whether a fitness professional makes a tape or CD from various songs on the radio or Internet, or from music he or she has purchased does not matter; the individual who uses that tape in a for-profit exercise class—legally speaking, a public performance—is in violation of copyright law.

Music volume also is an important consideration. Do not assume that because many older adults have diminished hearing, you should turn the volume up loudly. Most seniors dislike loud music, and those with some degree of deafness will not necessarily benefit from the increased volume. Seniors with uncorrected impairments will have a very difficult time hearing any of your instruction because of the loud music. Those with hearing aids may be most troubled by loud music because the aid magnifies all sounds, producing an uncomfortable mixture of music, voices, and background noise. The most effective strategy is to play the music at a moderate volume, watch for your students' response, and ask them how well they can hear the rhythm. Soon you will be able to easily recognize the volume appropriate to each class.

Be aware that when you are giving a lot of verbal instruction, such as explaining a new exercise, it is best to turn the music off so that it does not compete with your voice. Trying to hear new instructions over music can be very frustrating for older clients, especially those who are new to the class and already anxious about learning new movements and patterns.

# PARTICIPANT RECRUITMENT

Before developing a plan for recruiting participants, first determine who you are trying to recruit. As outlined in the beginning of this chapter, the term "senior exerciser" encompasses individuals from a broad range of functional abilities and exercise needs. Facility, staffing, and financial considerations will largely determine the type of programming you can provide and, thus, the type of senior you target.

## Facility

Facility type, size, and location, as well as accessibility for anyone with functional impairments, are significant factors in determining who you will be programming for. The type of equipment available for classes and the existing atmosphere of a facility also are important considerations.

### TYPE

Facility type is an obvious consideration. Exercise programming for skilled nursing and assisted-living facilities would consist of classes primarily for older adults in the dependent and frail categories. Senior residence facilities catering to the independent older adult and senior citizen centers may require exercise programming that meets the needs of frail to physically fit seniors. Fitness facilities catering to the general public would most likely provide programming for seniors from the independent to the more physically fit and elite categories of function.

### SIZE

Facility size largely determines your programming options. Sizes range from very large facilities with access to extensive equipment, to small fitness centers with very little equipment. In senior housing complexes, an exercise facility can range from one small room to a whole wellness center complete with a swimming pool, weight room, and aerobics room.

### LOCATION AND ACCESSIBILITY

The facility's location also is important. Facilities in a central area that can easily be reached on foot or by public transportation have the advantage of attracting older adults who no longer drive. In contrast, hard-to-reach facilities, regardless of the amenities offered, will be underutilized by a large percentage of seniors. Similarly, facilities in high-crime areas are not likely to attract a large percentage of senior participants.

Equally as important as an accessible location is the accessibility of the facility itself to those with mobility impairments.

Parking areas that are far from the building or facilities with excessive stairs make it difficult for many seniors in the lower range of the independent category to participate in programs. Poorly maintained parking lots and sidewalks, and areas where snow and ice are a problem also serve as a barrier to participation. Parking and environmental obstacles can make it impossible for older adults from the frail and dependent categories to access your program.

## EQUIPMENT AND FACILITY SYSTEMS

Equipment options within the facility are a consideration when programming for seniors. Resistance-training machines should be fully adjustable to body size and allow for increasing resistance by small increments (2½ pounds or less). Weight machines without these features not only pose an increased risk of injury to older adults, but can be especially intimidating to many older women as well.

Exercise facilities lacking appropriate heating or cooling systems can pose a hazard to seniors whose bodies often do not regulate heat as efficiently as those of younger adults. Evaluating these aspects of the facility in advance allows you to make the necessary adjustments for safe programming.

## ATMOSPHERE

One often-overlooked aspect of facility appropriateness is the existing atmosphere within a facility. Some facilities are oriented toward a younger clientele. These types of facilities do not provide a comfortable atmosphere for older adults, especially those who are trying exercise for the first time in many years and already feel like they do not belong there.

Another aspect of appropriateness concerns the times the facility is available for programming. To some degree, the times your programs are offered determine the type of seniors you will attract. Some seniors are early risers and love to get up and complete their exercise before proceeding with the rest of their day. Others prefer to exercise later in the day. To reach the largest percentage of seniors, offer both early morning and early afternoon classes if possible. The most critical component of scheduling is that it is consistent, allowing seniors to rely on a specific time and day for their program choice.

Evaluating the advantages and limitations of a facility helps you identify what types of programs are appropriate within that environment, and for which segments of the senior population you can provide safe and effective programming.

## Staffing

Staff training and staff/participant ratios also must be primary considerations when determining the level of programming you will provide. Meeting the needs of clients in the physically frail to physically dependent categories requires a highly trained staff with a thorough knowledge of limitations, as well as appropriate expectations for this group. The staff/participant ratio must be small enough to provide close supervision. This type of programming is most common to senior housing, such as assisted-living facilities and skilled nursing facilities.

Programs striving to meet the needs of the independent, physically fit, and elite categories of seniors are most common to community-based fitness facilities. Programs for these segments of the population allow for larger staff-to-participant ratios. However, as the instructor, you must be aware of the range of abilities common to seniors within these three categories. Of special importance is the broad range of functional abilities and limitations of seniors classified as functionally independent. Some functionally independent seniors are very close to being physically fit. However, others will walk into your class with no obvious functional impairments but who, in fact, have significantly diminished levels of balance, coordination, strength, and flexibility. This is the group of older adults that is at the highest risk for injury. Administering appropriate pre-assessments and using senior-safe activities and teaching styles throughout your programming is an important safeguard for preventing injuries.

## Cost

Facility and staffing considerations are largely responsible for determining the cost of senior programming. Many times, the cost of the program plays a vital role in determining who will be attending your classes. Evaluating population demographics in your area with regard to numbers of seniors, average incomes, and percentage of seniors within each economic category will help you determine realistic expectations for program recruitment.

# MARKETING STRATEGIES

After careful consideration of all the elements described previously, you can determine which segments of the senior population you can provide programming for. Once these market segments are identified, begin developing marketing strategies.

A large part of marketing your program is developing cooperative relationships with other individuals and organizations that work daily to provide a variety of services to the seniors in your community. Develop mutually beneficial relationships with senior services and health professional networks in your area.

## Senior Services

A very beneficial step you can take to market a senior exercise program is to become an integral part of the senior services network in your community. This includes senior centers, area agencies on aging, county offices on aging, and a wide range of senior support services that vary dramatically from community to community. It is a good practice to make easily available both general information about the benefits of exercise and specific information about your program throughout this senior services network. Look for ways to include information about this network in your own promotional materials, such as the availability of a senior transportation service as a way to get to your program. A safe and effective exercise program will be a welcome addition to the network of services for seniors.

## Health Professionals

An important part of your network should be area physicians, physical therapists, and orthopedic specialists. Utilize their expertise and request their input on program components. Seek their advice on such things as the level of aerobic conditioning appropriate to seniors with heart- and lung-related restrictions, and on the safety of specific exercises for special muscle and joint conditions. Establish a relationship of trust and reliability within this network. This is an ongoing process that takes time and careful attention to detail, but offers a great deal in return. Adequately involving area health professionals increases your program's safety and credibility. It also increases participation through direct referrals from these health professionals (Van Norman, 1995). Literature from numerous health-related disciplines strongly supports the belief that the right kind of exercise can improve many aspects of health (Spirduso, Francis, & MacRae, 2005; American College of Sports Medicine, 2003; Schilke, 1991; Blair, 2001; Chandler, 1996). Therefore, if area health professionals know you have a safe, effective program, they will be motivated to refer patients to your classes.

If you live in an area with close access to a college or university, it is a good practice to include its health and fitness professionals in your network. This relationship can be mutually beneficial, offering you access to current information in the field of exercise and aging, and providing research faculty an opportunity to involve your group in appropriate research projects.

## Focusing Your Marketing Efforts

When developing a marketing strategy for your program, you must obviously consider where to focus your marketing efforts. If you are programming for a residence facility, your market is already established because it is usually limited to on-site residents. In this instance, you must identify the range of functional abilities and needs within the resident population, and analyze how facility operations, such as meal schedules and medication distribution, support or restrict implementation of exercise programs. When developing programming that meets functional needs, remember to identify and program for your clients' interests. The compliance rate among seniors engaging in self-chosen activities is significantly higher than for those engaging in non-choice activities (Mills et al., 1997).

In community-based programs, you must find the senior consumer. Analyze where seniors do business, where their health needs are met, and where they congregate socially in your community. After locating the senior consumer, develop a marketing plan to ensure your materials are readily available to them.

### BUSINESSES

An effective strategy for marketing is to identify businesses that cater to older adults, such as clothing and shoe stores, gift shops, book stores, novelty shops, and barbers or hair designers. Look for businesses taking special care to be friendly and accommodating to seniors. Determine which restaurants draw a large number of older customers. Some restaurants cater to older adults with discounts and senior nights, offering additional discounts and extra special service. Some older cafés may be long-time favorites of seniors. In addition, identify a grocery store that is within walking distance to senior housing or shopping complexes offering one-stop shopping. Many seniors without personal transportation frequent stores where they can be dropped off for a few hours to take care of all their needs in one place (Van Norman, 1995).

### HEALTHCARE PROVIDERS

Consider where a high percentage of the older adults in your community are likely to have their health needs met. Seniors consume a high percentage of prescription drugs sold, so it is important to identify which drugstores cater to seniors. Look for one with a convenient location or one offering delivery service. If possible, identify the doctors who have a large senior clientele. They will include internists, family practice doctors, those who specialize in arthritis, and doctors who have been in the community for many years. Most doctors' offices have a bulletin board where notices can be posted. If you have a good relationship with area physicians, many will go a step further and place posters in examining rooms or hand out your materials when recommending exercise (Van Norman, 1995).

### SOCIAL AND RECREATION NETWORK

Determine where the seniors in your community socialize and recreate. Senior centers, social clubs, city recreation centers, golf courses, special community events, and night clubs with social dance music are likely choices. Determining where seniors go to enjoy themselves will help you target your marketing. A large number of seniors also socialize through volunteer work. Identify community organizations specifically designed to offer volunteer work, as well as other volunteer opportunities such as museums, hospitals, and churches.

## DEVELOPING RELEVANT MESSAGES

As previously discussed in this chapter, messages designed to reach potential senior clients must be relevant to them personally. Messages about your program that focus primarily on exercise and broad terms of wellness will only speak to that small percentage of seniors who consider themselves "exercisers." Therefore, when developing your media messages, determine who you are trying to reach and what issues pertaining to physical function and health are relevant to them. Since the largest number of seniors can be classified as functionally independent, it seems appropriate that many of your messages should focus on maintaining an independent lifestyle.

## HIGHLIGHTING ACTIVITIES OF INTEREST

An additional aspect of recruiting senior exercise participants is determining which types of activities they are most likely to participate in (Mills et al., 1996). A large number of senior programs consist of a group-based class, or a variety of such classes, led by an instructor. These programs attract seniors who either prefer group exercise or do not really have a preference for exercising (group or individual). The benefit of social interaction in group settings has been consistently reported (Spirduso, Francis, & MacRae, 2005). A study by Mills et al. (1997), however, points out that there also is a significant percentage of seniors who prefer to exercise on an individual basis. This study reflects that a similar degree of individual preferences for type of exercise appears in all age categories. Regardless of age, some people prefer group activities while others prefer individualized ones. This is a very simple but important point to consider when developing your programs and beginning recruitment procedures.

To reach those who prefer individualized experiences, your recruitment materials must highlight ways in which this type of activity will be used in your program. Note that activities suggested for meeting the needs of different levels of functional ability include both individualized and group activities. Some seniors may participate in group activities but will appreciate the opportunity to work individually; others may simply not participate because of a lack of individualized programming. An effective strategy for reaching these seniors is to ensure that your promotional messages emphasize how activities such as circuit training, strength training, and station formats can be either group-oriented or individualized. Even walking programs can be individualized. They can promote walking together at a set time and place, but also can be structured to allow individuals to walk on their own, keeping track of their progress through a cumulative minutes or miles program. Their progress can be recorded both individually and in the group's record.

## USING THE MEDIA

Newspapers, television, and radio can play a role in helping you reach the senior consumer. Newspaper editors have found that their most loyal readers are the older adult population and are responding with a significant increase in the coverage of aging issues that are personally relevant to seniors. Older television viewers' preference for news, sports, talk shows, and classic movies has begun to change the programming focus of cable television from entertainment only to a mix of entertainment, news, and lifestyle. The radio industry also is taking notice that older listeners are significantly more likely to listen to all-news formats, news/talk formats, easy-listening, and nostalgia programs.

These are important considerations when determining where to spend advertising dollars and how to utilize the media's focus on senior issues to promote your program. Television footage of seniors exercising in your program and personal interviews with seniors who want to talk about what exercise has done for them personally work very well to generate interest in your program.

# COMPLIANCE AND MOTIVATION

Many seniors are motivated to begin an exercise program due to a physician's advice. Many others will be motivated by a noticeable loss of physical abilities and a desire to regain full function (Strain, 1996). Regardless of their reasoning, they will join a program that addresses their individual needs and be motivated to continue a program if they experience noticeable improvements in physical capacities or an overall feeling of well-being (Barry & Eathorne, 1994). If you have a well-balanced program, clients will achieve noticeable results. Solicit feedback from your group on how they feel about their progress. Determine what improvements they notice in endurance, strength, flexibility, overall mobility, and well-being. Refer to Chapter 4 for appropriate pre- and post-assessments to track an individual's progress.

Another important element to consider when trying to motivate seniors to begin and maintain an exercise program is their individual stage of change. Behavioral researchers James Prochaska and Bess Marcus (1994) created the highly regarded "stages of change" theory identifying five hierarchical stages that individuals typically go through when forming a new habit or changing a behavior. An individual's stage of change will determine what messages are relevant to them, and what programs will best meet their needs. Refer to Table 7.7 for a summary of these stages and general approaches to reaching older adults at each stage. Chapter 2 provides more detailed coverage of the stages-of-change model.

## Goals and Rewards

An effective strategy for motivating seniors to continue involvement is to develop a program of mini-goals and a system of rewards, prizes, and mini-celebrations for reaching those goals. Chapter 2 includes a discussion of specific strategies for setting goals. Consider giving T-shirts and certificates of honor for regular attendance. Efforts to reward participation can provide the extra motivation a person sometimes needs to make exercise part of their healthy lifestyle.

When developing rewards systems it is important to make goals achievable for all participants, regardless of functional ability. A goal of walking 10 miles per week, for example, may be easy for some seniors, but impossible for others. Therefore, keeping track of the time spent walking may be more appropriate if you are providing programming for seniors from a range of functional abilities. Using the time-spent format works well for many forms of physical activity, including seated functional-based work and vigorous aerobics.

Having a time limit to reach rewards (one month, for example) may pose difficulty for some seniors. Design your goal system so that rewards are given for reaching benchmarks of time spent, regardless of how long it takes an individual to reach the benchmark. You can combine this basic reward system with a series of extra rewards for additional accomplishments.

Finally, when designing your goals and rewards, you need to give some thought to how much time it will take to track or record individual progress. If the recording of individual progress is left to the instructor, it becomes a time-intensive project. Consider developing a system that allows each individual to

Table 7.7

The Stages of Change and Corresponding Approaches for Increasing Physical Activity

| A PATTERN TO CHANGE | MATCHING THE STAGE |
|---|---|
| **Pre-contemplation (not ready to change)**<br>✓ Not intending to or ready to change<br>✓ May not understand the consequences of the behavior or advantages of making the change<br>✓ May be resistant to change<br>✓ May view the pros of the negative behavior as greater than the cons | ✓ Help by giving tidbits of information to spark interest<br>✓ Information must be personally relevant<br>✓ Use table tents, flyers, information cards<br>✓ Information must be available to them in the general course of their day (i.e., they don't have to go out of their way to receive it)* |
| **Contemplation (thinking about it)**<br>✓ Some knowledge of the consequences or advantages of the change<br>✓ Pros and cons of change are judged to be about equal<br>✓ Intending to or thinking about change but may not know how to get started | ✓ Provide information on physical activity at easily accessible locations*<br>✓ Attach informational "mini" sessions to regularly occurring activities (e.g., lunch)<br>✓ Determine what is personally relevant and address physical activity from that perspective |
| **Preparation (have decided to change; beginning the change process)**<br>✓ Have determined the pros outweigh the cons<br>✓ Intend to make a change within a month<br>✓ Have begun the change process | ✓ Provide introductory sessions: slide show and/or guest speaker<br>✓ Provide resources that allow clients/residents to "try it on their own"<br>✓ Organize a workshop, have a sample class, and/or air sessions on facility's T.V. network, and post in newspaper<br>✓ Have books, brochures, videos, and other activity opportunities easily available* |
| **Action (making changes)**<br>✓ Taking action on a regular basis (e.g., attending a class, eating nutritiously)<br>✓ Tend to feel empowered and in control of life<br>✓ At the greatest risk for relapse | ✓ Have regular classes<br>✓ Provide ongoing easy access, self-directed opportunities (e.g., videos, DVDs)<br>✓ Emphasize goal setting<br>✓ Provide encouragement/reinforcement, and ongoing positive messages |
| **Maintenance (sustaining the changes)**<br>✓ Have sustained the change for at least six months (e.g., walking daily, quit smoking)<br>✓ Old behavior has terminated and prevention of relapse is important<br>✓ Behavior change becomes part of the person's lifestyle | ✓ Continue goal setting<br>✓ Provide continual access to a variety of opportunities<br>✓ Give reinforcement and rewards<br>✓ Track progress and improvements |

* For information about the Activities of the Week Series, contact Kay Van Norman at (406) 587-0786 or go to www.seniorsunlimit.com.

record their own progress in an exercise log, a group chart, or both.

## Social and Emotional Motivation

A healthy lifestyle involves physical, mental, and social/emotional well-being. It is beneficial to design a program that strives to improve as many of these areas as possible. Setting a positive tone within your program begins with the first phone call a senior consumer makes to your program. Project professionalism in a friendly, interested manner, providing the information that is requested, and asking important questions about the caller in return. Ask them about their current level of physical condition, if they are now, or have recently been, involved in a regular exercise program, and what health and fitness goals they hope to achieve. It also is important to ask them what types of activities they are most interested in, and which they feel most comfortable participating in.

There are many reasons why someone may attend an exercise program. They may wish to improve their aerobic condition, strength in their legs and/or upper body, balance and coordination to prevent falls, or flexibility for decreased pain and increased mobility. Their goals may also be less specific, such as improving their overall appearance and health, or improving their social life. Knowing what a person is hoping to accomplish will help you determine how your program can best meet their needs. This exchange of information should be conversational rather than interrogative. When you have gathered the necessary information, explain how your program can help them accomplish their goals. If you offer a variety of classes, suggest the ones that will best meet their needs. Be prepared to visit with the client as long as necessary to obtain the needed information and to get to know a little something about the per-

son who is about to become part of your family of senior exercisers.

Making this first phone call to inquire about an exercise program is a big step for many older adults. A large part of your marketing program is designed to initiate this first step. If a potential client's phone call is met with impatience or indifference, they will not be motivated to visit or participate in your program.

When the senior arrives in class for the first time, give them a warm welcome and introduction to the class to generate a feeling of belonging among participants. Knowing clients' names and something specific about each one, such as a special interest or talent, reinforces a sense of belonging. Whenever possible, take time to visit before and after classes with your students. Also make time within the class for exchanges between instructor and participants and among participants. Generating a feeling of belonging to something special is key to motivating seniors to continue an exercise program (Van Norman, 1995).

## EQUIPMENT: BALANCING NEEDS WITH COST

Senior exercise programs housed within an existing fitness facility, university setting, or large wellness center within a senior housing complex will usually allow access to a wide range of equipment. It is ideal to have weight machines, aerobic machines, pool access, and specialized fitness rooms to support program development and implementation. However, a large percentage of senior exercise programs exist within a small fitness facility, a designated corner of a senior citizens' center, or a senior housing facility's activities room. Either in the absence of equipment or just for fun and variety, there are a number of inexpensive items that can be utilized in an exercise class for older adults.

## Tactile Manipulatives

Bean bags, Koosh™ balls, and gel balls are wonderful props to use in chair exercise classes. They are light and easy to handle, have an interesting feel, and can be easily squeezed in one hand. Another advantage is that they are easy to toss up in the air and catch, as they will not bounce off a person's hands like a tennis or foam ball. Gel balls rolled up and down the legs and arms, and in between the hands, provide tactile stimulation and help increase circulation, which can be especially beneficial in classes for dependent or frail seniors. These balls can also be used to exercise the feet, and can be rolled back and forth with the sole of the foot to provide a wonderful foot massage. The participants can attempt to pick up a bean bag or Koosh ball from the floor by gripping it with their toes, promoting foot and toe mobility. You can also have seniors pinch the gel balls between their fingers and thumb to improve pinch grip. Lack of foot mobility is identified as a contributor to falls, and pinch grip is closely associated with the ability to perform BADL (Spirduso, Francis, & MacRae, 2005).

Even something as simple as a newspaper can be used to improve hand agility. Have seniors hold up a half-sheet of newspaper by the corner with their right hand, and use the fingers of that hand to draw the newspaper into a ball. Then have seniors transfer the newspaper ball into their left hand and use only that hand to smooth out the newspaper ball.

Sponges of various sizes and shapes also can be used to squeeze and grip. Place a large sponge under the armpit, squeezing it flat against the body to work the shoulder and upper-arm muscles; or squeeze it between the knees to work the inner thigh muscles. Sponges can also be used as a prop to contract the abdominal muscles by asking seniors to flatten the sponge between

their back and the chair back. Clients also may squeeze or wring the sponges in their hands, or roll and squeeze them with their feet and toes. They also are a good prop for promoting ankle flexion. Have seniors place their toes on the sponge (heels on the floor), and then raise the ball of the foot and toes off of the sponge by flexing the ankle. Utilizing the sponge as a prop gives seniors a concrete image of what it means to flex the ankle, and often results in increased performance of the desired action.

## Manipulatives that Promote Range of Motion

An object such as a wooden dowel, old necktie, or other piece of cloth can be used as an aid in promoting range of motion. For example, have seniors grasp a wooden dowel, tie, or cloth in both hands and press it out in front of them (at shoulder level, horizontal to the floor), then straight overhead, and gently behind the head. Using this type of manipulative helps many seniors perform a larger range of motion than is achieved with simple verbal instructions of *raise your arms overhead* or *pull your shoulder blades together*.

By focusing on the specific functional needs of older adults, you can identify everyday items that can be used to promote these functions.

## Resistance Exercise Equipment

In the absence of weight machines, resistance bands and hand-held weights are useful for promoting strength. In addition, they are valuable for providing entry-level resistance work for those unable or unwilling to use the machines.

Resistance bands are stretchy bands that come in a variety of strengths, from light to heavy resistance. They can be ordered from most fitness supply catalogs, and are used to help develop both upper- and lower-body strength. A resistance band approximately 3 feet long works well for both upper- and lower-body exercises. When working on upper-body strength, use care to keep the elbow next to, or in front of, the body. Having the elbow behind the body while performing strength moves involving the shoulder joint can create impingement of the shoulder joint, a painful condition for a senior exerciser. In addition, ensure that your participants understand that the wrist must be held in a neutral position (not hyperflexed or hyperextended) when performing the exercises. Refer to Chapter 3 for additional high-risk exercises and Chapter 5 for specific exercise sequences.

Light ankle/wrist weights also are very useful for chair-based senior exercise classes. Ankle/wrist weights are more versatile than hand-held weights because they can be strapped on the ankle or around the wrist, or held in the hand. Variable weights can be used individually or added together for increased resistance, and work well for most seniors involved in chair exercise.

Research has demonstrated that even very frail seniors can safely participate in resistance training (Fiatarone et al., 1994). These studies utilized resistance-training machines and had participants perform sets lifting 80% of their one-repetition maximum. Another study by Fielding et al. (2002) highlights the dramatic difference between strength training and power training in older adults. Adding the element of speed to the standard progressive-resistance strength-training protocols had dramatic results. The improvements in peak power with power training were 84% greater for the leg press and 34% greater for knee extension when compared to standard strength training in older women. In addition, it appears that improvement in lower-extremity peak power may exert a greater influence on age-associated reductions in

physical function than other exercise. Therefore, programs having access to strength-training equipment that facilitates power training (e.g., Keiser Pneumatic Resistance Equipment) should use power-training protocols to improve peak power in older adults. Please note that standard weightstack equipment does not allow for safe power training with older adults due to the forces of mass (iron weights) and acceleration.

While you may not have access to resistance-training machines, resistance bands and weights provide opportunities for participants to challenge and improve their strength. In the absence of resistance equipment, you can use small plastic soda bottles filled with sand, or other household items such as soup cans, for resistance. Avoid partially filled containers that allow the contents to fall or slosh back and forth during use, and strongly emphasize the importance of proper joint alignment. Holding onto these objects may be awkward and movement of the contents can place undue stress on joints. Chapter 6 includes workouts utilizing various forms of resistance.

## Water-based Equipment

There is a variety of water-based equipment used to aid in flotation, including water bells, long foam noodles, and kick boards. Water bells and foam noodles are easy to hold in the hand and can be placed under the armpits. This is advantageous in programs serving seniors with severe arthritis in the hands. In the absence of a budget for equipment, milk jugs also work well for flotation. It is not advisable for seniors with severe arthritis to use the jugs, however, as gripping the small handles can aggravate their condition.

There also is a growing variety of resistance equipment designed for strength work in water. Water gloves and hand-held paddles can be used for upper-body exercises. Using ankle weights in the water for older adult classes is not recommended because it is difficult to monitor proper alignment under water. Adding weight while performing exercises increases the risk of injury to participants who are not always performing the exercises with proper alignment. This is a case where it is useful to weigh the benefits of adding the weights against the possible risks.

# CONCLUSION

Exercise programming for older adults is a rapidly growing field within the exercise and wellness professions. The knowledge base of research and practice is growing daily. In addition to available resources, there also are growing networks of professionals focused on senior exercise. Providing programming for this population is both challenging and rewarding. The challenge lies in carefully planning programs that balance the special needs of seniors with their fitness needs, and in keeping pace with the ongoing research relevant to this field. As a fitness professional working with older adults, you have a responsibility to continue reviewing research in the area of exercise and aging, and to determine what it means to the practitioner. In addition, it is beneficial to participate in the growing networks of senior exercise specialists to share program ideas and strengthen your professionalism.

Those who work with older adults, from the physically dependent through physically elite categories, can also gain a true sense of satisfaction. It is very rewarding working with dependent and frail seniors to help them maintain the dignity that comes with self-care, and to help guide independent older adults to a lifestyle that includes the physical activity necessary to maintain a positive quality of life. Working with the physically fit and elite older adults to help them attain a goal can also provide a sense of accomplishment, as well as wonderful role models for the aging. Few fields provide such an opportunity for positively impacting the lives of others and, at the same time, gaining personal inspiration.

# REFERENCES AND SUGGESTED READING

American College of Sports Medicine (2003). *ACSM's Exercise Management for Persons with Chronic Disease and Disabilities* (2nd ed.). Champaign, Ill.: Human Kinetics.

American Senior Fitness Association. (1995). *Senior Fitness Instructor, Personal Trainer, and Long-term Care Training Manuals.* New Smyrna Beach, Fla.

Barry, H.C. & Eathorne, S.W. (1994). Exercise and aging: Issues for the practitioner. *Sports Medicine,* 78, 2, 357–376.

Binder, E.F. et al. (1994). Effects of a group exercise program on risk factors for falls in frail older adults. *Journal of Aging and Physical Activity,* 2, 25–37.

Blair, S. et al. (2001). *Active Living Every Day: 20 Steps to Lifelong Vitality.* Champaign, Ill.: Human Kinetics.

Bonelli, S. (2001). *Aquatic Exercise.* San Diego: American Council on Exercise.

Carter, W.B. et al. (1991). Participation of older adults in health programs and research: A critical review of the literature. *The Gerontologist,* 31, 5, 584–592.

Chandler, J.M. (1996). Understanding the relationship between strength and mobility in frail older persons: A review of the literature. *Topics in Geriatric Rehabilitation,* 11, 3, 20–37.

Chandler, J.M. et al. (1996). The fear of falling syndrome: Relationship to falls, physical performance and activities of daily living in frail older persons. *Topics in Geriatric Rehabilitation,* 11, 3, 55–63.

Chodzko-Zajko, W. (Ed.). *Journal of Physical Activity and Aging.* Champaign, Ill.: Human Kinetics.

Fiatarone, M.A. et al. (1994). Exercise training and nutritional supplementation for physical frailty in very elderly people. *New England Journal of Medicine,* 330, 25, 1769–1775.

Fielding, R. et al. (2002). High-velocity power training increases skeletal peak power in older adult women. *Journal of American Geriatric Society,* 50, 4, 665–672.

Foldvari, M. et al. (2000). Association of muscle power with functional status in community dwelling elderly women. *Journal of Gerontology: Medical Sciences,* 554, 3, M1–8.

Frishkorn, P.H. (1994). Functional assessment as a reimbursement mechanism. *Topics in Geriatric Rehabilitation,* 10, 1, 67–71.

Gladwin, L. (1996). Stretching: A valuable component of functional mobility training in activities. *Adaptation & Aging,* 20, 3, 37–47.

Grant, L.D. (1996). Aspects of ageism on individual and health care providers' responses to healthy aging. *Health and Social Work,* 21, 1, 9–15.

Hellman, E.A., Williams, M.A., & Thalken, L. (1996). Modifications of the 7-day activity interview for use among older adults. *The Journal of Applied Gerontology,* 15, 1, 116–131.

Hubley-Kozey, C.L., Wall, J.C. & Hogan, D.B. (1995). Effects of a general exercise program on plantarflexor and dorsiflexor strength and power of older women. *Topics in Geriatric Rehabilitation,* 10, 3, 45–60.

Lewis, C.B., Lindsay, T. & Scott, C. (1996). Functional assessment in the psychosocial realm. *Topics in Geriatric Rehabilitation,* 11, 4, 64–83.

Markides, K. (Ed.). *Journal of Aging and Health.* SAGE Periodicals Press.

Mills, K.M. et al. (1996). Factors associated with enrollment of older adults into a physical activity promotion program. *Journal of Aging and Health,* 8, 1, 96–113.

Mills, K.M. et al. (1997). Consideration of older adults' preferences for format of physical activity. *Journal of Aging and Physical Activity,* 5, 50–58.

Perkins-Carpenter, B. (1993). *How to Prevent Falls.* New York: St. Martin's Press.

Prochaska, J.O. & Marcus, B.H. (1994). The transtheoretical model: Application to exercise. In R.K. Dishman (Ed.) *Advances in Exercise Adherence* (161–179). Champaign, Ill.: Human Kinetics.

CHAPTER SEVEN
Exercise Programming and Leadership

Resnick, B.M. (1991). Geriatric motivation: Clinically helping the elderly to comply. *Journal of Gerontological Nursing,* 17, 5, 17–20.

Rickli, R. & Jones, J. (2001). *Senior Fitness Test Kit.* Champaign, Ill.: Human Kinetics.

Ryan, J.W. & Spellbring, A.M. (1996). Implementing strategies to decrease risk of falls in older women. *Journal of Gerontological Nursing,* 22, 12, 25–31.

Schaller, K.J. (1996). Tai Chi Chih: An exercise option for older adults. *Journal of Gerontological Nursing,* 22, 10, 12–17.

Schilke, J.M. (1991). Slowing the aging process with physical activity. *Journal of Gerontological Nursing,* 17, 6, 4–8.

Shephard, R.J. (1993). Exercise and aging: Extending independence in older adults. *Geriatrics,* 48, 5, 61–64.

Spirduso, W., Francis, K.L., & MacRae, P.G. (2005). *Physical Dimensions of Aging* (2nd ed.). Champaign, Ill.: Human Kinetics.

Spirduso, W. & Asplund, L.A. (1995). Physical activity and cognitive function in the elderly. *Quest,* 47, 395–410.

Strain, L.A. (1996). Lay explanations of chronic illness in later life. *Journal of Aging and Health,* 8, 1, 3–26.

Tibbitts, M. (1996). Patients who fall: How to predict and prevent injuries. *Geriatrics,* 51, 9, 24–31.

Toomey, T.C. & Seville, J.L. (1994). Assessing functional impairment in elderly patients with chronic pain. *Topics in Geriatric Rehabilitation,* 10, 1, 58–66.

Van Norman, Kay (1995). *Exercise Programming for Older Adults.* Champaign, Ill.: Human Kinetics.

Welch, G. (1995). Stabilization: An integral part of real life function. *The Senior Fitness Bulletin,* 2, 2.

For further information on home-based exercise brochures, health education curriculums, or the Permission to M.O.V.E. (Motivation, Opportunity, Verification & Education) campaign, call Kay Van Norman at (406) 587-0786 or go to www.seniorsunlimit.com.

# APPENDIX

## FUNCTIONAL
## Ability Tests

# The Senior Fitness Test Items—Brief Overview

From R.E. Rikli and C.J. Jones, *Senior Fitness Test Manual*, pages 19–22.
© 2004 by Roberta E. Rikli and C. Jessie Jones.
Reprinted with permission from Human Kinetics (Champaign, Ill.).

## 30-Second Chair Stand

**Purpose:** To assess lower-body strength, needed for numerous tasks such as climbing stairs, walking, and getting out of a chair, tub, or car. Also reduces the chance of falling.

**Description:** Number of full stands that can be completed in 30 seconds with arms folded across chest.

## Arm Curl

**Purpose:** To assess upper-body strength, needed for performing household and other activities involving lifting and carrying things such as groceries, suitcases, and grandchildren.

**Description:** Number of biceps curls that can be completed in 30 seconds holding a hand weight of 5 lb (2.27 kg) for women; 8 lb (3.63 kg) for men.

## 6-Minute Walk

**Purpose:** To assess aerobic endurance—important for walking distances, stair climbing, shopping, sightseeing while on vacation, etc.

**Description:** Number of yards/meters that can be walked in 6 minutes around a 50-yard (45.7-meter) course. (5 yards = 4.57 meters.)

## 2-Minute Step Test

**Purpose:** Alternate aerobic-endurance test, for use when space limitations or weather prohibit giving the 6-minute walk test.

**Description:** Number of full steps completed in 2 minutes, raising each knee to a point midway between the patella (kneecap) and iliac crest (top of hip bone). Score is number of times right knee reaches the required height.

## Chair Sit-and-Reach

**Purpose:** To assess lower-body flexibility, which is important for good posture, for normal gait patterns, and for various mobility tasks such as getting in and out of a bathtub or car.

**Description:** From a sitting position at front of chair, with one leg extended and hands reaching toward toes, the number of inches (cm) (+ or −) between extended fingers and tip of toe.

## Back Scratch

**Purpose:** To assess upper-body (shoulder) flexibility, which is important in tasks such as combing one's hair, putting on overhead garments, and reaching for a seat belt.

**Description:** With one hand reaching over the shoulder and one up the middle of the back, the number of inches (cm) between extended middle fingers (+ or -).

## 8-Foot Up-and-Go

**Purpose:** To assess agility/dynamic balance, important in tasks that require quick maneuvering such as getting off a bus in time, or getting up to attend to something in the kitchen, to go to the bathroom, or to answer the phone.

**Description:** Number of seconds required to get up from a seated position, walk 8 feet (2.44 m), turn, and return to seated position.

## Height and Weight

**Purpose:** To assess body weight relative to body height, because of the importance of weight management for functional mobility.

**Description:** Involves measuring height and weight, then using a conversion table to determine body mass index (BMI).

## SFT Means and Standard Deviations for 60-, 70-, and 80-Year-Olds

| Test Item | 60–69 yrs | 70–79 yrs | 80–89 yrs | $p^{\dagger}$ |
|---|---|---|---|---|
| | n=32 91% female (SD) | n=96 84% female (SD) | n=62 81% female (SD) | |
| Chair stand (# in 30 sec) | 14.0 (2.4) | 12.9 (3.0) | 11.9 (3.6) | .013* |
| Arm curl (# in 30 sec) | 19.8 (4.1) | 18.2 (3.9) | 16.5 (4.1) | .007* |
| 6-min walk (total yards) | 677.8 (95.0) | 621.0 (82.4) | 550.1 (86.7) | .0001* |
| 2-min step (# in 2 min) | 100.4 (9.0) | 92.6 (16.0) | 83.5 (22.6) | .0001* |
| Chair sit-and-reach (inches from toe) | -0.4 (5.4) | -0.4 (6.2) | -3.3 (6.0) | .018** |
| Back scratch (inches from middle fingers) | 1.0 (2.0) | -0.4 (3.0) | -1.8 (4.4) | .0009* |
| 8-ft up-and-go (seconds) | 5.2 (0.6) | 6.1 (1.2) | 7.1 (2.0) | .0001* |

SD=standard deviation

Mean ages of the 60-, 70-, and 80-year-old groups were 65.9 (3.5), 75.1 (2.9), and 83.3 (3.0), respectively.

† Significance level of ANOVA F ratios.

* ANOVA and post hoc analyses revealed that all three ages groups differed significantly.

** The 80-year-olds were significantly different from the 60- and 70-year olds, but the 60- and 70-year-olds did not differ from each other.

From R.E. Rikli and C.J. Jones, Development and Validation of a Functional Fitness Test for Community-Residing Older Adults, in the *Journal of Aging and Physical Activity,* 7, 2, page 141, Table 5. © 1999 by Human Kinetics. Reprinted with permission from Human Kinetics (Champaign, Ill.).

# Fullerton Advanced Balance Scale

From D.J. Rose, *Fallproof!*, pages 66–71.
© 2003 by Deborah J. Rose.
Reprinted with permission from Human Kinetics (Champaign, Ill.).

The Fullerton Advanced Balance Scale is designed to measure changes in multiple dimensions of balance in higher functioning community-dwelling older adults.

## Test Administration Instructions for the Fullerton Advanced Balance (FAB) Scale

### 1. Stand with feet together and eyes closed

**Purpose:** Assess ability to use ground cues to maintain upright balance while standing with reduced base of support
**Equipment:** Stopwatch
**Testing procedures:** Demonstrate the correct test position and then instruct the participants to move the feet independently until they are together. If some participants are unable to achieve the correct position due to lower extremity joint problems, encourage them to bring their heels together even though the front of the feet are not touching. Have participants adopt a position that will ensure their safety as the arms are folded across the chest and they prepare to close the eyes. Begin timing as soon as the participant closes the eyes. (Instruct participants to open the eyes if they feel so unsteady that a loss of balance is imminent.)
**Verbal instructions:** "Bring your feet together, fold your arms across your chest, close your eyes when you are ready, and remain as steady as possible until I instruct you to open your eyes."

### 2. Reach forward to retrieve an object (pencil) held at shoulder height with outstretched arm

**Purpose:** Assess ability to lean forward to retrieve an object without altering the base of support; measure of stability limits in a forward direction
**Equipment:** Pencil and 12-inch ruler
**Testing procedures:** Instruct the participant to raise the preferred arm to 90° and extend it with fingers outstretched. (Follow with a demonstration of the correct action.) Use the ruler to measure a distance of 10 inches from the end of the fingers of the outstretched arm. Hold the object (pencil) horizontally and level with the height of the participant's shoulder. Instruct the participant to reach forward, grasp the pencil, and return to the initial starting position without moving feet, if possible. (It is acceptable to raise the heels as long as the feet do not move while reaching for the pencil.) If the participant is unable to reach the pencil within 2–3 seconds of initiating the forward lean, indicate to the participant that it is okay to move the feet in order to reach the pencil. Record the number of steps taken by the participant in order to retrieve the pencil.
**Verbal instructions:** "Try to lean forward to take the pencil from my hand and return to your starting position without moving your feet from their present position." After allowing 2–3 seconds of lean time: "You can move your feet in order to reach the pencil."

### 3. Turn 360° in right and left directions

**Purpose:** Assess ability to turn in a full circle in both directions in the fewest number of steps without loss of balance
**Equipment:** None
**Testing procedures:** Verbally explain and then demonstrate the task to be performed, making sure to complete each circle in four steps or less and pause briefly between turns. Instruct the participant to turn in a complete circle in one direction, pause, and then turn in a complete circle in the opposite direction. Count the number of steps taken to complete each circle. Allow for a small correction in foot position before a turn in the opposite direction is initiated.

**Verbal instructions:** "Turn around in a full circle, pause, and then turn in a second full circle in the opposite direction."

### 4. Step up, onto, and over a 6-inch bench

**Purpose:** Assess ability to control center of gravity in dynamic task situations; also a measure of lower-body strength and control

**Equipment:** 6-inch-high bench (18- by 18-inch stepping surface)

**Testing procedures:** Verbally explain and demonstrate the step up, onto, and over the bench in both directions before the participant performs the test. Instruct the participant to step onto the bench with the right foot, swing the left leg directly up and over the bench, and step off the other side, then repeat the movement in the opposite direction with the left leg leading the action. During performance of the test, watch to see that the participant's trailing leg (a) does not make contact with the bench or (b) swing around, as opposed to directly over, the bench.

**Verbal instructions:** "Step up onto the bench with your right leg, swing your left leg directly up and over the bench, and step off the other side. Repeat the movement in the opposite direction with your left leg as the leading leg."

### 5. Tandem walk

**Purpose:** Assess ability to dynamically control center of mass with an altered base of support

**Equipment:** Masking tape

**Testing procedures:** Verbally explain and demonstrate how to perform the test correctly before the participant attempts to perform it. Instruct the participant to walk on the line in a tandem position (heel-to-toe) until you tell them to stop. Allow the participant to repeat the test one time if unable to achieve a tandem stance position within the first two steps. The participant may elect to step forward with the opposite foot on the second trial. Score as interruptions any instances where the participant (a)

takes a lateral step away from the line when performing the tandem walk or (b) is unable to achieve correct heel-to-toe position during any step taken along the course. Do not ask the participant to stop until 10 steps have been completed.

**Verbal instructions:** "Walk forward along the line, placing one foot directly in front of the other such that the heel and toe are in contact on each step forward. I will tell you when to stop."

### 6. Stand on one leg

**Purpose:** Assess ability to maintain upright balance with a reduced base of support.

**Equipment:** Stopwatch

**Testing procedures:** Instruct the participant to fold the arms across the chest, lift the preferred leg off the floor, and maintain balance until instructed to return the foot to the floor. Begin timing as soon as the participant lifts the foot from the floor. Stop timing if the legs touch, the preferred leg contacts the floor, or the participant removes the arms from the chest before 20 seconds have elapsed. Allow the participant to perform the test a second time with the other leg if they are unsure as to which is the preferred limb.

**Verbal instructions:** "Fold your arms across your chest, lift your preferred leg off the floor (without touching other leg), and stand with your eyes open as long as you can."

### 7. Stand on foam with eyes closed

**Purpose:** Assess the ability to maintain upright balance while standing on a compliant surface with eyes closed

**Equipment:** Stopwatch; two Airex pads, with a length of nonslip material placed between the two pads and an additional length of nonslip material between the floor and first pad if the test is being performed on an uncarpeted surface

**Testing procedures:** Instruct the participant to step onto the foam pads without assistance, fold the arms across the chest, and close the eyes when ready. (Demonstrate the correct standing position on foam.) Make sure the position adopted ensures the safety of the participant. Position the foam pads close to a wall in all cases and in a corner of the room if the participant appears unsteady. Begin timing as soon as the eyes close. Stop the trial if the participant (a) opens the eyes before the timing period has elapsed, (b) lifts the arms off the chest, or (c) loses balance and requires manual assistance to prevent falling. (Instruct participants to open their eyes if they feel so unsteady that a loss of balance is imminent.)

**Verbal instructions:** "Step up onto the foam and stand with your feet shoulder-width apart. Fold your arms over your chest, and close your eyes when you are ready. I will tell you when to open your eyes."

### 8. Two-footed jump for distance

**Purpose:** Assess upper- and lower-body coordination and lower-body power

**Equipment:** 36-inch ruler

**Testing procedures:** Instruct the participant to jump as far but as safely as possible while maintaining a two-footed stance. Demonstrate the correct movement prior to the participant performing the jump. (Do not jump much more than twice the length of your own feet when demonstrating.) Observe whether the participant leaves the floor with both feet and lands with both feet. Use the ruler to measure the length of the foot and then multiply by two to determine the ideal distance to be jumped.

**Verbal instructions:** "Try to jump as far but as safely as you can with both feet."

### 9. Walk with head turns

**Purpose:** Assess ability to maintain dynamic balance while walking and turning the head

**Equipment:** Metronome set at 100 beats per minute

**Testing procedures:** After first demonstrating the test, allow the participant to practice turning the head in time with the metronome while standing in place. Encourage the participant to turn the head at least 30° in each direction (e.g., "Turn your head to look into each corner of the room."). Observe how far the participant is able to turn the head during the standing head turns. A 30° head turn is required during the walking trial. Instruct the participant to walk forward while turning the head from side to side and in time with the auditory tone. Begin counting steps as soon as the participant deviates from a straight path while walking or is unable to turn the head the required distance to the timing of the metronome.

**Verbal instructions:** "Walk forward while turning your head from left to right with each beat of the metronome. I will tell you when to stop."

### 10. Reactive postural control

**Purpose:** Assess ability to efficiently restore balance following an unexpected perturbation

**Equipment:** None

**Testing procedures:** Instruct the participant to stand with his or her back to you. Extend your arm with the elbow locked and place the palm of your hand against the participant's back between the scapula. Instruct the participant to lean back slowly against your hand until you tell him or her to stop. Quickly flex your elbow until your hand is no longer in contact with the participant's back at the moment you estimate that a sufficient amount of force has been applied to require a movement of the feet to restore balance. You may actually begin releasing your hand while you are still giving the instructions. This release should be unexpected, so do not prepare the participant for the moment of release.

**Verbal instructions:** "Slowly lean back into my hand until I ask you to stop."

# Score Sheet for
# Fullerton Advanced Balance (FAB) Scale

Name:_____ Date of Test:_____

### 1. Stand with feet together and eyes closed

(   )   0   Unable to obtain the correct standing position independently
(   )   1   Able to obtain the correct standing position independently but unable to maintain the position or keep the eyes closed for more than 10 seconds
(   )   2   Able to maintain the correct standing position with eyes closed for more than 10 seconds but less than 30 seconds.
(   )   3   Able to maintain the correct standing position with eyes closed for 30 seconds but requires close supervision
(   )   4   Able to maintain the correct standing position safely with eyes closed for 30 seconds

### 2. Reach forward to retrieve an object (pencil) held at shoulder height with outstretched arm

(   )   0   Unable to reach the pencil without taking more than two steps
(   )   1   Able to reach the pencil but needs to take two steps
(   )   2   Able to reach the pencil but needs to take one step
(   )   3   Can reach the pencil without moving the feet but requires supervision
(   )   4   Can reach the pencil safely and independently without moving the feet

### 3. Turn 360° in right and left directions

(   )   0   Needs manual assistance while turning
(   )   1   Needs close supervision or verbal cueing while turning
(   )   2   Able to turn 360° but takes more than four steps in both directions
(   )   3   Able to turn 360° but unable to complete in four steps or fewer in one direction
(   )   4   Able to turn 360° safely taking four steps or fewer in both directions

### 4. Step up, onto, and over a 6-inch bench

(   )   0   Unable to step up onto the bench without loss of balance or manual assistance
(   )   1   Able to step up onto the bench with leading leg, but trailing leg contacts the bench or leg swings around the bench during the swing-through phase in both directions
(   )   2   Able to step up onto the bench with leading leg, but trailing leg contacts the bench or swings around the bench during the swing-through phase in one direction
(   )   3   Able to correctly complete the step up and over in both directions but requires close supervision in one or both directions.
(   )   4   Able to correctly complete the step up and over in both directions safely and independently

### 5. Tandem walk

(   )   0   Unable to complete 10 steps independently
(   )   1   Able to complete the 10 steps with more than five interruptions
(   )   2   Able to complete the 10 steps with five or fewer interruptions
(   )   3   Able to complete the 10 steps with two or fewer interruptions
(   )   4   Able to complete the 10 steps independently and with no interruptions

## 6. Stand on one leg

( ) 0 Unable to try or needs assistance to prevent falling
( ) 1 Able to lift leg independently but unable to maintain position for more than 5 seconds
( ) 2 Able to lift leg independently and maintain position for more than 5 but less than 12 seconds
( ) 3 Able to lift leg independently and maintain position for more than 12 but less than 20 seconds
( ) 4 Able to lift leg independently and maintain position for the full 20 seconds

## 7. Stand on foam with eyes closed

( ) 0 Unable to step onto foam or maintain standing position independently with eyes open
( ) 1 Able to step onto foam independently and maintain standing position but unable or unwilling to close eyes
( ) 2 Able to step onto foam independently and maintain standing position with eyes closed for at least 10 seconds
( ) 3 Able to step onto foam independently and maintain standing position with eyes closed for more than 10 seconds but less than 20 seconds
( ) 4 Able to step onto foam independently and maintain standing position with eyes closed for 20 seconds

## 8. Two-footed jump for distance

( ) 0 Unable to attempt or attempts to initiate two-footed jump, but one or both feet do not leave the floor
( ) 1 Able to initiate two-footed jump, but one foot either leaves the floor or lands before the other
( ) 2 Able to perform two-footed jump, but unable to jump farther than the length of their own feet
( ) 3 Able to perform two-footed jump and achieve a distance greater than the length of their own feet
( ) 4 Able to perform two-footed jump and achieve a distance greater than twice the length of their own feet

## 9. Walk with head turns

( ) 0 Unable to walk 10 steps independently while maintaining 30° head turns at an established pace
( ) 1 Able to walk 10 steps independently but unable to complete required number of 30° head turns at an established pace
( ) 2 Able to walk 10 steps but veers from a straight line while performing 30° head turns at an established pace
( ) 3 Able to walk 10 steps in a straight line while performing head turns at an established pace but head turns less than 30° in one or both directions
( ) 4 Able to walk 10 steps in a straight line while performing required number of 30° head turns at established pace.

## 10. Reactive postural control

( ) 0 Unable to maintain upright balance; no observable attempt to step; requires manual assistance to restore balance
( ) 1 Unable to maintain upright balance; takes fewer than two steps and requires manual assistance to restore balance
( ) 2 Unable to maintain upright balance; takes fewer than two steps, but is able to restore balance independently
( ) 3 Unable to maintain upright balance; takes one to two steps, but is able to restore balance independently
( ) 4 Unable to maintain upright balance but able to restore balance independently with only one step

# Interpretation of the Individual Test Items on the Fullerton Advanced Balance (FAB) Scale for Possible Underlying Impairments

| Item | Possible impairments | Recommended exercises |
|---|---|---|
| 1. Stand with feet together and eyes closed | 1. Weak hip abductors/adductors<br>2. Poor COG control<br><br>3. Poor use of somatosensory cues | Lateral weight shifts against resistance; side leg raises against gravity/resistance<br>Seated/standing balance activities emphasizing weight shifts in multiple directions<br>Standing balance activities with eyes closed (controlled sway in A-P and lateral directions) |
| 2. Reach forward to object | 1. Reduced limits of stability<br>2. Reduced ankle ROM<br>3. Fear of falling<br>4. Lower-body muscle weakness | Seated/standing COG control activities<br>Ankle circles, heel lifts, and drops from height<br>Confidence-building activities—high success<br>Wall sits; LB exercises with resistance |
| 3. Turn in a full circle | 1. Poor dynamic COG control<br><br>2. Possible vestibular impairment (e.g., dizziness)<br>3. Lower-body weakness | Standing weight-transfer activities; gait pattern enhancement (turns, directional changes)<br>Head and eye movement coordination exercises<br><br>LB exercises with resistance; emphasize hip and knee flexion; hip abduction/adduction |
| 4. Step up and over | 1. Poor dynamic COG control<br>2. Lower-body weakness<br><br>3. Reduced ROM at ankle, knee, hip | Seated/standing balance activities emphasizing backward weight shifts<br>LB exercises with resistance (own body/resistance band; emphasize sustained unilateral stance positions)<br>Flexibility exercises emphasizing hip/knee/ankle flexion; seated and standing |
| 5. Tandem walk | 1. Poor dynamic COG control<br><br>2. Poor use of vision<br>3. Weak hip abductors/adductors | Standing/moving COG control activities; emphasize A-P control during weight shifts<br>Activities emphasizing gaze-stabilization techniques<br>Side leg raise against gravity/resistance; lateral weight shift and lunge activities |
| 6. Stand on one leg | 1. Poor COG control<br>2. Lower-body muscle weakness<br><br>3. Poor use of vision | Standing A-P weight shifts and transfers; reduced BOS activities<br>LB exercises with resistance (body/resistance band); emphasize hip abductors/adductors<br>Activities emphasizing gaze stabilization |
| 7. Stand on foam with eyes closed | 1. Poor use of vestibular inputs for balance<br>2. Lower-body muscle weakness<br><br>3. Heightened fear of falling when vision absent | Seated/standing activities performed with reduced/absent vision on altered surfaces<br>LB exercises with resistance (body/resistance band); emphasize quadriceps, gastrocnemius/soleus muscles<br>Confidence-building activities with progressive reduction in availability of vision |
| 8. Two-footed jump | 1. Poor dynamic COG control<br>2. Poor upper- and lower-body coordination<br>3. Lower-body muscle weakness | Standing/moving COG activities emphasizing leaning away from and back to midline<br>Selected exercises to improve UB and LB coordination; multiple task activities<br>LB exercises with resistance (body/resistance band) performed at progressively faster speeds |
| 9. Walk with head turns | 1. Possible vestibular impairment<br><br>2. Poor use of vision<br>3. Poor dynamic COG control | Head and eye movement coordination exercises; gait pattern enhancement (turns, directional changes)<br>Activities emphasizing gaze stabilization<br>Standing/moving activities with head turns; progressively increase speed and frequency of head turns |
| 10. Reactive postural test | 1. Absent postural strategy (i.e., step)<br>2. Poor COG control<br><br>3. Lower-body muscle weakness | Activities emphasizing step strategy (i.e., resistance band release activity)<br>Standing COG control activities; volitional stepping activities in multiple directions<br>LB exercises with resistance; emphasize hip and knee flexion; hip abduction/adduction. |

Note: A-P = anterior-posterior direction; BOS = base of support; COG = center of gravity; LB = lower body; UB = upper body.

# Test Administration Instructions for Multidirectional Reach Test (MDRT)

From D.J. Rose, *Fallproof!*, pages 63–66. © 2003 by Deborah J. Rose. Reprinted with permission from Human Kinetics (Champaign, Ill.).

**Purpose:** To measure the distance a person is able or willing to lean in a forward, backward, and lateral direction.
**Equipment:** Yardstick; wall

### Forward reach
- Position yardstick on wall at height of acromion.
- Instruct the individual to stand in a comfortable position with feet shoulder-width apart.
- Instruct the individual to raise one arm in front to shoulder height (hand extended, palm turned to face medially) and not to touch the yardstick.
- Instruct the individual to reach forward as far as possible without raising the heels from the floor. Record the location of the middle fingertip.
- Now instruct the individual to stop reaching and return to the starting position.
- Subtract the end number from the starting position number to obtain length reached.
- Pause before the next trial.
- Provide on practice trial before the start of the three test trials.

### Backward reach
Repeat all instructions, but this time ask the individual to lean backward as far as possible without raising the toes from the floor. Record the location of the middle fingertip.

### Lateral reach to the right
- Position yardstick on wall at height of acromion.
- Instruct the individual to stand in a comfortable position with feet shoulder-width apart.
- Instruct the individual to raise one arm horizontally to shoulder height (hand extended, palm turned to face medially) and not to touch the yardstick.
- Instruct the individual to reach sideways to the right as far as possible. Record the location of the middle fingertip.
- Now instruct the individual to stop reaching and return to the starting position.
- Subtract the end number from the starting position number to obtain the number of inches reached.
- Pause before the next trial.
- Provide one practice trial before the start of the three test trials.

### Lateral reach to the left
Repeat all previous instructions, but this time ask the individual to reach sideways to the left as far as possible. Record the location of the middle fingertip.

# Scoring Form for Multidirectional Reach Test (MDRT)

## FORWARD REACH

### Distance reached

Trial 1_____

Trial 2_____

Trial 3_____

Mean:_____

### Movement strategy

hip_____ ankle_____ trunk rotation_____
scapular protraction_____ other_____
hip_____ ankle_____ trunk rotation_____
scapular protraction_____ other_____
hip_____ ankle_____ trunk rotation_____
scapular protraction_____ other_____

## BACKWARD REACH

### Distance reached

Trial 1_____

Trial 2_____

Trial 3_____

Mean:_____

### Movement strategy

hip_____ ankle_____ trunk rotation_____
scapular protraction_____ other_____
hip_____ ankle_____ trunk rotation_____
scapular protraction_____ other_____
hip_____ ankle_____ trunk rotation_____
scapular protraction_____ other_____

## LATERAL REACH TO THE RIGHT

### Distance reached

Trial 1_____

Trial 2_____

Trial 3_____

Mean:_____

### Movement strategy

hip_____ ankle_____ trunk rotation_____
scapular protraction_____ other_____
hip_____ ankle_____ trunk rotation_____
scapular protraction_____ other_____
hip_____ ankle_____ trunk rotation_____
scapular protraction_____ other_____

## LATERAL REACH TO THE LEFT

### Distance reached

Trial 1_____

Trial 2_____

Trial 3_____

Mean:_____

### Movement strategy

hip_____ ankle_____ trunk rotation_____
scapular protraction_____ other_____
hip_____ ankle_____ trunk rotation_____
scapular protraction_____ other_____
hip_____ ankle_____ trunk rotation_____
scapular protraction_____ other_____

# Multidirectional Reach Test (MDRT) Reference Values

On the basis of recommendations forwarded by Newton (2001), the following values for each direction can be used as the basis for evaluating an individual's performance:

| | | |
|---|---|---|
| **Forward direction** | Above average | >12.2 in. |
| (Mean: 8.9 in.) (SD: ± 3.4 in.) | Below average | <5.6 in. |
| **Backward direction** | Above average | >7.6 in. |
| (Mean: 4.6 in.) (SD: ± 3.1 in.) | Below average | <1.6 in. |
| **Right lateral direction** | Above average | >9.4 in. |
| (Mean: 6.2 in.) (SD: ± 3.0 in.) | Below average | <3.8 in. |
| **Left lateral direction** | Above average | >9.4 in. |
| (Mean: 6.6 in.) (SD: ± 2.9 in.) | Below average | <3.8 in. |

# Berg Balance Scale

Source: Berg, K.O. et al. (1992). Measuring balance in the elderly: Validation of an instrument. *Canadian Journal of Public Health*, 2, S7–S11. Reprinted with permission.

Name: _____ Date of Test: _____

### 1. Sit to stand

Instructions: "Please stand up. Try not to use your hands for support."

Grading: Please mark the lowest category that applies.

(   ) 0 Needs moderate or maximal assistance to stand

(   ) 1 Needs minimal assistance to stand or to stabilize

(   ) 2 Able to stand using hands after several tries

(   ) 3 Able to stand independently using hands

(   ) 4 Able to stand with no hands and stabilize independently

### 2. Standing unsupported

Instructions: "Please stand for 2 minutes without holding onto anything."

Grading: Please mark the lowest category that applies.

(   ) 0 Unable to stand 30 seconds unassisted

(   ) 1 Needs several tries to stand 30 seconds unsupported

(   ) 2 Able to stand 30 seconds unsupported

(   ) 3 Able to stand 2 minutes with supervision

(   ) 4 Able to stand safely for 2 minutes

If person is able to stand 2 minutes safely, score full points for sitting unsupported (item 3). Proceed to item 4.

### 3. Sitting with back unsupported with feet on floor or on a stool

Instructions: "Sit with arms folded for 2 minutes."

Grading: Please mark the lowest category that applies.

(   ) 0 Unable to sit without support for 10 seconds

(   ) 1 Able to sit for 10 seconds

(   ) 2 Able to sit for 30 seconds

(   ) 3 Able to sit for 2 minutes under supervision

(   ) 4 Able to sit safely and securely for 2 minutes

### 4. Stand to sit

Instructions: "Please sit down."

Grading: Please mark the lowest category that applies.

(   ) 0 Needs assistance to sit

(   ) 1 Sits independently, but has uncontrolled descent

(   ) 2 Uses back of legs against chair to control descent

(   ) 3 Controls descent by using hands

(   ) 4 Sits safely with minimal use of hands

## 5. Transfers

Instructions: "Please move from chair to chair and back again." (Person moves one way toward a seat with armrests and one way toward a seat without armrests.) Arrange chairs for pivot transfer.

Grading: Please mark the lowest category that applies.

( ) 0 Needs two people to assist or supervise to be safe
( ) 1 Needs one person to assist
( ) 2 Able to transfer with verbal cueing and/or supervision
( ) 3 Able to transfer safely with definite use of hands
( ) 4 Able to transfer safely with minor use of hands

## 6. *Standing unsupported with eyes closed

Instructions: "Close your eyes and stand still for 10 seconds."

Grading: Please mark the lowest category that applies.

( ) 0 Needs help to keep from falling
( ) 1 Unable to keep eyes closed for 3 seconds but remains steady
( ) 2 Able to stand for 3 seconds
( ) 3 Able to stand for 10 seconds with supervision
( ) 4 Able to stand for 10 seconds safely

## 7. *Stand unsupported with feet together

Instructions: "Place your feet together and stand without holding on to anything."

Grading: Please mark the lowest category that applies.

( ) 0 Needs help to attain position and unable to hold for 15 seconds
( ) 1 Needs help to attain position, but able to stand for 15 seconds with feet together
( ) 2 Able to place feet together independently, but unable to hold for 30 seconds
( ) 3 Able to place feet together independently and stand for 1 minute with supervision
( ) 4 Able to place feet together independently and stand for 1 minute safely

*The following items are to be performed while standing unsupported.*

## 8. *Reaching forward with outstretched arm

Instructions: "Lift your arm to 90°. Stretch out your fingers and reach forward as far as you can." (Examiner places a ruler at end of fingertips when arm is at 90°. Fingers should not touch the ruler while reaching forward. The recorded measure is the distance forward that the fingers reach while the person is in the most forward lean position.)

Grading: Please mark the lowest category that applies.

( ) 0 Needs help to keep from falling
( ) 1 Reaches forward, but needs supervision
( ) 2 Can reach forward more than 2 inches safely
( ) 3 Can reach forward more than 5 inches safely
( ) 4 Can reach forward confidently more than 10 inches

9. *Pick up object from the floor from a standing position

Instructions: "Please pick up the shoe/slipper that is placed in front of your feet."

Grading: Please mark the lowest category that applies.

( ) 0 Unable to try/needs assistance to keep from losing balance or falling

( ) 1 Unable to pick up shoe and needs supervision while trying

( ) 2 Unable to pick up shoe, but comes within 1–2 inches and maintains balance independently

( ) 3 Able to pick up shoe, but needs supervision

( ) 4 Able to pick up shoe safely and easily

10. * Turn to look behind over left and right shoulders while standing

Instructions: "Turn your upper body to look directly over your left shoulder. Now try turning to look over your right shoulder."

Grading: Please mark the lowest category that applies.

( ) 0 Needs assistance to keep from falling

( ) 1 Needs supervision when turning

( ) 2 Turns sideways only, but maintains balance

( ) 3 Looks behind one side only; other side shows less weight shift

( ) 4 Looks behind from both sides and weight shifts well

11. * Turn 360°

Instructions: "Turn completely in a full circle. Pause, then turn in a full circle in the other direction."

Grading: Please mark the lowest category that applies.

( ) 0 Needs assistance while turning

( ) 1 Needs close supervision or verbal cueing

( ) 2 Able to turn 360° safely but slowly

( ) 3 Able to turn 360° safely to one side only in less than 4 seconds

( ) 4 Able to turn 360° safely in less than 4 seconds to each side

12. * Place alternate foot on bench or stool while standing unsupported

Instructions: "Place each foot alternately on the bench (or stool). Continue until each foot has touched the bench (or stool) four times." (Recommend use of 6-inch-high bench.)

Grading: Please mark the lowest category that applies.

( ) 0 Needs assistance to keep from falling/unable to try

( ) 1 Able to complete fewer than two steps; needs minimal assistance

( ) 2 Able to complete four steps without assistance, but with supervision

( ) 3 Able to stand independently and complete eight steps in more than 20 seconds

( ) 4 Able to stand independently and safely and complete eight steps in less than 20 seconds

**13. * Stand unsupported with one foot in front**

Instructions: "Place one foot directly in front of the other. If you feel that you can't place your foot directly in front, try to step far enough ahead that the heel of your forward foot is ahead of the toes of the other foot." (Demonstrate this test item.)

Grading: Please mark the lowest category that applies.

(   ) 0 Loses balance while stepping or standing

(   ) 1 Needs help to step, but can hold for 15 seconds

(   ) 2 Able to take small step independently and hold for 30 seconds

(   ) 3 Able to place one foot ahead of the other independently and hold for 30 seconds

(   ) 4 Able to place feet in tandem position independently and hold for 30 seconds

**14. * Standing on one leg**

Instructions: "Please stand on one leg as long as you can without holding onto anything."

Grading: Please mark the lowest category that applies.

(   ) 0 Unable to try or needs assistance to prevent fall

(   ) 1 Tries to lift leg, unable to hold 3 seconds, but remains standing independently

(   ) 2 Able to lift leg independently and hold up to 3 seconds

(   ) 3 Able to lift leg independently and hold for 5 to 10 seconds

(   ) 4 Able to lift leg independently and hold more than 10 seconds

Total score_____/56

**Note:** Perform only items 6 though 14 (*) in the modified version of the scale. Maximum score for modified version is 36 points.

**Score Interpretation:**

0–20: Wheelchair bound

21–40: Walking with assistance

41–56: Independent

# Interpretation of Individual Test Item Results on the Berg Balance Scale (BBS)

| Item | Possible Impairments | Recommended exercises |
|---|---|---|
| 1. Sit to stand | 1. Lower- and/or upper-body weakness<br>2. Poor dynamic COG control<br>3. Abnormal weight distribution | Wall sits; UB and LB exercises with resistance (quadriceps, biceps/triceps, hip abductors/adductors)<br>Seated/standing balance activities emphasizing forward weight shifts<br>Standing balance activities with eyes closed (controlled sway in A-P and lateral directions) |
| 2. Stand for 2 minutes | 1. Poor gaze stabilization<br>2. Lower-body weakness<br>3. Abnormal weight distribution in standing | Teach gaze fixation and stabilization techniques<br>Wall sits; LB exercises with resistance<br>COG standing balance activities |
| 3. Sit for 2 minutes | 1. Poor trunk stabilization and/or UB weakness<br>2. Abnormal perception of true vertical | UB exercises with resistance (own body); seated balance activities on compliant surfaces<br>Standing against wall with eyes closed; somatosensory cues |
| 4. Stand to sit | 1. Poor dynamic COG control<br><br>2. Lower- and/or upper-body weakness<br>3. Poor trunk flexibility | Seated/standing balance activities emphasizing backward weight shifts<br>UB and LB exercises with resistance (own body/resistance band; emphasize eccentric component)<br>Flexibility exercises emphasizing trunk rotation/flexion; seated and standing |
| 5. Transfer (chair to chair) | 1. Poor dynamic control of COG<br>2. Lower- and/or upper-body weakness | Seated/standing balance activities emphasizing multidirectional weight shifts<br>UB and LB exercises with resistance |
| 6. Stand with eyes closed (10 sec) | 1. Poor use of somatosensory inputs; visual dependency and/or fear of falling<br>2. Lower-body weakness | Seated/standing balance activities with eyes closed; verbally emphasize use of surface cues<br><br>Wall sits; LB exercise with resistance |
| 7. Stand with feet together (1 min) | 1. Poor COG control<br>2. Weak hip abductors/adductors | Standing balance activities with reduced BOS<br>Lateral leg raises/weight shifts against resistance |
| 8. Standing forward reach | 1. Poor dynamic COG control (reduced limits of stability)<br>2. Lower-body weakness<br><br>3. Reduced ankle ROM | Seated/standing COG activities emphasizing leaning away from and back to midline<br>LB exercises with resistance (body/resistance band); emphasize dorsiflexors; gastrocnemius/soleus muscles<br>Flexibility exercises (emphasize dorsiflexion) |

Note: A-P = anterior-posterior direction; BOS = base of support; COG = center of gravity; LB = lower body; UB = upper body.

| Item | Possible Impairments | Recommended exercises |
|---|---|---|
| 9. Pick up object | 1. Poor dynamic COG control | Seated/standing COG activities emphasizing leaning away from and back to midline |
| | 2. Poor upper- and lower-body flexibility | Selected exercises to improve UB and LB flexion |
| | 3. Lower-body weakness | LB exercises with resistance (body/resistance band) |
| | 4. Vestibular impairment (dizziness) | Head and eye movements; habituation exercises |
| 10. Turn to look behind | 1. Poor dynamic COG control | Standing weight shifts in lateral direction |
| | 2. Poor neck and/or trunk flexibility | Selected exercises emphasizing rotation of neck, shoulders, and hips |
| | 3. Lower-body weakness | LB exercises with resistance; ball movement exercises in standing position |
| 11. Turn in a circle | 1. Poor dynamic COG control | Standing weight transfer activities; gait pattern enhancement (turns, directional changes) |
| | 2. Possible vestibular impairment (e.g. dizziness) | Head and eye movement coordination exercises |
| | 3. Lower-body weakness | LB exercises with resistance; emphasize hip and knee flexion; hip abduction/adduction |
| 12. Dynamic toe touch | 1. Poor dynamic COG control | Standing weight shifts in lateral/A-P directions |
| | 2. Lower-body weakness | LB exercises with resistance; emphasize hip and knee flexion; hip abduction/adduction |
| 13. Tandem stance | 1. Poor static and dynamic COG control | Standing A-P weight shifts and transfers; reduced BOS activities |
| | 2. Lower-body weakness | LB exercises with resistance (body/resistance band); emphasize hip abductors/adductors |
| | 3. Poor gaze stabilization | Practice focusing on visual targets in front of and at head height during standing and moving activities |
| 14. Stand on one leg | 1. Poor static and dynamic COG control | Standing A-P weight shifts and transfers; reduced BOS activities |
| | 2. Lower-body weakness | LB exercises with resistance (body/resistance band); emphasize hip abductors/adductors |
| | 3. Poor gaze stabilization | Practice focusing on visual targets during standing and moving activities |

Note: A-P = anterior-posterior direction; BOS = base of support; COG = center of gravity; LB = lower body; UB = upper body.

# glossary

# Glossary

*adiposity* The state of being fat; fatness; obesity.

*allergens* Substances capable of inducing allergy or specific hypersensitivity.

*angina pectoris* Pain originating from the heart that is characterized by a substantial "pressure" sensation within the chest, commonly radiating down the arm, up into the jaw, or to another site. Generally caused by decreased blood flow through the coronary arteries supplying oxygen to the myocardium (heart muscle) due to partial occlusion from plaque or clot formation or spasm of the artery itself. Often aggravated or induced by exercise or stress (emotional or environmental).

*articular cartilage* Cartilage covering the ends of the bones inside diarthroidial joints; allows the ends of the bones to glide without friction.

*ataxia* Failure of muscular coordination; irregularity of muscular action.

*atherosclerosis* A specific form of arteriosclerosis characterized by the accumulation of fatty material on the inner walls of the arteries, causing them to harden, thicken, and lose elasticity.

*atrophy* A wasting away; a diminution in the size of a cell, tissue, organ, or part.

*attending* A nonverbal communication skill that gives acknowledgement through posture, eye contact, and gestures. It entails being attentive through physical attention and putting the speaker at ease.

*autoimmune disease* Any of a group of disorders in which tissue injury is associated with the body's responses to its own constituents; they may be systemic (e.g., systemic lupus erythematosus) or organ-specific (e.g., autoimmune thyroiditis).

*autonomic nervous system* The portion of the nervous system concerned with regulation of cardiac muscle, smooth muscle, and glands; the self-controlling nervous system.

*biological age* A means of measuring age that focuses on biological, rather than chronological, processes; examines various biological processes and their effects on behavior.

*calcification* A process in which calcium builds up in tissue, causing it to harden. This can be a normal (e.g., in bone tissue) or abnormal (e.g., in arteries) process.

*carcinogen* Any cancer-producing substance.

*cardiac output (CO)* The amount of blood pumped by the heart per minute; usually expressed in liters of blood per minute.

*catecholamine* One of a group of similar compounds having a sympathomimetic action (mimicking the effects of impulses conveyed by the sympathetic nervous system).

*chronic obstructive pulmonary disease (COPD)* A condition, such as asthma, bronchitis, or emphysema, in which there is a chronic obstruction of air flow.

*chronological age* The length of time—in years or months since birth—a person has lived.

*cirrhosis* A disease of the liver in which normal cells in the liver are replaced by scar tissue. This condition results in the failure of the liver to perform many of its usual functions.

*cognitive* Pertaining to, or characterized by, that operation of the mind by which we become aware of objects of thought or perception; includes all aspects of perceiving, thinking, and remembering.

*congestive heart failure* A clinical syndrome due to heart disease and characterized by sodium and water retention, resulting in edema and breathlessness. The congestion can occur in the lungs, in the peripheral circulation, or both.

*costochondral*   Relating to the costal cartilages (i.e., of the ribs).

*costovertebral*   Relating to the ribs and the bodies of the thoracic vertebrae with which they articulate.

*covalent bond*   A chemical bond in which electrons can be shared, such as the peptide bonds in proteins.

*degenerative changes*   The process of declining from a higher to a lower level of effective functioning or overall essential quality.

*degenerative joint disease*   A non-infectious, progressive disorder of the weightbearing joints. The majority of degenerative joint disease is the result of mechanical instabilities or aging-related changes within the joint.

*dementia*   A deteriorative mental state characterized by absence of, or reduction in, intellectual faculties; may be caused by disease or trauma.

*demyelinization*   The destruction or removal of the myelin sheath of a nerve or nerves.

*diabetes*   A disease of carbohydrate metabolism in which an absolute or relative deficiency of insulin results in an inability to metabolize carbohydrates normally. See *type 1 diabetes* and *type 2 diabetes*.

*diaphragmatic breathing*   A deep, relaxing breathing technique that helps COPD patients improve their breathing capacity.

*disability*   The inability to perform certain essential movements, such as dressing, walking, bathing, and climbing stairs.

*dopamine*   An inhibitory neurotransmitter secreted by neurons that are located in the substantia nigra of the basal ganglia.

*dyspnea*   Shortness of breath, resulting in difficult or labored breathing.

*dystrophy*   Any disorder arising from defective or faulty nutrition, especially the muscular dystrophies.

*edema*   The presence of abnormally large amounts of fluid in the intercellular tissue spaces of the body.

*empathetic response*   A response based on the understanding of a person's experience from their perspective; it should acknowledge and increase the awareness of their experience and therefore make them more open to learning.

*exercise prescriptions*   Written directions for the administration of exercise programs with the intent of addressing or treating a specific medical condition. It is beyond a fitness professional's scope of practice to prescribe exercise.

*extrinsic asthma*   Form of asthma related to a specific allergen.

*forced expiratory volume*   The percentage of vital capacity that can be expired in one second; provides an indication of expiratory power and overall resistance to air movement in the lungs.

*free-radical oxidation*   A mechanism of cellular aging in which a highly unstable molecule of oxygen (i.e., a free-radical) with an uneven number of electrons in its outer shell attempts to link up with other molecules, thereby causing a series of destructive chain reactions; possible outcomes include reduced elasticity in the skin and declines in flexibility and range of motion.

*functional age*   A measure of aging using various indications beyond chronological age; these indices include biological age, social age, and psychological age.

*functional limitation*   A restriction in certain physical or mental tasks that can be the result of an impairment.

*gerontologist*   A specialist in the scientific study of the clinical, biological, historical, and sociological problems of aging.

*Hayflick limit*   Finite number of times that a cell is able to reproduce. Suggests that cellular aging is, at least to some degree, preprogrammed.

*heart-rate reserve (HRR)* The reserve capacity of the heart; the difference between maximal heart rate and resting heart rate. It reflects the heart's ability to increase the rate of beating and cardiac output above resting level to maximal intensity.

*homeostasis* A tendency toward stability in the normal body states achieved by a system of control mechanisms activated by negative feedback.

*hypercholesterolemia* An excess of cholesterol in the blood.

*hyperglycemia* An abnormally high content of glucose in the blood.

*hyperlipidemia* An excess of lipids in the blood that could be primary, as in disorders of lipid metabolism, or secondary, as in uncontrolled diabetes.

*hypokalemia* A deficiency of potassium in the blood.

*impairment* A decrease in strength or function; can be anatomical or structural in nature.

*intrinsic asthma* Form of asthma not related to a specific allergen.

*Karvonen method* A method of determining target heart rate that uses heart-rate reserve (maximal heart rate minus resting heart rate).

*kyphosis* Abnormally increased convexity of the curvature of the thoracic spine (hunchback).

*lactic acid* A by-product of anaerobic glycolysis known to cause localized, acute muscle fatigue.

*liposoluble* Able to be dissolved in fats.

*Major Histocompatibility Complex (MHC)* A group of genes that code for certain proteins that are found on the surface of cells and help the immune system to recognize foreign substances. MHC proteins are found in all higher vertebrates. In human beings the complex is also called the human leukocyte antigen (HLA) system.

*maximal oxygen consumption (VO₂max)* The point at which oxygen consumption plateaus with an additional workload; represents a person's capacity for the aerobic synthesis of ATP.

*maximum voluntary ventilation* A dynamic test of ventilatory capacity that requires rapid and deep breathing for 15 seconds (extrapolated to one minute).

*neoplastic* Pertaining to any new and abnormal growth; specifically when the growth is uncontrolled and progressive.

*neurotransmitter* A substance that transmits nerve impulses across a synapse (e.g., acetycholine, norepinephrine).

*obesity* An excessive accumulation of body fat. Usually defined as more than 20% above ideal weight, or >25% body fat for men and >32% body fat for women; also can be defined as a Body Mass Index (BMI) of >30 kg/m², or a waist girth of >40 inches (102 cm) in men and >35 inches (89 cm) in women.

*open kinetic chain (exercises)* Exercises in which a muscle or muscle group is isolated to function alone.

*orthostatic hypotension* A progressive disorder that includes abnormally low blood pressure and symptoms of weakness or fainting upon rising to an erect position; usually occurs after prolonged bed rest; also known as postural hypotension.

*ossification* The formation of bone.

*osteoarthritis* An abnormal condition of the joint characterized by erosion of articular cartilage. See also *primary osteoarthritis* and *secondary osteroarthitis.*

*osteoarthrosis* See *osteoarthritis.*

*osteophytes* Bone spurs; the result of deterioration of the articular cartilage, causing a tremendous amount of pain.

*osteoporosis* A disorder in which bone density decreases and susceptibility to fracture increases; primarily affects women past menopause.

*paresthesia* An abnormal sensation such as numbness, prickling, or tingling.

*pathology* Anatomic or functional manifestations of a disease.

*peripheral* Situated away from the center or central structure.

*phase II cardiac-rehabilitation program* Begins once the patient is released from the hospital; goals during this phase include improvements in capacity for physical work, clinical status, and pychosocial well-being. Hospital-based exercises are performed under the supervision of nurses and exercise specialists, usually three times per week on an outpatient basis.

*phase III cardiac-rehabilitation program* Upon completion of phase II, exercise is performed at home or in a gymnasium and supervised by nurses or exercise specialists with a goal of increasing exercise tolerance; duration or workout can be 30 to 45 minutes.

*postural hypotension* See *orthostatic hypotension*.

*primary osteoarthritis* Osteoarthritis of unknown origin; the most common form of the disease.

*psychological age* A measurement of aging based on an individual's abilities of mental and cognitive functioning, including self-esteem, self-efficacy, learning, memory, and perception.

*pursed-lips breathing* A breathing technique that increases the amount of air taken in through the damaged tissues of the lungs (e.g., in COPD patients) and reduces the incidence of dyspnea.

*relative age* The extent to which an individual is aging faster or slower than an average person of the same age.

*residual volume* The volume of air that remains in the lungs when an individual exhales as deeply as possible.

*rhabdomyolysis* The breakdown of muscle fibers resulting in the release of muscle fiber contents into the circulation. Some of these are toxic to the kidney and frequently result in kidney damage.

*rheumatic disease* Any of a variety of disorders marked by inflammation, degeneration, or metabolic derangement of the connective tissue structures of the body, especially the joints and related structures (e.g., rheumatoid arthritis, lupus, fibromyalgia).

*rheumatic disease* A general term applied to a wide variety of conditions affecting cartilage and other connective tissues; usually inflammatory and frequently autoimmune in nature (e.g., rheumatoid arthritis and lupus).

*sciatica* A syndrome characterized by pain radiating from the back into the buttock and into the lower extremity along its posterior or lateral aspect, most commonly caused by prolapse of the intervertebral disk. Also refers to pain anywhere along the course of the sciatic nerve.

*secondary osteoarthritis* Osteoarthritis resulting from an injury or a mechanical derangement of the joint.

*self-efficacy* Self-confidence in one's ability to perform a certain task.

*senescence* The process or condition of growing old.

*shoulder impingement* A shoulder-joint injury that arises from the continual use of the arm(s) above the horizontal plane; commonly occurs in the supraspinous muscle at the acromion and coracoacromial ligament.

*social age* Considers aging in terms of what is and is not socially acceptable behavior for a person of a particular age group.

*syncope* A transient state of unconsciousness during which a person collapses to the floor as a result of lack of oxygen to the brain; commonly known as fainting.

*total peripheral resistance (TPR)* The resistance to the passage of blood through the small blood vessels, especially arterioles.

*type 1 diabetes* Form of diabetes caused by the destruction of the insulin-producing beta cells in the pancreas, which leads to little or no insulin secretion; generally develops in childhood and requires regular insulin injections; also known as insulin-dependent diabetes mellitus (IDDM) and childhood-onset diabetes.

*type 2 diabetes* Most common form of diabetes; typically develops in adulthood, is characterized by a reduced sensitivity of the insulin target cells to available insulin, and is usually associated with obesity; also known as non-insulin-dependent diabetes mellitus (NIDDM) and adult-onset diabetes.

*vagus nerve* The tenth cranial nerve; parasympathetic, general sensory nerve.

*Valsalva maneuver* Increase of intrathoracic pressure by forcible exhalation effort against a closed glottis.

*vital capacity* The total volume of air that can be voluntarily moved in one breath, from full inspiration to maximum expiration, or vice versa.

# index

# Index

and strength training, 83, 185

*See also* osteoarthritis; rheumatoid arthritis

Arthritis Foundation PACE program, 17

articular cartilage, 81

artifact, 109

assessment

battery, 101

body composition, 108–113

of functional strength and ability, 101, 120–121

heart rate, 113–114

physical, 39, 101, 119–121

pre-exercise interview, 118–119

Specifit™ Walking Test, 119–120

tests of function, 121–123

*See also* pre-exercise screening

assisted living facilities, 229, 236

asthma, 75–78

attacks during exercise, 75

causes of, 75

coughing, 76

exercise guidelines, 76–78

medications to treat, 76

shortness of breath, 75–76

symptoms of, 75–76

what to do if client is having an attack, 79

wheezing, 76

Atenolol, 92

atherosclerosis, 11, 72

athletes, older, 103

attending skills, 48

attitudes toward exercise, 28, 113

auditory disorders, suggestions for working with clients with, 90–91

autoimmune disease, 6, 81

**B**

Baby Boomer generation, aging of, 3

back pain, acute, 84–85

balance, medications and substances affecting, 107

balance/coordination exercise, 132, 139, 173–176

for clients with Parkinson's disease, 90

for functional fitness, 178

one-legged stand, 174–175

safety, 175–176

Balanos, G. M., 114

ballet arc, chair-seated, 148

ballistic movements, 194

ballistic stretching, 137

ball play, 173

balls, 145

Barke, C. R., 31

base steps, 151

basic activities of daily living (BADL), 103, 221–222, 224, 227, 229, 243

bean bags, 243

beclomethasone diproprionate, 76

behavioral change

stages of, 240

strategies, 32–33

*See also* health change behavior, theories of

behavioral contract, 40

behavioral cues, 42–43

behaviors vs. outcomes, 39

bent-knee lift, aquatic exercise, 167

Berg Balance Scale, 123, 260–265

beta-adrenergic agents, 76

beta-agonist, 76

beta blockers, 73, 87, 92, 107, 115

biceps curl, chair-seated, 144

biceps stretch, standing, 160

biceps/triceps strengthener, aquatic exercise, 166

bicycle ergometer, 84

biological age, 4, 102

biological theories

cellular theories, 5–6

control theories, 6–7

genetic theories, 6

biomarkers of aging, 102

Birren, J. E., 4

bitolterol, 76

blood glucose levels, 86–87

blood lipids, 11

blood pressure

checking in clients with coronary heart disease, 73

classification of for adults age 18 and older, 110

defined, 108

and diuretics, 92

monitoring for clients with hypertension, 74

and physical activity, 10

blood pressure screening, 108–110